PREFACE TO THE SECOND EDITION

In an age when so many dental textbooks have a multiplicity of authors, I was pleased to have the opportunity, in 1976, to draw together my own thoughts on fluorides in caries prevention. One reviewer wrote that he hoped the book would be kept up to date, but added that it would be 'a labour of Hercules'. I was delighted when Andrew Rugg-Gunn agreed to join me in attempting the Second Edition, and hope that our efforts have produced a more comprehensive summary of the effects of fluoride on dental caries.

One of the major developments in fluoride therapy since the publication of the First Edition has been the increasing use of combinations of types of fluoride used to prevent caries, either as part of the care of the individual patient or in community preventive schemes. This aspect has been expanded in this edition and examples given of fluoride-based schemes which have been implemented at the community level in some areas of the world. The number of countries operating water fluoridation schemes has expanded and these are now brought together in a new chapter.

PREFACE TO THE FIRST EDITION

Any clinical therapy must have a firm rational basis for its application. If a supposed caries-inhibitory agent is to be used clinically, its effectiveness must be confirmed by carefully controlled clinical trials, the results of which have been confirmed by several independent investigators. In addition, dentists, although being predominantly concerned with the effects of treatment at the individual dentist–patient level, also have the responsibility of appreciating the effectiveness of measures designed to reduce the prevalence of dental caries within the community.

The main aim of this book is to present the evidence concerning the clinical effectiveness of fluoride, in its various forms, as a caries-inhibitory agent. The first four chapters of the book are concerned with the systemic administration of fluoride; the next five chapters consider the effect of fluoride applied topically in toothpaste, prophylactic paste, solutions, gels, varnishes and mouth rinses. The final three chapters are concerned with the physiology and toxicity of fluoride and with the possible mechanisms by which fluoride exerts its caries-preventive effect.

A DENTAL PRACTITIONER HANDBOOK
SERIES EDITED BY DONALD D. DERRICK, DDS, LDS RCS

FLUORIDES IN CARIES PREVENTION

JOHN J. MURRAY

PhD, MChD (Leeds), FDS RCS (Eng.)

*Professor and Head
Department of Child Dental Health
Dental School
University of Newcastle upon Tyne*

*Formerly Reader and Honorary Consultant
Department of Children's Dentistry
Institute of Dental Surgery
Eastman Dental Hospital*

ANDREW J. RUGG-GUNN

RD, PhD, BDS, FDS RCS (Edin.)

*Reader in Preventive Dentistry
Departments of Child Dental Health and Oral Biology
Dental School
University of Newcastle upon Tyne*

Second Edition

WRIGHT·PSG

BRISTOL LONDON BOSTON
1982

Published by:
John Wright & Sons Ltd, 823–825 Bath Road,
Bristol BS4 5NU, England
John Wright PSG Inc., 545 Great Road, Littleton,
Massachusetts 01460, USA

First edition, 1976
Second edition, 1982

British Library Cataloguing in Publication Data
Murray, John J.
    Fluorides in caries prevention.—2nd ed.—
    (A Dental practitioner handbook)
    1. Dental caries—Prevention
    2. Water—Fluoridation
    I. Title II. Rugg-Gunn, Andrew J. III. Series
    617.6'01 RK52

ISBN 0 7236 0644 7

Library of Congress Catalog Card Number: 82–50758

Typeset and printed in Great Britain by
John Wright & Sons (Printing) Ltd at The Stonebridge Press, Bristol

ACKNOWLEDGEMENTS TO THE FIRST EDITION

I would like to express my gratitude to Professor D. Jackson, of the University of Leeds Dental School, for the training he gave me whilst I was Research Fellow in his department. The first four chapters of this book have been influenced by his teaching. Secondly, I thank Professor G. B. Winter, my present Head of Department, for stimulating my interest in all forms of topical fluoride therapy, and for encouraging me to carry out clinical trials in this field. My thanks go also to two former postgraduate students in the Department of Children's Dentistry at the Institute of Dental Surgery, Miss D. M. Bennett and Miss L. H. McAllan; their reviews of the literature on topical fluorides and fluoride toothpastes form the basis of the appropriate chapters in this book.

I am indebted to many Editors who have given me permission to reproduce material; in particular to Mr J. A. Donaldson, Editor of the *British Dental Journal,* for allowing me to reproduce my article on the 'History of Water Fluoridation', which was first published in the *Journal* in 1973. I am grateful to Mr R. I. Nairn for permission to use some of the material from a review article on topical fluorides which was published in the *Dental Practitioner* in 1972. My thanks go also to the Editors of *Archives of Oral Biology, British Dental Journal, Caries Research, Community Health, Fluoride Drinking Water, Journal of the American Dental Association, Journal of Dental Research, Journal of Pathology and Bacteriology, Community Dentistry and Oral Epidemiology,* and to Blackwell Scientific Publications, Professor I. J. Møller, Charles C. Thomas, Publishers, University of Chicago Press, and the World Health Organisation for permission to reproduce illustrations. Appropriate acknowledgement is made under each illustration in the text.

Finally, this book could not have been written without the help and encouragement of my wife Valerie, who has endured patiently my surveys in fluoride and non-fluoride areas. To her, and to our son Mark, I dedicate this book.

Institute of Dental Surgery, 1975   *J. J. M.*

ACKNOWLEDGEMENTS TO THE SECOND EDITION

We are extremely grateful to Area Dental Officers for providing information on water fluoridation schemes, and to Dr L. Shaw and Mr L. Ness for their help in producing summary tables on sodium monofluorophosphate and stannous fluoride toothpaste trials.

ACKNOWLEDGEMENTS

We are grateful to the Editors of *Community Dentistry and Oral Epidemiology, Scandinavian Journal of Dental Research, Acta Odontologica Scandinavica, Helvetica Odontologica Acta* and the *British Dental Journal* for permission to reproduce illustrations.

Our thanks go also to Mrs J. Young who has been responsible for most of the secretarial work involved in producing the manuscript for the Second Edition, to Miss A. M. Crumbley, Librarian, Newcastle Dental School, for help with the references and to Dr John Gillman of John Wright & Sons Ltd, for his patience and encouragement.

Finally we dedicate this book to Valerie, Diane and our children.

J. J. M.
A. R.-G.

CONTENTS

CHAPTER 1

A HISTORY OF WATER FLUORIDATION

COLORADO STAIN

The history of fluoridation is more than 70 years old. It started with the arrival of Dr Frederick McKay in Colorado Springs, Colorado, USA, in 1901, the year following his graduation from the University of Pennsylvania Dental School. He soon noticed that many of his patients, particularly those who had lived in the area all their lives, had an apparently permanent stain on their teeth, which was known to the local inhabitants as 'Colorado Stain'. McKay checked the lecture notes he had saved from dental school but found nothing to describe such markings, nor could he find any reference to them in any of the available scientific literature. He called the stain 'mottled enamel' and said that it was characterized by:

Minute white flecks, or yellow or brown spots or areas, scattered irregularly or streaked over the surface of a tooth, or it may be a condition where the entire tooth surface is of a dead paper-white, like the colour of a china dish. (McKay, 1916a.)

The first systematic endeavour to investigate this lesion was made by the Colorado Springs Dental Society in 1902.

At that time it was generally supposed that a limited area of territory, measured by a comparatively short radius of miles, was the only area affected, and as a first step toward defining its limits, a series of letters were addressed to dentists practising in various portions of the Rocky Mountain region. The answers received brought very little information of value and the matter of further investigation was allowed to rest for the next six years. (McKay, 1916a.)

In 1905, McKay moved to St Louis to practise orthodontics. He stayed there for three years, during which time he never saw a case of mottled enamel, whereas in Colorado Springs he saw cases every day. He returned to Colorado in 1908 and the stain problem struck him with more force than ever. At the May 1908 meeting of the El Paso County Odontological Society McKay revived the question. After hearing his talk, the society sent him, together with a patient whose teeth bore the markings of the stain, to the annual meeting in June of the State Dental Association in Boulder. McKay exhibited the patient and, though dentists showed a passing interest in the problem, he learned of similar conditions in several other towns. The dentists in these towns, unimpressed by an almost universal condition, had not bothered to report the stain (Minutes of Colorado Springs Dental Society, 1908).

By showing an actual case of Colorado Stain to dentists from all over the State, McKay scattered the seeds of interest beyond the borders of his

1

recently adopted home. As a result of the meeting in Boulder, McKay decided that, firstly, he needed help from a recognized dental research worker and, secondly, he needed to define the exact geographical area of the stain—the endemic area. To attain his first objective he approached one of America's foremost authorities on dental enamel, Dr Greene Vardiman Black, Dean of the Northwestern University Dental School in Chicago. At first Black thought that McKay was mistaking the stain for something else. He could scarcely believe there could be a dental lesion affecting so many people which still remained unmentioned in the dental literature. Black asked that some of the mottled teeth be sent to him for examination (Black, 1916). He agreed to attend the Colorado State Dental Association meeting in July 1909, and promised to spend some weeks in Colorado Springs before the annual meeting.

In preparation for this visit, and as a first step in mapping out the entire endemic area, McKay and a fellow townsman, Dr Isaac Binton, examined the children in the public schools of Colorado Springs. In all they inspected 2945 children and discovered to their complete astonishment that 87·5 per cent of the children native to the area had mottled teeth (McKay, 1916a). For the first time investigators had statistical data detailing the prevalence of the lesion in the community. This new information was given to Black when he arrived in Denver, in June 1909, to tour the Colorado Springs area. Black addressed the State Dental Association meeting: he described the histological examination of the lesion and recounted his personal observations noted during the several weeks he had been touring the Rocky Mountain area. His interest, together with his authority and prestige, raised the study of the problem from the status of a local curiosity to that of an investigation meriting the earnest concern of all dental research workers. Black's histological findings were published in a paper entitled: 'An endemic imperfection of the enamel of the teeth heretofore unknown in the literature of dentistry' (Black, 1916).

THE ENDEMIC AREA

Despite Black's involvement other dentists were unimpressed and showed little enthusiasm for carrying on the investigation. It was left to McKay to sustain the study by his persistent interest. His Colorado Springs survey had shown that almost 9 out of 10 of the native children had mottled teeth: he began searching for other endemic areas. His travels took him up and down the creek valleys of the mountainous region and out onto the nearby plains. He examined children living in Pueblo, Maniton, La Junta, Cripple Creek, Woodland Park and Great Mountain Falls. A few trips convinced McKay that the phenomenon called 'mottling' was much more widespread than he had thought. Slowly, too, McKay began to get help from other dentists in the country. As a result of a short article by Dr Black in the newspaper *Dental Brief*, a Dr W. H. Arthur wrote a letter to the newspaper describing the condition in a town in one of the Southern States on the Atlantic seaboard. The letter was brought to the notice of Dr McKay by a dental nurse, Mrs Mayhall, and he immediately wrote to Dr Arthur requesting information. The reply, dated 18 April 1912, described the classic picture of mottled enamel: the condition was confined to a 'small circumscribed geographical area, it was confined exclusively to children and young people born in the territory, but not to any set or class of people'. (McKay, 1916b.)

Another dentist, Dr Rice, reported the stain at Smavillo, Texas, and donated two incisor teeth from that district which exactly corresponded in appearance with those from previously studied districts (McKay, 1916c). McKay was greatly helped by Dr Joseph Murphy, medical supervisor of the US Indian Service, who instructed his field dentists to examine and report on the prevalence of mottling among the Indians in all schools under his jurisdiction. From as far away as Tacoma, Washington, Rapid City, South Dakota and Mojave City, Arizona, McKay received reports which broadened the boundaries of the endemic areas (McKay, 1916d).

The horizons were broadened still further when, in 1912, McKay discovered that people from parts of Naples in Italy also had stained teeth. He came across an article written in 1902 by Dr J. M. Eager, a United States Marine Hospital Service surgeon stationed in Italy, who reported that a high proportion of certain Italian emigrants embarking at Naples had a dental peculiarity known locally as *denti di Chiaie* (Eager, 1902). Some of these Italians had ugly brown stains on their teeth; others had a fine horizontal black line crossing the incisor teeth. McKay heard that a young doctor, Dr J. F. McConnell from Colorado Springs, was planning a holiday in Italy, and asked him to examine some Naples children and report back. The doctor was familiar with the stain in Colorado Springs and wrote back from Naples that there was no doubt that the mottled teeth in Naples were the same as those being investigated by McKay (McKay, 1916c).

MOTTLED ENAMEL AND DENTAL CARIES

Throughout this period the energy and enthusiasm which kept McKay going was generated by a desire to find out the cause of mottling so that some means might be found of preventing the unsightly stains on people's teeth. The histological investigations by Black (1916) showed that in mottled teeth there was a failure of the cementing substance of the enamel. One would have expected that imperfect, hypocalcified enamel would have decalcified more readily than normal enamel. However, throughout his investigations, McKay was struck by the fact that caries experience

3

was no higher in mottled teeth. In 1916 he wrote:

This mottled condition, in itself, does not seem to increase the susceptibility of the teeth to decay, which is perhaps contrary to what might be expected, because the enamel surface is much more corrugated and rougher than normal enamel. (McKay, 1916a.)

This contradiction must have been in the back of McKay's mind throughout the whole period of his research. He expressed it more forcibly in a paper to the Chicago Society on 17 April 1928:

Mottled enamel is a condition in which the enamel is most obviously and unmistakably defective. In fact it is the most poorly calcified enamel of which there is any record in dental literature. If the chief determining factor governing the susceptibility to decay is the integrity or perfection of the calcification of enamel, then by all the laws of logic this enamel is deprived of the one essential element for its protection. . . . In spite of this the outstanding fact is that mottled enamel shows no greater susceptibility to the onset of caries than does enamel that may be considered to have been normally or perfectly calcified. This statement is made as a result of extensive observations and examinations of several thousand cases during the past years. . . . My testimony has been supplemented by that of others, who report that these mottled enamel cases, in the various districts, are singularly free from caries. One of the first things noted by Dr Black during his first contact with an endemic locality was the singular absence of decay, and it can hardly be said that his faculty for observations was superficial. (McKay, 1928.)

MOTTLED ENAMEL: AETIOLOGICAL FACTORS

Yet in the forefront of McKay's mind all the time was the desire to determine the cause of mottled enamel. He established that the occurrence of mottled enamel was localized in definite geographical areas. Within these endemic areas a very high proportion of children were affected; only children who had been born and lived all their lives in an endemic area had mottled enamel; children who had been born elsewhere and brought to the district when 2 to 3 years of age were not affected. The condition was not affected by home or environment factors; families whether rich or poor were affected. This factor tended to eliminate diet as an aetiological factor. McKay observed that three cities in Arkansas, where mottling occurred, although separated from each other by some miles, all received their water supply from one source, Fountain Creek. This, together with many other reports, led him to believe that something in the water supply was responsible for mottled enamel.

Even from the very beginning of the notice taken of this lesion and before any definite steps were taken to study it, the sentiment of both the profession and the laity in the areas of susceptibility was that the water was in some way responsible. Indeed it was hardly possible to mention this condition without at once encountering a question, and often a dogmatic assertion, indicating the water as the cause. (McKay, 1916b.)

4

Further evidence supporting the water-supply hypothesis came from a dentist, Dr O. E. Martin, practising in Britton, South Dakota. On reading McKay's 1916 article in the *Dental Cosmos*, he felt that McKay's description of mottling sounded suspiciously like the blemishes he had seen on certain local children and asked for McKay's advice. McKay visited Britton in October 1916. He discovered that in 1898 Britton had changed its water supply from individual shallow wells to a deep-drilled artesian well. Without exception, McKay found that all those who had passed through childhood prior to the changing of the water supply had normal teeth, while natives who had grown up in Britton since 1898 had mottling. He concluded that some mysterious element in the water supply was responsible (McKay, 1918).

So convinced was he that something in the water supply was responsible for causing mottling, that McKay persuaded a community to change its water supply solely because of the existence of a dental abnormality. The town was Oakley, Idaho, a tiny frontier village 75 miles north-west of Great Salt Lake. In 1908 the community had constructed a pipeline from a warm spring 5 miles out of town. A few years after they began using the water from this source, people began to notice that their children's teeth had a peculiar brownish discoloration. In contrast, children in neighbouring communities seemed to have normal teeth. By 1923, the mothers of the town were so concerned that, with the help of the local dentist, they initiated a survey of children attending the local schools. They found that every child who had been born and lived in the town since 1908 had mottled teeth (McKay, 1925). The mothers of the town demanded action. They appointed a committee and appealed to Dr McKay to visit the town to support them in their efforts to raise a 35 000-dollar bond issue to change the water supply. Several influential townspeople thought the water theory was absurd. They asked the proponents that if they were so certain the present water supply was the cause of the mottling, how could they predict that a different supply would not do the same thing? McKay gave a lecture on his findings in other areas to a mass meeting in the community. Recalling the incident some years later he wrote:

It was a source of regret to be unable to give any definite answer to the most important question; of a proper substitute for the then existing water supply at Oakley, but I did state that the most valuable and conclusive evidence that could be obtained would be to locate individuals who had spent the years of enamel development in contact with a contemporary source of a new supply. The condition of their enamel would determine the question more definitely than any other means at our disposal. (McKay, 1933.)

Located near Oakley was Carpenter Spring, which had a different water supply; 4 children raised on this water had normal teeth free from brown stain. This meagre information was sufficient to sway the officials of Oakley and they voted to lay a new pipeline to bring water from Carpenter Spring, which was opened on 1 July 1925. The climax came $7\frac{1}{2}$ years later in February 1933 when McKay again examined the teeth of Oakley children. Of 24 children born in Oakley following the change in water supply, none had any brown stain in those permanent teeth which had erupted (McKay, 1933).

A similar occurrence was reported in the town of Bauxite, a community formed in 1901 to provide homes for employees of the Republic Mining and Manufacturing Company, a subsidiary of the Aluminium Company of America (ALCOA). The first domestic water supply to Bauxite came from shallow wells and springs, but in 1909 a new source of water was obtained from a 297-foot well. A practising dentist, Dr F. L. Robertson, of nearby Benton, reported to the State Board of Health that the younger citizens of Bauxite seemed to have badly stained teeth, whereas children living in Benton had normal teeth. The State health officer made a formal request to the US Public Health Service in Washington to examine the children living in Bauxite and Benton. In 1928 the US Public Health Service asked Dr McKay to accompany Dr Gromer Kempf, one of their medical officers, to carry out the examinations. They found that no mottling occurred in people who grew up on Bauxite water prior to 1909, but all native Bauxite children who used the deep-well water after that date had mottled teeth. No individual whose enamel developed during residence in Benton had mottled teeth. They reported that the standard water analysis of Bauxite water 'throws little light whatever on the probable causal agent' (Kempf and McKay, 1930). Another piece of evidence had been gathered, but McKay seemed no closer to the solution.

MOTTLED ENAMEL AND FLUORIDE CONCENTRATION IN THE DRINKING WATER

The answer was now close at hand. In New Kensington, Pennsylvania, the chief chemist of ALCOA, Mr H. V. Churchill, read Kempf and McKay's paper and was greatly disturbed. Certain people in the United States were condemning the use of aluminium-ware for cooking. ALCOA mined most of its aluminium supply from Bauxite: if the story of the stain in Bauxite got into the hands of those who claimed that aluminium cooking utensils caused poisoning, ALCOA would have to reply to the charge. When Churchill received a sample of Bauxite water he instructed Mr A. W. Petrey, head of the testing division of the ALCOA laboratory, to look for traces of rare elements—those not usually tested for. Petrey ran a spectrographic analysis and noted that fluoride was present in Bauxite water at a level of 13·7 parts per million (ppm). Churchill wrote to McKay on 20 January 1931:

> We have discovered the presence of hitherto unsuspected constituents in this water. The high fluorine content was so unexpected that a new sample was taken with extreme precautions and again the test showed fluorine in the water. (Churchill, 1931a.)

6

He also asked McKay to send samples of water from other endemic areas with a 'minimum of publicity'. McKay quickly arranged for dentists in Britton, South Dakota, Oakley, Idaho and Colorado Springs to send samples of the water in their areas. The results of these analyses were published in 1931 (*see below*).

Location of sample	Fluorine as fluoride parts per million
Deep Well, Bauxite, Ark.	13·7
Colorado Springs, Colo.	2·0
Well near Kidder, S.Dak.	12·0
Well near Lidgerwood, N.Dak.	11·0
Oakley, Idaho	6·0

Churchill emphasized the fact that no precise correlation between the fluoride content of these waters and the mottled enamel had been established. All that was shown was the presence of a hitherto unsuspected common constituent of the waters from the endemic areas (Churchill, 1931b).

Confirmation of Churchill's findings came from a husband and wife team, working at the Arizona Agricultural Experiment Station, Dr Margaret Cammack Smith, head of the nutrition department, and Howard V. Smith, agricultural chemist. They observed that mottled enamel occurred in residents of St David and decided to try to produce mottled enamel experimentally in rats. Their first experiment, with ordinary diet and water taken from St David, was a failure. In their next experiment they concentrated St David water to one-tenth of its original volume by boiling and within a week a difference was noted—the rats' incisor teeth lost translucency. Within a month the enamel was 'strikingly dull, white in appearance and pitted' (Smith, 1931). A review of the literature revealed that a report had been written in 1925 on the effect of additions of fluorine to the diet of rats on the quality of their teeth (McCollum et al., 1925). The Arizona workers then carried out further experiments, feeding sodium fluoride to rats in amounts equalling 0·025, 0·1 and 0·5 per cent of the diet. The characteristic enamel defects which developed in the rats were so strikingly similar to those produced by the feeding of the residue from St David water that no one could fail to associate the two (Smith, 1931). An analysis of St David water supply was carried out and showed that the fluoride concentration was 3·8–7·2 ppm. Further analyses of 185 public and private water supplies in Arizona were carried out—the fluoride concentration varied from 0·0 to 12·6 ppm fluoride (Smith and Smith, 1931).

An abstract of Churchill's work appeared on 10 April 1931 in the *Industrial and Engineering Chemistry, News Edition*. His complete report was published in the September issue of the journal. Only 3 weeks after Churchill's preliminary report had been published, Margaret Cammack Smith presented her findings to the Tucson Dental Association at a dinner on 2 May 1931. After nearly 30 years, the solution to McKay's problem had been solved by two independent workers, reaching the same conclusion within a few days of one another.

MOTTLED ENAMEL IN THE UNITED KINGDOM

McKay's work had not gone unnoticed in the United Kingdom. Reference to McKay's and Black's articles in *Dental Cosmos* of 1916 had been made in the fifth edition of Colyer's *Dental Surgery and Pathology* (London, Longmans) which was required reading for all dental students of that time. One such dental student was Norman Ainsworth.

Having read this [account of mottled teeth] as a dental student I regret to say that I forgot it, together with a great many other paragraphs in that volume, immediately after qualifying. When I was a student in Middlesex Hospital in 1921, I chanced to be given charge of a girl patient, aged 15, in one of the surgical wards and noticed that her teeth showed a very unusual appearance. They were curiously opaque and flecked with brownish black spots. It appeared that many other people in her home town, Maldon, Essex, were affected in the same way, and it was generally supposed that the drinking water was responsible. I fear that I had already forgotten Rocky Mountain mottled teeth, but the condition was so unusual that I made a mental note that I would look for a chance to verify the girl's statements. A year later I undertook a tour of council schools in various parts of England and Wales for the Dental Diseases Committee of the Medical Research Council, and remembering the incident I arranged that Maldon should be included. (Ainsworth, 1933.)

The MRC report was published in 1925 (*Special Report Series* No. 97). Ainsworth examined 4258 children aged 2–15 years attending 36 schools in England and Wales. He visited two schools in Maldon, examining 202 children aged 5–15 years. His results showed that, taking all children, the percentage of permanent teeth with dental caries was 13·1 per cent. Considering Maldon children only, the percentage was 7·9 per cent. Ainsworth was particularly interested in the prevalence of mottling in Maldon children. He recorded that of 134 children who were lifelong residents of Maldon, 125 showed mottling. He concluded:

The distribution of the stain . . . points to an outside origin for the stain, either atmospheric or in the water, since these are precisely the surfaces most exposed to air and fluid in the acts of speaking and drinking respectively. My own view, and it is little more than a guess, is that the cause of both mottling and stain will be found in some quality or impurity of the drinking water not ascertainable by ordinary analytical methods. (Ainsworth, 1928.)

At this time Ainsworth had not read Black and McKay's (1916) accounts of mottled teeth in America. When he did so he knew that 'the similarity between my own description and theirs is so striking in every detail as to leave no reasonable doubt that the conditions are identical' (Ainsworth, 1933).

Ainsworth read the reports by Churchill showing that water from endemic areas contains fluorides in quantities varying from 2 to 13 ppm and wanted to test the Maldon water fluoride concentration.

I will not weary you with the last stage. Public authorities are slow-moving bodies, and in the end I paid a surprise visit to Maldon with a car and a crate of Winchester quart bottles. They were filled at the various pumping stations in the district and, as a control, one from the drinking water of Witham, a town a few miles distant, which I had already found to be immune, though the water supply was declared exactly similar by the county analyst. The National Physical Laboratory, at my request, had already worked out a method of measuring minute quantities of fluorine in water, and they found that they could be reasonably sure by using de Boer's colorimetric method of attaining an accuracy of 0·1 part per million. Using this method, they tested the five samples and reported that, whereas Witham water contained 0·5 parts of fluorine per million, the water from the four endemic areas contained 4·5–5·5 parts per million. (Ainsworth, 1933.)

The significance of Ainsworth's contribution was that he gave statistical data showing that caries experience in a fluoride area was lower than average. McKay had stressed that mottled teeth had a caries rate no higher than normal teeth.

'SHOE LEATHER SURVEY'

The study of the relationship between fluoride concentration in drinking water, mottled enamel and dental caries was given an impetus by the decision of Dr Clinton T. Messner, Head of the US Public Health Service, in 1931, to assign a young dental officer, Dr H. Trendley Dean, to pursue full-time research on mottled enamel. Dean was responsible for the research unit within the US Public Health Service and was the first dental officer of the service to be given a non-clinical assignment. His first task was to continue McKay's work and to find the extent and geographical distribution of mottled enamel in the United States. He sent a questionnaire to the secretary of every local and state dental society in the country asking if mottled enamel existed in their areas and if so how extensive was it and from what source was the drinking water obtained. Out of 415 questionnaires distributed 207 replied. In cases where Polk's Dental Register (1928) failed to show a dentist practising in a county, the questionnaire was sent to the county health officer, and in a few cases to local physicians. In all 1197 of these individual questionnaires were sent and 632 replies were received. As a result of this investigation Dean reported that there were 97 localities in the country where mottled enamel was said to occur and this claim had been confirmed by a dental survey. There were a further 28 areas referred to in the literature where mottled enamel was said to be endemic but no confirmatory dental surveys had yet been carried out, and there were 70 areas which had been reported by questionnaires but which had not yet been confirmed by extensive surveys (Dean, 1933).

Many of these confirmatory surveys were carried out by Dean himself. He started in Courtland, Virginia, and then followed with examinations in North Carolina, Tennessee and Illinois. Dean and his colleagues referred to the investigations as 'shoe leather epidemiology'. His travels gave Dean a very clear picture of the variations in mottling which could occur. He developed a standard of classification of mottling in order to record quantitatively the severity of mottling within a community (Dean, 1934) so that he could relate the fluoride concentration in the drinking water to the severity of mottling in a given area. His aim was to find out the 'minimal threshold' of fluorine—the level at which fluorine began to blemish the teeth. He showed conclusively that the severity of mottling increased with increasing fluoride concentration in the drinking water (Dean and Elvove, 1936; Dean, 1936). His results are expressed diagrammatically in *Fig*. 1. He concluded that:

> From the continuous use of water containing about one part per million, it is possible that the very mildest form of mottled enamel may develop in about 10 per cent of the group. In waters containing 1·7 or 1·8 parts per million the incidence may be expected to rise to 40 or 50 per cent, although the percentage distribution of severity would be largely of the 'very mild' and 'mild' types. (Dean, 1936.)

Dean continued his studies into the relationship between the severity of mottled enamel and the fluoride concentration in the water supply. He presented additional evidence to show that amounts of fluoride not exceeding 1 ppm were of no public health significance (Dean and Elvove, 1936). On 25 October 1938, in conjunction with Frederick McKay, he summarized the knowledge of mottled enamel in a paper to the Epidemiology Section of the American Public Health Association. He reported

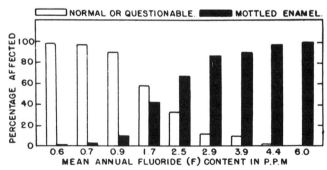

Fig. 1. The prevalence of mottled enamel in areas with differing concentrations of fluoride in the water supply. (From Dean, 1936.) (*Reproduced from 'Fluoride Drinking Waters', edited by McClure F. J., by kind permission of the US Department of Health, Education and Welfare, 1962.*)

that in the United States there were now 375 known areas, in 26 states, where mottled enamel of varying degrees of severity was found. He also stated that the production of mottled enamel had been halted at Oakley, Idaho, Bauxite, Arkansas, and Andover, South Dakota, simply by changing the water supply, which contained high concentrations of fluoride, to one whose fluoride concentration did not exceed 1 ppm. This information was 'the most conclusive and direct proof that fluoride in the domestic water is the primary cause of human mottled enamel' (Dean and McKay, 1939). The publication of this information brought to a successful conclusion McKay's search for the cause of mottled enamel which began in Colorado Springs in 1902 and lasted for almost 40 years.

DENTAL CARIES PREVALENCE IN NATURAL FLUORIDE AREAS

The story of fluoridation now entered a new and, from a public health point of view, a most important phase. Dean was aware of the reports from the literature that there may be an inverse relationship between the level of mottling and the prevalence of caries in a community. He knew of McKay's observations, first made in 1916, that mottled enamel was no more susceptible to decay than normal enamel. He had read Ainsworth's report in 1933 that caries experience in the high fluoride area was markedly lower than caries experience in all other districts examined. During his study to determine the minimum threshold of mottling, Dean had, in some cities, also examined the children for dental caries. Taking a selected sample of 9-year-old children, he found that of 114 children who had continuously used a domestic water supply comparatively low in fluoride (0·6–1·5 ppm) only 5, or 4 per cent, were caries-free. On the other hand, of the 122 children who had continuously used domestic water containing 1·7–2·5 ppm fluoride, 27 (22 per cent) were caries-free. He concluded: 'Inasmuch as it appears that the mineral composition of the drinking water may have an important bearing on the incidence of dental caries in a community, the possibility of partially controlling dental caries through the domestic water supply warrants thorough epidemiological-chemical study.' (Dean, 1938.)

To test further the hypothesis that an inverse relationship existed between endemic dental fluorosis and dental caries, a survey of four Illinois cities was planned. The cities were Galesburg and Monmouth (water supply contained 1·8 and 1·7 ppm fluoride respectively), and the nearby cities of Macomb and Quincy (water supply contained 0·2 ppm F). Altogether 885 children, aged 12–14 years, were examined. The results were clear: caries experience in Macomb and Quincy was more than twice as high as that in Galesburg and Monmouth (Dean et al., 1939).

This study paved the way for a much larger investigation of caries experience of 7257 12–14-year-old children from 21 cities in four states. The results are shown diagrammatically in *Fig.* 2 and depict with startling clarity the association between increasing fluoride concentration in the drinking water and decreasing caries experience in the population. Furthermore this study showed that near maximal reduction in caries experience occurred with a concentration of 1 ppm F in the drinking water. At this concentration fluoride caused only 'sporadic instances of the mildest forms of dental fluorosis of no practical aesthetic significance' (Dean et al., 1942).

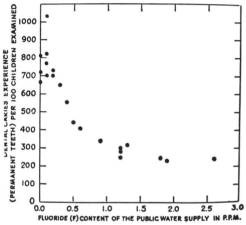

Fig. 2. The relation between caries experience of 7257 12–14-year-old white schoolchildren of 21 cities in the USA and the fluoride content of the water supply. (From Dean et al., 1942.) (*Reproduced from 'Fluoride Drinking Waters', edited by McClure F. J., by kind permission of the US Department of Health, Education and Welfare, 1962.*)

In Great Britain a natural fluoride area was discovered as a result of children being evacuated from an industrial area because of the Second World War. In 1941 Robert Weaver was told by Mr Irvine, Senior School Dentist for Westmorland, that children evacuated to the Lake District from South Shields, on the mouth of the River Tyne, 'had remarkably good teeth—much better than those of the local children'. Weaver, who was a dentist in the Ministry of Education, visited Westmorland, examined 117 evacuees (average age 11 years) and found the mean for decayed, missing or filled (DMF) teeth was 1·7. Weaver (1944) reported:

Bearing in mind the work which had been done in America, I got in touch with Dr Campbell Lyons, Medical Officer of Health for South Shields, and asked him if he would have the town's water analysed for fluorine. He did so, and a preliminary analysis suggested that the fluorine content might be as much as two parts per million. It was obvious that the conditions were such as to make possible a perfectly controlled investigation since North Shields, on the opposite bank of the River Tyne has an entirely different water supply. [The River Tyne at this part varies in width from 350 to 500 yards and the two communities are linked by a ferry.]

At Weaver's request Dr Dawson, the Medical Officer of Health for the North Shields area, arranged for the water to be analysed and this showed a fluorine content of less than 0·25 ppm. Subsequently Weaver (1944) examined 1000 children on each side of the River Tyne. He reported that the mean dmft in 5-year-old children was 6·6 in North Shields and 3·9 in South Shields; the comparable figures for 12-year-old children were 4·3 and 2·4 DMF teeth. Weaver's observations were extremely important because he focused attention on the deciduous dentition as well as the permanent dentition.

DENTAL CARIES PREVALENCE IN ARTIFICIALLY FLUORIDATED AREAS

a. Grand Rapids–Muskegon Study

The fluoridation story now entered the final phase. The crucial step was to see if dental caries could be reduced in a community by adding fluoride at 1 ppm to a fluoride-deficient water supply. The US Public Health Service was ready to embark on such an experiment. In December 1942 the service began talks with city officials of two cities in the Lake Michigan area, Grand Rapids and Muskegon. Extensive field and laboratory studies were carried out on the physiological effects of fluoride ingestion and it was concluded that not only was a fluoride concentration of 1 ppm the best for caries control, but also it was well within the limits of safety (Moulton, 1942).

In view of this information both city councils agreed in August 1944 to conduct the experiment, which would be carried out by Dr Dean, in conjunction with the Michigan State Health Department and the University of Michigan Dental School. It was decided that Grand Rapids would be the experimental town and that Muskegon would be the control town. In September 1944 Dean and his co-workers, Francis Arnold, Philip Jay and John Knutson, began the dental examinations of 19 680 Grand Rapids children and 4291 Muskegon children aged 4–16 years. All were continuous residents of the two cities. These baseline studies showed that caries experience in the deciduous and permanent dentitions in Grand Rapids was similar to that of Muskegon (Dean et al., 1950). The method used to measure caries experience was to count the number of decayed, missing and filled teeth for each child—the DMF index (Klein et al., 1938). In addition 5116 children continuously resident in the natural fluoride area of Aurora, Illinois (F = 1·4 ppm), were examined to provide

13

further baseline information. On 25 January 1945 sodium fluoride was added to the Grand Rapids water supply. This was an historic occasion, because for the first time a permissible quantity of a beneficial dietary nutrient was added to the communal drinking water.

The effects of $6\frac{1}{2}$ years of fluoridation in Grand Rapids were reported by Arnold et al. in 1953. The results were clear: caries experience of 6-year-old Grand Rapids children was almost half that of 6-year-old Muskegon children (*Table* 1). The city officials of Muskegon, convinced of the efficacy of fluoridation, decided to fluoridate their own water supply in July 1951, so from this date Muskegon could no longer be used as a control town.

Table 1. Mean def in Grand Rapids and Muskegon, 1951 (*Arnold et al., 1953*)

| | Grand Rapids | | Muskegon | |
Age	No. of children	Mean def	No. of children	Mean def
4	168	2·13	63	4·46
5	853	2·27	351	5·25
6	750	2·98	294	5·67

The only control left for Grand Rapids was a retrospective comparison with baseline data. Results after 10 years of fluoridation (Arnold et al., 1956) and 15 years of fluoridation (Arnold et al., 1962) are recorded in *Fig.* 3. They indicate that caries experience in 15-year-old Grand Rapids children had fallen from 12·48 DMF teeth per mouth in 1944 to 6·22 DMF teeth per mouth in 1959, a reduction of approximately 50 per cent. Furthermore, caries experience in the fluoridated community of Grand Rapids was very similar to that occurring in the natural fluoride area of Aurora. This was the experimental proof that the previously observed inverse relationship between fluoride in drinking water and dental caries experience was a cause and effect relationship.

The feelings that Trendley Dean and his co-workers had when they started the Grand Rapids experiment were recalled in a recent article by John Knutson (1970):

It is now 25 years ago that the late Trendley Dean and I journeyed by train from Washington, D.C., to Grand Rapids, Michigan, to be joined by Philip Jay for a meeting with the mayor to gain his approval for a water fluoridation experiment.... There were no signs of apprehension or daring or of pioneering. There were no implications or inferences that we were being foolhardy in subjecting a population of 160,000 people to a procedure which might have either short or long-range hazards. We were merely replicating nature's best, based on an extensive background of study data in nature's laboratory, a laboratory which was extremely large. In the United States alone, some seven million people in 1,900 communities had throughout life used drinking water which was naturally fluoridated with a fluoride concentration of 0·7 ppm or greater. We knew what too

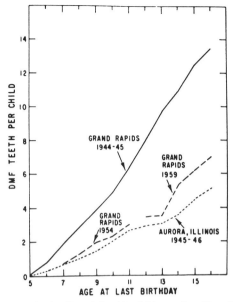

Fig. 3. Dental caries in Grand Rapids children after 10 and 15 years of fluoridation. (From Arnold et al., 1962.) (*Copyright by the American Dental Association. Reprinted by permission.*)

much did, we knew what too little did, we knew what the optimum amount was and we had assurance that one part per million fluoride in the drinking water had the same biological effect whether it got there from flowing over rocks or from a feeding machine.

b. Newburgh–Kingston Study

In addition to the Grand Rapids–Muskegon study two other fluoridation studies were carried out in the United States. On 2 May 1945 sodium fluoride was added to the drinking water of Newburgh, on the Hudson river. The town of Kingston, situated 35 miles away from Newburgh, was chosen as a control town. This study was directed by David B. Ast, Chief of the Dental Bureau, State of New York Department of Health. Baseline studies were carried out in the two communities in 1944–1946 (Ast et al., 1950). Clinical examinations after 10 years of fluoridation were carried out in 1954–1955 (Ast et al., 1956). They reported that whilst caries experience in 10–12-year-old Kingston children had changed little from 1945 (23·1 per cent of teeth were carious) to 1955 (26·3 per cent), in contrast in similarly aged Newburgh children over the 10-year period the DMF rate had fallen from 23·5 per cent to 13·9 per cent, thus confirming the caries-inhibitory property of fluoride drinking water.

15

c. Evanston–Oak Park Study

A third American fluoridation experiment began in January 1946 in Evanston, Illinois; the nearby community of Oak Park acted as the control town. Drs J. R. Blayney, I. N. Hill and S. O. Zimmerman of the University of Chicago Memorial Dental Clinic conducted the study and their findings after 14 years of fluoridation in Evanston were published in 1967 (Blayney and Hill, 1967). Whereas the DMF values of 14-year-old Evanston children fell from 11·66 to 5·95 between 1946 and 1960 (a reduction of 49 per cent), no change was observed in the DMF values of 14-year-old Oak Park children over the intervening years. Here again was experimental proof of the caries-inhibitory property of fluoride in drinking water at a concentration of 1 ppm. The Evanston–Oak Park study presented the most detailed data of all the fluoridation studies. In an introduction to the report Dr F. A. Arnold, jun., Chief Dental Officer, United States Public Health Service wrote:

Here in a single report are data on the effect of water fluoridation on dental caries so completely documented that the article is virtually a textbook for use in further research. It is an important scientific contribution towards betterment of the dental health of our nation. It is a classic in this field. (Arnold, 1967.)

Yet the strength of the experimental proof of the caries-inhibitory property of fluoride drinking water lies not only in the conclusion of one study but also in the fact that the three American studies, carried out by different investigators in different parts of the country, reached similar conclusions: addition of 1 ppm fluoride in the drinking water reduced caries experience by approximately 50 per cent.

d. Canadian Study (Brantford, Sarnia and Stratford)

In Canada a project was undertaken in Brantford, Ontario, where fluoride was added to the water supply in June 1945. The community of Sarnia was established as the control town; in addition the community of Stratford, where fluoride was naturally present in the drinking water at a level of 1·3 ppm, was used as an auxiliary control. After 17 years of fluoridation in Brantford, caries experience was similar to that occurring in the natural fluoride area of Stratford and was 55 per cent lower than in the control town of Sarnia (Hutton et al., 1951; Brown and Poplove, 1965).

e. Dutch study (Tiel–Culemborg)

The caries-inhibitory action of fluoride in drinking water is not uniform: fluoride inhibits smooth-surface caries much more than pit and fissure caries. Investigation of this selective property of fluoride was an important component of the Dutch study, instituted in 1953 in Tiel and Culemborg.

16

This study was designed to assess the preventive effect of fluoride drinking water on the anatomical siting of caries attack: approximal surfaces, free smooth surfaces (buccal and lingual) and pit and fissure sites. In March 1953 the drinking water in Tiel was fluoridated at a level of 1·1 ppm. Culemborg, with a fluoride concentration of 0·1 ppm, was to serve as a control. Baseline examinations of 11–15-year-old children were carried out in 1952. There were no significant differences between Tiel and Culemborg data at the beginning of the investigation (Backer Dirks et al., 1961).

The examinations in 1969 provided data on 15-year-old children who had been born within the first year after the introduction of fluoridation 16 years previously (Kwant et al., 1973). Approximal cavities were established from radiographs only; caries in pits and fissures and on free smooth surfaces was determined clinically. The 135 Culemborg 15-year-olds had a mean of 25·8 carious sites or surfaces compared with 11·3 carious sites or surfaces in the 147 Tiel 15-year-olds. Over all the sites there was, therefore, 56 per cent less caries in Tiel (*Table* 2). The percentage

Table 2. Mean Number of Pit and Fissure, Approximal and Smooth-surface Cavities in 15-year-old Children, born in 1954 and examined in 1969, in Tiel and Culemborg (*Kwant et al., 1973*)

	No. of children	Pit and fissure	Approximal	Free smooth-surface	Total
Culemborg	135	12·0	10·1	3·6	25·8
Tiel	147	8·3	2·5	0·5	11·3
Difference		3·7	7·6	3·1	14·5
% Difference		31	75	86	56

reduction was highest (86 per cent) in the free smooth surfaces (buccal and lingual) and least (31 per cent) in the pit and fissure sites. A 75 per cent reduction was observed for approximal surfaces, which amounted to a difference of 7·6 approximal surfaces per child between Tiel and Culemborg. The number of teeth which had been extracted due to caries was 85 per cent less in Tiel 15-year-olds (1·55 extractions per child) compared with Culemborg 15-year-olds (0·23 extractions per child).

Kwant et al. (1974) reported on the effect of lifelong water fluoridation in 17- and 18-year-olds. The authors pointed out that direct comparisons between the inhabitants of the two towns were becoming more difficult in the older age groups since the number of extractions had a considerable bearing on the results. In Culemborg, 17- and 18-year-olds had had six times as many teeth extracted as in Tiel. The difference in the number of cavities between the 17-year-olds born in 1954 and examined in 1971 in Tiel and Culemborg was 19 cavities per person, or 53 per cent fewer cavities in Tiel. For the 18-year-olds, born in 1953, the difference was 17 cavities per person or 48 per cent fewer cavities in Tiel.

The epidemiological evidence from this well-conducted Dutch study indicates that adequate ingestion of fluoride at an early stage of enamel formation is important in preventing pit and fissure caries, but is of less importance as far as smooth-surface caries is concerned.

f. New Zealand Study (Hastings)

The effectiveness of fluoridation was also demonstrated in a study carried out in Hastings, New Zealand. This was a retrospective study: baseline examinations were carried out in 1954; further examinations were carried out in 1964 after 10 years of fluoridation (Ludwig, 1965) and in 1970 after 16 years' fluoridation (Ludwig, 1971). The mean DMFT of 15-year-old children fell from 16·8 in 1954 to 8·5 in 1970, a reduction of 8·3 teeth or 49 per cent. This study, like the Dutch study, also demonstrated the selective caries-inhibitory action of fluoride on different tooth surfaces. In these 15-year-old children, free smooth-surface caries was reduced by 87 per cent (a difference of 3·3 surfaces between 1954 and 1970), approximal caries by 73 per cent (a difference of 14·7 surfaces) and occlusal surface caries by 39 per cent (a difference of 7·2 surfaces).

The effect of fluoridation in Hastings on the cost of a dental public health programme has been reported by Denby and Hollis (1966). There was a 45 per cent increase in the number of children that could be treated by a dental nurse and a decrease in the cost of the General Dental Benefits programme.

g. British Studies

In Great Britain the studies by Weaver (1944) had shown that caries experience in South Shields (natural fluoride content 1·4 ppm) was approximately 50 per cent lower than in North Shields (fluoride content 0·25 ppm), thus confirming Dean's findings in Galesburg and Monmouth, Macomb and Quincy (Dean et al., 1939).

In addition, Weaver (1950) carried out a second investigation in 1949, in the North-East of England, including a survey of West Hartlepool children, where fluoride content of the water supply was 2 ppm. He examined 500 5-year-old children and reported that the mean dmft was 1·76 and that 53·6 per cent of the children were caries-free. A similar number of 12-year-old children were examined: the mean DMF was 0·96 and 59·8 per cent were caries-free. He commented: 'There can be few, if any, other areas in this country where the average DMF figure for unselected 12-year-old children is less than 1, as it was found to be in West Hartlepool.'

Forrest (1956) studied 324 12–14-year-old children in other parts of Britain with concentrations of fluoride in the drinking water varying from 0·9 to 5·8 ppm. She compared the caries prevalence with 259 children of the same age in non-fluoride areas. Caries was markedly lower in the high-fluoride regions.

A further study of areas with varying concentrations of fluoride in drinking water was carried out by James (1961), who examined 1027 children aged 11–13 years from three areas in East Anglia: Norwich and Yarmouth (Norfolk) (F = 0·17–0·2 ppm), Chelmsford (intermittent fluoride content) and Colchester (F = 1·2–2 ppm). Children from Colchester were further divided into 'continuous' and 'non-continuous' residents. This study showed that the DMF of those children continuously resident in the high-fluoride area was less than half that of corresponding children in the low-fluoride area. Children aged 11–13 years who were continuous residents of Colchester had nearly double the proportion of sound first permanent molars found in the non-continuous residents.

In 1952 the British Government sent a mission to the United States of America and Canada to study fluoridation in operation. The mission concluded that fluoridation of water supplies was a valuable health measure but recommended that in this country fluoride should be added to the water supplies of some selected communities before its general adoption was considered (Report of the United Kingdom Mission, 1953). The selected communities chosen were Watford, Kilmarnock and part of Anglesey. Fluoride was added to these drinking waters in 1955–1956. Sutton, Ayr and the remaining part of Anglesey acted as the control towns. The results after 5 years of fluoridation (Department of Public Health and Social Security, 1962) showed that caries experience in 5-year-old children was 50 per cent lower in the fluoride areas than the non-fluoride areas (*Table* 3). In spite of this, fluoridation was discontinued in Kilmarnock in 1962, on the instructions of the local council. However, dental examinations continued to be carried out in all areas and the findings after 11 years' fluoridation were reported in 1969 (*Table* 4). The report confirmed the main findings of 1962, that fluoridation of water supplies is a highly effective method of reducing dental decay.

In addition to demonstrating the beneficial effects of fluoridation, the Report also confirmed its complete safety. 'During the eleven years under review, medical practitioners reported only two patients with symptoms which they felt might have been associated with fluoridation. Careful investigation in both instances failed to attribute the symptoms to the drinking of fluoridated water.' (Report of the Committee on Research into Fluoridation, 1969.) The Government is so confident of the safety of water fluoridation that it is prepared to give unlimited indemnity to any local authority in respect of actions for damages based on alleged harm to health resulting from fluoridation. In the Republic of Ireland, where fluoridation of community water supplies has been mandatory since 1964,

Table 3. Number of Children examined and Mean dmft in 1956 and 1961 for each Year Age Group in Study Areas and Control Areas
(Department of Public Health and Social Security, 1962)

| | Study areas | | | | Control areas | | | |
| | 1956 | | 1961 | | 1956 | | 1961 | |
Age	No. of children	Mean dmf	No. of children	Mean dmf	No. of children	Mean dmf	No. of children	Mean dmf
3*	450	3·80	388	1·29	297	3·53	329	3·32
4*	591	5·39	468	2·31	334	5·18	295	4·83
5†	785	5·81	531	2·91	461	5·66	374	5·39
6†	883	6·49	615	4·81	566	6·32	432	6·22
7†	952	7·06	593	6·05	577	7·08	446	6·89

* Full dentition. † Canines and molars only.

Table 4. Number of Children examined and Mean DMF in Study and Control Areas (Department of Public Health and Social Security, 1969)

| | Study areas | | | | | Control areas | | | | |
| | 1956 | | 1967 | | | 1965 | | 1967 | | |
Age	No. of children	Mean DMF	No. of children	Mean DMF	Per cent difference	No. of children	Mean DMF	No. of children	Mean DMF	Per cent difference
8	806	2·1	378	1·2	43	499	2·2	204	2·0	8
9	780	2·8	395	1·8	36	491	2·8	229	2·7	3
10	636	3·4	356	2·4	31	460	3·5	213	3·3	5
8–10	2222	2·8	1129	1·8	36	1450	2·8	646	2·7	5

legal action has already been taken. After a lengthy case lasting 65 days before Mr Justice Kenny in the Irish High Court, the Judge held that the amount of fluoride ingested at a concentration of 1 ppm in the drinking water did not involve any risk to health and concluded that the fluoridation of the public water supplies was not a violation of constitutional rights. His judgement was subsequently upheld in the Supreme Court of the Republic of Ireland. In the United Kingdom the decision to fluoridate the public water supplies is taken by individual local authorities. In 1971 approximately 5 per cent of the total population in this country had the benefit of fluoridated drinking water (Parliamentary News, 1971), and by 1980 approximately 10 per cent of the population were drinking fluoridated drinking water. There are now fluoridation schemes in parts of 24 Area Health Authorities in England and Wales, but Birmingham and Newcastle remain the only major towns which have been fluoridated for 10 or more years. The number of fluoridation plants and the population served in the various Area Health Authorities are given in *Table* 5. Surveys have been carried out in Great Britain of natural and artificially fluoridated areas (*see map*).

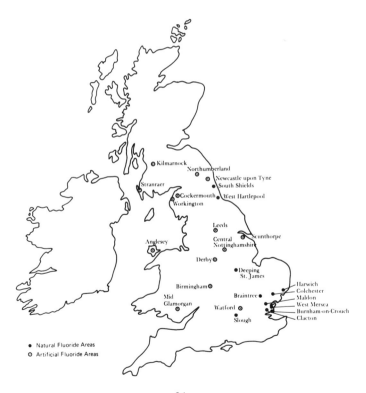

21

Table 5. Details of Fluoridation Plants in 22 English Area Health Authorities

AHA	Date scheme(s) introduced	No. of fluoridation plants	Population served by each plant	Type of plant (acid/powder)	Comments
Bedfordshire	10/1972	Bedford	117 200	Fluosilicic acid	Approx. 184 800 out of total pop. of 490 000 Grafham water—either untreated or mixed with fluoridated water from time to time
	3/1973	Meppershall	20 600		
	5/1974	Pulloxhill	11 500		
	6/1973	Dunton }	35 500		
	1/1973	Newspring }			
Birmingham	6/1964	Elan Valley }	1 197 000	Powder	
	9/1967	Trimpley }			
Bradford	6/1972		2600	Acid	Approx. 200 households in Esholt receive F water as overflow from Leeds Aireborough Plant
Buckinghamshire	1974	Radnage	1300 children	Acid	
Cheshire	4/1975		127 500	Acid	
Cumbria	10/1969	Cornhow	50 000	Sodium silica fluoride powder	
	11/1972	Ennerdale	60 000	Hydrofluosilicic acid	
Derbyshire	1970–1971	Stanley Moor	20 825	Acid	Two naturally fluoridated sources in Derbyshire, at Lowtown and Cubley
		Lindway	1050		
		Homesford	126 157		
		Washgreen	12 720		
		Belper Meadows	12 735		
		Little Eaton	330 422		
		Stanton	11 905		
	1975	Budby	40 545		

22

Durham	4/1970	Honey Hill	127036	Acid	
Gateshead	1970	Honey Hill	32000	Acid	Water from Horsley Reservoir supplements supplies from Whittle Dene and Throckley; acid to be added to it shortly
	10/1968	{ Whittle Dene, Throckley	192000	Powder	
Hereford and Worcester	1968	Sugarbrook	40000	Powder	
	1969	Wildmoor	20000		
	1971	Bellington	30000		
	1973	Burcot	25000		
	1973	Washingstocks	25000	} Acid	
	1974	Web Heath	30000		
	1977	Brockhill	25000		
Hertfordshire	5/1956	Grove	11000, 67000 }	Acid	
Humberside	5/1968	Winterton Holmes	32340	Powder	
	6/1969	Barrow	97250		
	1972	Immingham	12190	} Acid	Not functioned since 1977
	1972	Barnoldby-le-Beck	1340		
Kirklees	8/1970, 11/1978, 6/1979			Acid	
Leeds	1968	Riva Reservoir	28000	Powder	
Newcastle	1968	Whittle Dene, Henderson Filters, { Throckley, Horsley	600000	Sodium silicofluoride	
	1980			Hydrofluosilicic acid	Changing to acid
North Tyneside	7/1968	Whittle Dene, Henderson Filters, { Throckley, Horsley	105000	Powder	
	1979–1980			Acid	

Table 5 (cont.)

AHA	Date scheme(s) introduced	No. of fluoridation plants	Population served by each plant	Type of plant (acid/powder)	Comments
Northumberland	1969	Gunnerton	36 000	Originally powder, changed to acid	
	1968	Whittle Dene / Throckley	60 000	Powder	
	1979	Horsley	35 000	Acid	
	1979	Alnwick/Berwick		Acid	
Nottingham	1971	(Water source, not plant) Amen Corner Bradmer Budby Caunton Chequer House Clay Lane Clipstone Edwinstowe Epperstone Far Baulker Farnsfield Fishpool Norman Hollow Rainworth Rushley Sunnyside	358 500	Hydrofluosilicic acid	Difficulty in maintaining level of fluoride
Oxfordshire	2/1972	Near Witney	30 000	Acid	Difficulty in maintaining level of fluoride

Sandwell	1964–1970	F water from Elan Valley and Trimpley plants (Birmingham)		Powder
Solihull	1964	No F plant in borough—F water supplied by Elan Valley and Trimpley plants (Birmingham)	180 000	Powder
Warwickshire	1968	Rugby	108 000	Powder
	1973	Campion Hills	72 000	Acid
	1974	Campion Terrace	52 000	Acid
	1971	Mill End	12 000	Acid
	1976	Haseley	9200	Acid
	1976	Heath End	8800	Acid
	1977	Thelsford	6800	Acid
	1974	Wellesbourne	6800	Acid
	1972	August/Ryon Hill	6400	Acid
	1971	Rowington	6000	Acid
	1972	Warwick Rd/Welcombe Fields	5600	Acid
	1977	Flowers Borehold	4400	Acid
	1970	Lillington	4400	Acid
	1971	Budbroke	3600	Acid
	1971	Shrewley	3600	Acid
	1970	Leicester Lane	2400	Acid
	1973	Alveston Hill	2000	Acid
	1971	Birmingham Road	2000	Acid
	1971	Whitnash	2000	Acid
	1977	Alcester Road	1200	Acid
	1968	Leek Wootton	520	Acid
		Total (Warwickshire)	319 720	

THE WORLD HEALTH ORGANISATION

Looking further afield, the World Health Organisation has always taken a keen interest in the effect of fluoridation on dental health. In 1958 they produced a first report by an expert committee on water fluoridation and concluded that drinking water containing about 1 ppm fluoride had a marked caries-preventive action and that controlled fluoridation of drinking water was a practicable and effective public health measure (WHO, 1958). In a later article, 'Fluoridation and dental health' (WHO, 1969), it was stated that as a result of the initial controlled fluoridation studies in America and Canada, further programmes were under way in more than 30 countries and territories serving over 120 million people.

In 1962 the World Health Organisation invited 29 experts to collaborate in the preparation of a monograph relating to the effects of fluoride on human health. The object of the monograph was to provide an impartial review of the scientific literature on the varied aspects of fluoridation and the many complex questions relating to the metabolism of fluorides and their use in medicine and public health (WHO, 1970). In a summary of the section on fluorides and general health, A. E. Martin (1970) stated that:

By their wide distribution in nature, their inevitable presence in man's food and drink and their consequent presence in the tissues of the human body, fluorides form a natural part of man's environment, yet when present in excess they are known to be harmful. Studies of the geographical distribution of dental mottling in the U.S.A. were begun during the early decades of the century and the identification of fluorides in water supplies in 1931 led to a comprehensive survey designed, in the first place, to find the threshold limit for the avoidance of dental fluorosis and, later, to ascertain the concentration in a water supply necessary for optimal dental protection. When the artificial fluoridation of water was first considered, this survey provided a useful starting point for a programme of specific epidemiological and experimental studies which, over the past three decades, has yielded a mass of data confirming the safety of fluoridation. This has been supplemented by independent studies from other countries which have provided further supplementary material for use in defining the upper limits of a safe fluoride intake. The results have shown that for the climatic, nutritional and environmental conditions under which the surveys have been carried out, a level of approximately 1 ppm fluoride in temperate climates has no harmful effects on the community. The margin of safety is such that it will cover any individual variation of intake to be found in such areas.

A report on fluoridation was submitted by the Director of WHO to the 22nd World Health Assembly, as a result of which the following resolution was adopted by the Assembly on 22 July 1969:

The World Health Organisation recommends member states to examine the possibility of introducing and where practicable to introduce fluoridation of those community water supplies where the fluoride intake from water and other sources for the given population is below optimal levels, as a proven public health measure; and where fluoridation of community water supplies is not practicable to study other methods of using fluorides for the protection of dental health. (WHO, 1969.)

This resolution was reaffirmed in the Report of the WHO Director General in 1975: 'Fluoridation of communal water supplies, where feasible, should be the cornerstone of any national programme of dental caries prevention.'

McKay would have been well pleased. His observations in Colorado Springs over 70 years ago, followed by his persistence in determining the cause of mottled enamel, had transcended national boundaries and resulted in the discovery of a public health measure, which would markedly reduce the prevalence of dental caries, being recommended to all member states of the World Health Organisation. The history of fluoridation must surely rank as one of the classic epidemiological studies of chronic disease in the history of medicine.

REFERENCES

Ainsworth N. J. (1928) Mottled teeth. *R. Dent. Hosp. Mag.* February.

Ainsworth N. J. (1933) Mottled teeth. *Br. Dent. J.* **60**, 233–250.

Arnold F. A. jun., (1967) Foreword to fluorine and dental caries. *J. Am. Dent. Assoc.* **74**, 230.

Arnold F. A. jun., Dean H. T. and Knutson J. W. (1953) Effect of fluoridated public water supplies on dental caries prevalence. Results of the seventh year of study at Grand Rapids and Muskegon, Mich. *Public Health Rep.* **68**, 141–148.

Arnold F. A. jun., Dean H. T., Jay P. and Knutson J. W. (1956) Effect of fluoridated public water supplies on dental caries prevalence. 10th year of the Grand Rapids–Muskegon Study. *Public Health Rep.* **71**, 652–658.

Arnold F. A., Likens R. C., Russell A. L. and Scott D. B. (1962) Fifteenth year of the Grand Rapids fluoridation study. *J. Am. Dent. Assoc.* **65**, 780–785.

Ast D. B., Finn S. B. and McCafferty I. (1950) The Newburgh–Kingston caries fluorine study. I, Dental findings after three years of water fluoridation. *Am. J. Public Health* **40**, 116–124.

Ast D. B., Smith D. J., Wacks B. and Cantwell K. T. (1956) Newburgh–Kingston caries-fluorine study XIV. Combined clinical and roentgenographic dental findings after ten years of fluoride experience. *J. Am. Dent. Assoc.* **52**, 314–325.

Backer Dirks O., Houwink B. and Kwant G. W. (1961) The results of $6\frac{1}{2}$ years of artificial fluoridation of drinking water in the Netherlands. The Tiel–Culemborg experiment. *Arch. Oral Biol.* **5**, 284–300.

Beal J. F. and Clayton M. (1981) Fluoridation: a clinical survey in Corby and Scunthorpe. *Publ. Hlth, Lond.* **95**, 152–160.

Black G. V. (1916) Mottled teeth. *Dent. Cosmos* **58**, 129–156.

Blayney J. R. and Hill I. N. (1967) Fluorine and dental caries. *J. Am. Dent. Assoc.* **74**, 233–302.

British Association for the Study of Community Dentistry (1980) Information service on epidemiological studies. *Proc. BASCD* **2** (1), 41–46.

Brown H. K. and Poplove M. (1965) Brantford–Sarnia–Stratford fluoridation caries study: final survey 1963. *J. Can. Dent. Assoc.* **31**, 505–511.

Chalmers Clarke J. H. (1954) The value of fluoridation of domestic water supplies in prevention of dental caries and sepsis. *Med. Off.* **92**, 39–43.

Chalmers Clarke J. H. and Mann J. E. (1960) Natural fluoridation and mottling of teeth in Lincolnshire. *Br. Dent. J.* 181–187.

Churchill H. V. (1931a) Letter to F. S. McKay in the McKay papers. Cited by McNeil (1957), p. 26.

Churchill H. V. (1931b) Occurrence of fluorides in some waters of the United States. *Ind. Eng. Chem.* **23**, 996–998.

Dean H. T. (1933) Distribution of mottled enamel in the United States. *Public Health Rep.* **48**, 704–734.

Dean H. T. (1934) Classification of mottled enamel diagnosis. *J. Am. Dent. Assoc.* **21**, 1421–1426.

Dean H. T. (1936) Chronic endemic dental fluorosis (mottled enamel). *J. Am. Med. Assoc.* **107**, 1269–1272.

Dean H. T. (1938) Endemic fluorosis and its relation to dental caries. *Public Health Rep.* **53**, 1443–1452.

Dean H. T. and Elvove E. (1936) Some epidemiological aspects of chronic endemic dental fluorosis. *Am. J. Public Health* **26**, 567–575.

Dean H. T., Arnold F. A. jun. and Elvove E. (1942) Domestic water and dental caries, V, additional studies of the relation of fluoride domestic waters to dental caries experience in 4,425 white children aged 12–14 years, of 13 cities in 4 states, *Public Health Rep.* **57**, 1155–1179.

Dean H. T., Arnold F. A. jun., Jay P. and Knutson J. W. (1950) Studies on mass control of dental caries through fluoridation of public water supply. *Public Health Rep.* **65**, 1403–1408.

Dean H. T., Jay P., Arnold F. A. jun. and Elvove E. (1939) Domestic water and the dental caries including certain epidemiological aspects of oral *L. acidophilus*. *Public Health Rep.* **54**, 862–888.

Dean H. T. and McKay F. S. (1939) Production of mottled enamel halted by a change in common water supply. *Am. J. Public Health* **29**, 590–596.

Denby G. C. and Hollis M. J. (1966) The effect of fluoridation on a dental public health programme. *N. Z. Dent. J.* **62**, 32–36.

Eager J. M. (1902) Abstract: chiaie teeth. *Dent. Cosmos* **44**, 300–301.

Fallon S. J. J. S. and Watson G. S. (1982) Survey of dental caries experience in 5- and 15-year-old Humberside schoolchildren. *Publ. Hlth Lond.* **96**, 15–19.

Forrest J. R. (1956) Caries incidence and enamel defects in areas with different levels of fluoride in the drinking water. *Br. Dent. J.* **100**, 195–200.

Hutton W. L., Linscott B. W. and Williams D. B. (1951) Brantford fluorine experiment. *Can. J. Public Health* **42**, 81.

James P. M. C. (1961) Dental caries prevalence in high and low fluoride areas of East Anglia. *Br. Dent. J.* **110**, 165–169.

Kempf G. A. and McKay F. S. (1930) Mottled enamel in a segregated population. *Public Health Rep.* **45**, 2923–2940.

Klein H., Palmer G. E. and Knutson J. W. (1938) Studies on dental caries: (1) Dental status and dental needs of elementary schoolchildren. *Public Health Rep.* **53**, 751–765.

Knutson J. W. (1970) Water fluoridation after 25 years. *Br. Dent. J.* **129**, 297–300.

Kwant G. W., Houwink B., Backer Dirks O., Groeneveld A. and Pot T. J. (1973) Artificial fluoridation of drinking water in the Netherlands; results of the

Tiel–Culemborg experiment after $16\frac{1}{2}$ years. *Netherl. Dent. J.* **80**, suppl. 9, 6–27.

Kwant G. W., Groeneveld A., Pot T. J. and Purdell Lewis D. (1974) Fluoridetoevoeging aan het drinkwater *V. Nederl. Tijds. Tandheelk.* **81**, 251–261.

Ludwig T. G. (1965) The Hastings Fluoridation Project V—Dental effects between 1954 and 1964. *N.Z. Dent. J.* **61**, 175–179.

Ludwig T. G. (1971) Hastings fluoridation project VI. *N.Z. Dent J.* **67**, 155–160.

McCollum E. V., Simmonds N., Becker J. E. and Bunting R. W. (1925) The effect of additions of fluoride to the diet of rats on the quality of their teeth. *J. Biol. Chem.* **63**, 553.

McKay F. S. (1916a) An investigation of mottled teeth (I). *Dent. Cosmos* **58**, 477–484.

McKay F. S. (1916b) An investigation of mottled teeth (II). *Dent. Cosmos* **58**, 627–644.

McKay F. S. (1916c) An investigation of mottled teeth (III). *Dent. Cosmos* **58**, 781–792.

McKay F. S. (1916d) An investigation of mottled teeth (IV). *Dent. Cosmos* **58**, 894–904.

McKay F. S. (1918) Progress of the year in the investigation of mottled enamel with special reference to its association with artesian water. *J. Natl Dent. Assoc.* **5**, 721–750.

McKay F. S. (1925) Mottled enamel: A fundamental problem in dentistry. *Dent Cosmos* **67**, 847–860.

McKay F. S. (1928) The relation of mottled teeth to caries. *J. Am. Dent. Assoc.* **15**, 1429–1437.

McKay F. S. (1933) Mottled teeth: The prevention of its further production through a change in the water supply at Oakley, Idaho. *J. Am. Dent. Assoc.* **20**, 1137–1149.

McNeil D. R. (1957). *The Fight for Fluoridation.* New York, OUP.

Martin A. E. (1970) In: *Fluorides and Human Health. WHO Monogr. Ser.* No. 59. Geneva, WHO, pp. 316–318.

Medical Research Council (1925) The incidence of dental disease in children. *Med. Res. Counc. Spec. Rep. Ser. (Lond.)* No. 97.

Minutes of Colorado Springs Dental Society (1908) Cited by McNeil D. R. (1957), p. 5.

Moulton F. R. (1942) *Fluorine and Dental Health.* Washington, DC, American Association for the Advancement of Science.

Department of Public Health and Social Security (1962) The results of fluoridation studies in the United States and the results achieved after five years. *Rep. Public Health Med. Subj. (Lond.)* No. 105.

Department of Public Health and Social Security (1969) Report of the Committee on Research into Fluoridation. The fluoridation studies in the United Kingdom and the results achieved after eleven years. *Rep. Public Health Med. Subj. (Lond.)* No. 122.

Parliamentary News (1971) Report of question in the House of Commons on 23 April, 1971. *Br. Dent. J.* **130**, 412.

Report of the Director General WHO (1975) 28th World Health Assembly, Geneva, May 1975.

Report of United Kingdom Mission (1953) *The Fluoridation of Domestic Water Supplies in North America*. London, HMSO.

Smith H. V. and Smith M. C. (1931) Mottled enamel in Arizona and its correlation with the concentration of fluorides in water supplies. *Bull. Ariz. Agric. Exp. Stn.* No. 32.

Smith M. C. (1931) Account of Tucson Dental Association meeting in Arizona. *Daily Star*, 3 May, 1931, cited by McNeil D. R. (1957), p. 34.

Weaver R. (1944) Fluorosis and dental caries on Tyneside. *Br. Dent. J.* **76**, 29–40.

Weaver R. (1950) Fluorine and wartime diet. *Br. Dent. J.* **88**, 231–239.

World Health Organisation (1958) Report of Expert Committee on Water Fluoridation. *WHO Tech. Rep. Ser.* No. 146.

World Health Organisation (1969) Fluoridation and dental health. *WHO Chron.* **23**, 505–512.

World Health Organisation (1970) *Fluorides and Human Health. WHO Monogr. Ser.* No. 59. Geneva, WHO.

BIBLIOGRAPHY

Dunning J. M. (1962) *Principles of Dental Public Health*. Cambridge, Mass., Harvard University Press.

McClure F. J. (ed.) (1962) *Fluoride Drinking Waters*. Bethesda, Md, US Department of Health Education and Welfare, National Institute of Dental Research.

McClure F. J. (1970) Water Fluoridation. Bethesda, Md, US Department of Health Education and Welfare National Institute of Dental Research.

McNeil D. R. (1957) *The Fight for Fluoridation*. New York, Oxford University Press.

World Health Organisation (1970) *Fluorides and Human Health. WHO Monogr. Ser.* No. 59. Geneva, WHO.

Young W. O. and Striffler D. F. (1964) *The Dentist, His Practice and His Community*. Philadelphia, Saunders.

CHAPTER 2

WATER FLUORIDATION AND CHILD DENTAL HEALTH

In the previous chapter attention was focused on results reported from fluoride and non-fluoride areas. The purpose of this chapter is to consider in greater detail the impact of water fluoridation on the dental needs of children.

THE DECIDUOUS DENTITION

1. The Pre-school Child

Very few studies have concentrated on the pre-school child. Tank and Storvick (1964) examined 132 children aged 1–6 years, born and brought up in Corvallis (1·0 ppm F in drinking water) and 114 children of similar age from Albany (fluoride-free). The examinations were carried out once a year for 5 years, so although a total of 246 children were involved in the study, some were examined more than once. The results showed that for each age group caries experience was lower in Corvallis than in Albany; combining all age groups, the mean caries rate was 56 per cent lower in the fluoride area than in the non-fluoride area. There was no difference between the communities in the number of erupted teeth at each year age group (*Table* 6).

Winter et al. (1971) reported the caries rate in 602 pre-school children aged 1–4 years in London, England, a low-fluoride area. The only study giving the caries experience of pre-school children from a high-fluoride

Table 6. Number of Erupted Teeth and Mean dmft in 1–6-year-old Children living in Albany (Fluoride-free) and Corvallis (1·0 ppm F)
(After Tank and Storvick, 1964)

Age in years at last birthday	No. of children examined		No. of erupted deciduous teeth		Mean dmft	
	Albany	Corvallis	Albany	Corvallis	Albany	Corvallis
1	36	96	11·2	11·3	0·14	0·08
2	50	73	17·9	18·1	1·26	0·59
3	53	66	20·0	20·0	4·25	1·44
4	53	52	20·0	20·0	5·51	2·31
5	24	28	19·4	19·4	6·00	3·29
6	13	27	16·5	17·6	7·77	3·19
All ages	229	322	17·5	17·7	4·16	1·82

area in Great Britain was carried out in Hartlepool (F = 1·5–2·0 ppm) by Atkinson in 1968 (Murray and Atkinson, 1971). Ten nursery schools and play groups in the town were visited to give elementary oral hygiene instruction to mothers and children. As part of this programme 448 children aged 2–5 years received a dental examination. The results of these two studies are compared in *Table 7* and show that the benefits of fluoridation are apparent even from the earliest years.

Table 7. Caries Experience of Pre-school Children in Hartlepool and London (*After Winter et al., 1971; Murray and Atkinson, 1971*)

Age in *years*	Hartlepool F = 1·5–2·0 ppm			London (F = 0·2 ppm)		
	No. of children	Mean dmf	Per cent caries-free	No. of children	Mean dmf	Per cent caries-free
1	—	—	—	172	0·04	98
2	45	0·2	93	173	0·8	82
3	148	0·6	77	146	1·4	64
4	223	1·0	63	110	3·1	42
5	32	1·3	50	—	—	—

2. The Primary School Child

The early fluoridation studies in America concentrated mainly on the permanent dentition. One of the first studies to highlight in detail the effect of water fluoridation on the deciduous dentition was that reported by Weaver (1944) in North Shields (F = 0·4 ppm) and South Shields (F = 1·4 ppm). The mean dmf was 41 per cent lower in South Shields than North Shields (3·9 dmf teeth as against 6·6 dmf teeth) and this difference seemed to be distributed fairly evenly throughout the various deciduous teeth (*Fig.* 4).

This observation was supported by a 'cradle to the grave' study carried out in Hartlepool in 1967–1970 (Murray, 1969a, b). Three thousand eight hundred and four children aged 3–18 years, being a stratified random sample of all children born and continuously resident in Hartlepool, were examined, including 500 5-year-old children. A sample of 527 5-year-old children from the low-fluoride town of York (F = 0·25 ppm) were also examined during the same period to provide a control. The mean dmf in Hartlepool was 64 per cent lower than in York (1·5 dmf teeth compared with 4·1 dmf teeth). The number of dmf teeth per 100 erupted teeth for each tooth type is given diagrammatically in *Fig.* 5. The percentage number of dmf teeth in York was 20·5; in Hartlepool it was 7·45, giving a York : Hartlepool ratio of 2·75 : 1. This ratio for all teeth is very similar to the ratios for deciduous molars and for maxillary incisors, which contribute approximately 95 per cent of the total dmf value, and show

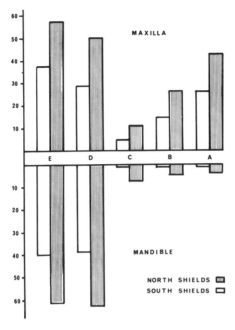

Fig. 4. Per cent caries experience in each tooth type in 5-year-old children from North and South Shields. (From Weaver, 1944.)

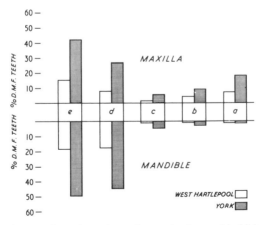

Fig. 5. Caries experience in each tooth type in 5-year-old children from Hartlepool and York. (From Murray, 1969a.) (*Reproduced by courtesy of the Editor, 'British Dental Journal'.*)

33

that deciduous molars and deciduous maxillary incisors benefit approximately equally from water fluoridation. Over half the Hartlepool 5-year-old children were caries-free (51·2 per cent) compared with less than a quarter of the York children (22·4 per cent) (*Fig.* 6). Twice as many deciduous molars had to be extracted in York (7·8 per cent) compared with Hartlepool (3·7 per cent).

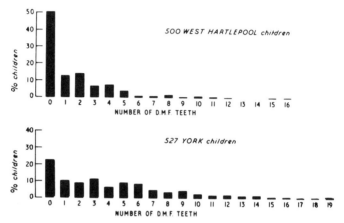

Fig. 6. The frequency distribution of dmf teeth in 5-year-old children from Hartlepool and York. (From Murray, 1969a.) (*Reproduced by courtesy of the Editor, 'British Dental Journal'.*)

The first city in the UK to fluoridate was Birmingham in 1964. In 1970, 5-year-olds from non-fluoridated Dudley had 5·1 deft compared with 2·5 deft in the 5-year-olds living in fluoridated Birmingham (Beal and James, 1971). In a later survey, Whittle and Downer (1979) observed that dmft scores for 4–5-year-old children living in fluoridated Birmingham were 54 per cent less than the dmft scores of 4–5-year-old children living in an area of non-fluoridated Salford, which had been matched with the Birmingham area on socioeconomic factors and dentist : population ratio. Rock et al. (1981) compared the dental health of 6–13-year-old children who had lived continuously in fluoridated Birmingham with children of the same age living in non-fluoridated Wolverhampton. Bitewing radiographs supplemented the clinical examination. The result for deciduous teeth in the 6–9-year-olds showed that the average Wolverhampton child had nearly twice as many decayed teeth, had the same number of filled teeth and had had four times as many teeth extracted because of decay, as the average child in Birmingham.

Half of the island of Anglesey was one of the original three test areas for fluoridation in the UK, commencing fluoridation in 1955. However, the non-fluoridated (control) half of Anglesey fluoridated in 1964, so that in a study conducted by Jackson, James and Wolfe (1975) in 1974, the mainland area of Bangor/Caernarvon was used as a control. This study was unique in that children from the fluoridated and non-fluoridated areas were brought to a central site and mixed before examination. The Anglesey 5-year-olds had 2·8 dmft, 38 per cent less than the Bangor/Caernarvon 5-year-olds (4.6 dmft).

Part of west Cumbria fluoridated in October 1969. The caries experience of 5-year-olds living in this area was compared with the caries experience of similarly aged children living in non-fluoridated Cumbria (Jackson, Gravely and Pinkham, 1975). Mean dmft scores for the two areas were 2·4 and 4·4 respectively, a difference in favour of the children living in fluoridated Cumbria of 46 per cent.

Similar results were observed in four districts of Leeds which fluoridated in 1968. A comparison of the caries experience of 5-year-old children living in these districts with the caries experience of similarly aged children in two neighbouring non-fluoridated areas, in 1979, revealed that the children in the former areas had 62 per cent less caries experience than the children in the non-fluoridated areas. Per 1000 children, there were 43 extracted deciduous teeth in the non-fluoridated areas compared with 11 in the fluoridated districts (Jackson et al., 1980).

The city of Newcastle and areas of Northumberland County fluoridated in June 1969. A total of 771 5-year-olds were included in a study conducted in 1975 where urban fluoridated Newcastle was compared with urban non-fluoridated Ashington, and rural fluoridated Northumberland compared with similar areas of Northumberland which were not fluoridated (Rugg-Gunn et al., 1977). The children in fluoridated Newcastle had 57 per cent less, and children in fluoridated Northumberland 67 per cent less caries experience (deft) compared with their non-fluoridated controls. Twenty-nine per cent of the Newcastle children were caries-free compared with only 11 per cent in Ashington, and 34 per cent of children in fluoridated Northumberland were caries-free compared with only 12 per cent in non-fluoridated Northumberland.

A unique feature of this study is that lifetime experiences of toothache and general anaesthetics for dental extractions were measured. Forty per cent of the Ashington 5-year-olds had suffered from toothache compared with 22 per cent of fluoridated Newcastle children, and 38 per cent of 5-year-olds in non-fluoridated Northumberland had had toothache compared with only 17 per cent in fluoridated Northumberland. General anaesthetic experience was 47 per cent less in Newcastle compared with Ashington and 68 per cent less in fluoridated compared with non-fluoridated Northumberland. The cost of treating the 5-year-olds was £5–6 per child more expensive (1976 NHS scale of fees) in the non-fluoridated areas compared with the fluoridated areas. The reduction in caries was greatest in the approximal surfaces, both in actual surfaces (2·5 per child) and percentage difference (75 per cent) (*Fig.* 7). The percentage reduction was lower for fissure sites (56 per cent) compared with free smooth surfaces (72 per cent), but was more important in absolute terms (a difference of 2·2 surfaces compared with 0·8 surfaces per child).

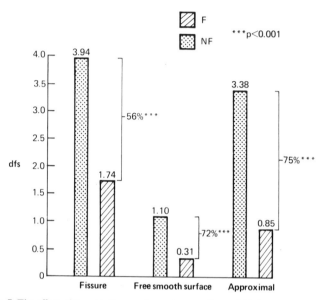

Fig. 7. The effect of fluoridation on the caries experience (dfs) for each surface type (fissure, approximal and free smooth surface) separately in the deciduous dentition of 5-year-old children in Newcastle and Northumberland. (From Rugg-Gunn et al., 1977.) (*Reproduced by courtesy of the Editor, 'British Dental Journal'.*)

Social class information was available for children in the above study. The differences in caries experience (deft) between children in the fluoridated and non-fluoridated areas were 26 per cent for social classes I and II, 60 per cent for social class III and 71 per cent for social classes IV and V (*Table* 8). Fluoridation appeared to particularly benefit lower social class children and remove intersocial class differences in dental caries experience (Carmichael et al., 1980).

In addition to the areas artificially fluoridated at 1·0 ppm the North-East of England contains communities receiving natural fluoride levels of 0·2 and 0·5 ppm F. The curve in *Fig.* 8 shows the relation between the caries experience of 5-year-old children living in four communities and their water fluoride levels (Rugg-Gunn et al., 1981). The slightly curved shape is very similar to those recorded for the permanent dentition by American dental epidemiologists (*Fig.* 9).

Table 8. Caries Experience (deft) for 5-year-olds in Fluoridated and Non-fluoridated Newcastle and Northumberland according to Social Class *(Carmichael et al., 1980)*

Social class	Area Fluoridated	Non-fluoridated	Difference (%)
I and II	2·5	3·4	0·9 (26)
III	2·4	6·0	3·6 (60)
IV and V	2·0	7·0	5·0 (71)

The effect of water fluoridation in reducing dental caries in the deciduous dentition should not be underestimated. Although in a sense deciduous teeth are 'temporary', approximately 30 per cent of all teeth that decay are deciduous teeth (Jackson, 1974). Thus a reduction in the caries experience of the deciduous dentition is a most important factor when the need for dental treatment in a community is considered. In addition it has important psychological and social benefits in that far fewer children in a fluoride area are exposed to the unfortunate sequelae of untreated dental caries—pain, sepsis, extraction of teeth—and so are likely to have a more positive attitude to dental treatment in later life.

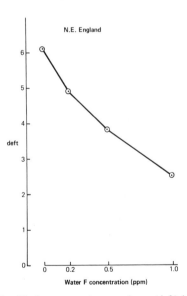

Fig. 8. The relationship between caries experience (deft) in 1038 5-year-old children living in 4 areas of North-East England and the fluoride concentration in their drinking water. (Rugg-Gunn et al., 1981.) *(Reproduced by courtesy of the Editor, 'British Dental Journal'.)*

37

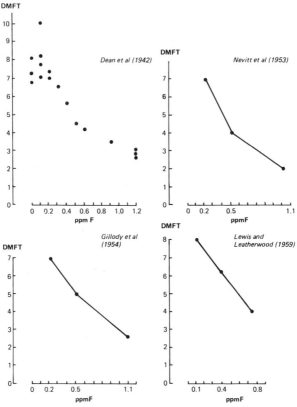

Fig. 9. The relationship between caries experience (DMFT) and water fluoride concentration (ppm F) in four American studies. (1) Dean et al., 1942; data shown refer to 5963 12- to 14-year-old children; (2) Nevitt et al., 1953; 318 12-year-old children; (3) Gillody et al., 1954; 311 13-year-old children; (4) Lewis and Leatherwood, 1959: 899 14-year-old children. (Rugg-Gunn et al., 1981.) (*Reproduced by courtesy of the Editor, 'British Dental Journal'*.)

THE PERMANENT DENTITION

The early studies by Dean and co-workers in Galesburg and Monmouth and Macomb and Quincy (Dean et al., 1939) stressed two important points about the effect of water fluoridation on the pattern of caries attack in the permanent dentition. Firstly, they observed a strikingly low amount of interproximal caries and, secondly, they reported that the mortality rate of first permanent molars was much lower in the fluoride areas (Galesburg 1·8 ppm and Monmouth 1·7 ppm) than in the non-fluoride areas (Macomb and Quincy 0·2 ppm) The data on which these two observations were based are summarized in *Tables* 9 and 10. This suggested that firstly, fluoride in drinking water had a greater caries-inhibitory effect on approximal or smooth surfaces than on pit and fissure caries and, secondly, that the rate of progression of a carious lesion is much slower in a fluoride area than in a non-fluoride area.

Table 9. Approximal Surface Caries in Maxillary Incisors of 12–14-year-old Children *(Galesburg and Monmouth and Macomb and Quincy) (Dean et al., 1939)*

	No. of children*	No. of approximal surfaces	No. of carious surfaces	Dental caries per 100 surfaces
Galesburg and Monmouth	342	2718	16	0·59
Macomb and Quincy	354	2814	251	9·00

* The children in this table include only those who have continuously used the municipal water supply throughout life.

Table 10. Mortality of First Permanent Molars in 12–14-year-old Children *(from Galesburg and Monmouth, and Macomb and Quincy), (Dean et al., 1939)*

	No. of children	No. of first permanent molars missing or extraction indicated	No. missing per 100 children examined	Per cent of those examined with one or more missing first permanent molars
Galesburg and Monmouth	467	56	12·0	8·6
Macomb and Quincy	418	292	70	35·4

Both these observations have been substantiated by subsequent studies. The Tiel–Culemborg water fluoridation experiment was designed specifically to assess the preventive effect of fluoridated drinking water on different tooth surfaces. The study's findings on fluoride's protective effect on all tooth surfaces has been presented previously on page 16 and in *Table* 2.

Backer Dirks (1974) compared the percentage distribution of the various types of carious surfaces in 15-year-old children from Holland and New Zealand (*Table* 11). He concluded that in the fluoridated towns, the relative importance of proximal and gingival lesions is markedly reduced, the pit and fissure lesions constituting more than 65 per cent of all cavities. Thus, not only was a reduction in the total number of cavities achieved, but also there was an important shift towards less complicated restorations. He calculated that if pit and fissure cavities are regarded as one

Table 11. Percentage Distribution of the various Types of Carious Surfaces in 15-year-old Children consuming Drinking Water with 0·1 or 1·0 ppm F (*Backer Dirks, 1974*)

	ppm F	Pits and fissures	Gingival lesions	Proximal lesions	Total
Culemborg	0·1	48·1	13·5	38·0	99·6
Tiel	1·0	73·2	4·5	22·3	100
Hastings, 1954	0·1	43·8	8·7	47·5	100
Hasting, 1970	1·0	65·5	2·9	31·6	100

treatment unit, gingival cavities as one unit, and the more time-consuming proximal cavities as $1\frac{1}{2}$ units, an assessment of the reduction in treatment time can be made (*Table* 12). These figures show the reduction in treatment time brought about by water fluoridation.

Table 12. Units of Time Necessary for Treatment of 15-year-old Children consuming Water with 0·1 or 1·0 ppm F (*Backer Dirks, 1974*)

	ppm F		Difference in treatment time (percentage)
	0·1	1·0	
Hasting, 1954–1970	62·7	22·9	63
Culemborg–Tiel	36·7	13·7	63

However, because the figures in *Table* 12 have only included time to treat caries, they are likely to be an overestimate of the saving in surgery time. Ast et al. (1970) reported that the chair time needed to provide examination, prophylaxis and corrective care was about $1\frac{1}{2}$ times more in non-fluoridated Kingston than in fluoridated Newburgh. Reductions in dental manpower required in fluoridated areas have been reported by Denby and Hollis (1966) in New Zealand and by Künzel (1976) in East Germany. Both these areas were fortunate, and perhaps unusual, in having sufficient manpower to meet the dental needs of the children. Denby and Hollis observed that the number of children who were able to be treated by a New Zealand dental nurse was 690 in fluoridated Hastings but only 475 in a non-fluoridated town. Künzel observed that the paedodontist : child ratio increased from 1 : 1659 in 1959 to 1 : 3208 in 1971 following the introduction of fluoridation in Karl-Marx-Stadt in 1959. The trend towards a requirement for simpler fillings in fluoridated areas was highlighted by Künzel (1976) who reported that single surface fillings were reduced by 52 per cent, and 2 or more surface fillings by 77 per cent in 6–18-year-olds after 12 years' fluoridation.

Backer Dirks (1974) also summarized data concerning the number of missing first permanent molars in fluoride and non-fluoride areas (*Table*

13) and concluded that in fluoride areas the number of extracted first molars is reduced by at least 75 per cent. He also pointed out that the baseline rate of extractions is very different in the three studies referred to, indicating that apart from dental caries the availability and type of dental treatment must also affect the rate of extractions.

Table 13. Number of Missing First Molars per 100 Children consuming Drinking Water with 0·1 or 1·0 ppm F

	Age	ppm F 0·1	ppm F 1·0	Per cent difference
Kingston–Newburgh	13/14	61	9	85
Evanston, 1946–1961	12/14	16	4	75
Culemborg–Tiel	15	44	2	95

Data for 15-year-old children in the Hartlepool–York study also confirmed these observations (Murray, 1969b). The mean DMF was 45 per cent lower in Hartlepool than York (5·0 as against 9·0). The distribution of DMF teeth in the two communities is shown diagrammatically in *Fig.* 10. The percentage number of DMF teeth for each tooth type is shown in *Fig.* 11. Approximately 95 per cent of first permanent molars in York were carious; the figure for Hartlepool was 65 per cent—a difference of approximately 30 per cent. Twice as many first molars had been extracted in York as in Hartlepool (17·9 per cent as against 8·7 per cent) in spite of the fact that the dentist : population ratio, and hence the availability of dental treatment, was much more favourable in York than it was in Hartlepool.

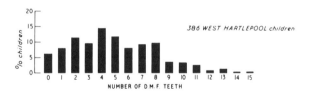

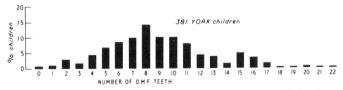

Fig. 10. The frequency distribution of DMF teeth in 15-year-old children from Hartlepool and York. (From Murray, 1969b.) (*Reproduced by courtesy of the Editor, 'British Dental Journal'.*)

41

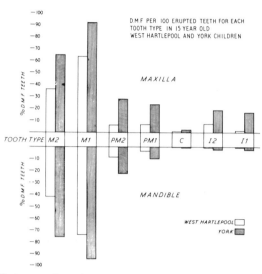

Fig. 11. Caries experience in each tooth type in 15-year-old children from Hartlepool and York. (From Murray, 1969b.) (*Reproduced by courtesy of the Editor, 'British Dental Journal'.*)

Maxillary incisors benefited more from exposure to fluoride than first molars and apparently maxillary central incisors were protected to a greater extent than maxillary lateral incisors. This apparent anomaly is because there are far more palatal pit lesions in lateral incisors than central incisors. When only approximal surfaces on these teeth were considered, there were 11 times more approximal lesions in York than in Hartlepool at 15 years of age (*Table* 14).

Table 14. Maxillary Incisor Approximal Caries in 15-year-old Children in Hartlepool (1·5–2·0 ppm F) and York (0·25 ppm F)

	No. of children	No. of DF sites	Per cent sites carious
Hartlepool	386	19	0·6
York	381	200	6·6

The greatly reduced occurrence of caries in incisor teeth in fluoridated areas has also been reported in other UK studies. Fifteen-year-old children in fluoridated Anglesey had 82 per cent fewer carious incisor teeth than children in fluoride-low control areas (Jackson, James and Wolfe, 1975). In addition, Whittle and Downer (1979) reported that the number of carious anterior teeth in 11–12-year-old children living in fluoridated Birmingham was 74 per cent less than in non-fluoridated Salford.

Thus, the effect of living in a fluoridated area is to reduce mean caries experience by 45 per cent, to markedly reduce the need to extract first permanent molars, and to virtually eliminate the need for approximal restorations in maxillary incisors.

REFERENCES

Ast D. B., Cons N. C., Pollard S. T. and Garfinkel J. (1970) Time and cost factors to provide regular, periodic dental care for children in a fluoridated and non-fluoridated area: final report. *J. Am. Dent. Assoc.* **80**, 770–776.

Backer Dirks O. (1974) The benefits of water fluoridation. *Caries Res.* **8**, Suppl. 2–15.

Beal J. F. and James P. M. C. (1971) Dental caries prevalence in 5 year old children following five and a half years of water fluoridation in Birmingham. *Br. Dent. J.* **130**, 284–288.

Carmichael C. L., Rugg-Gunn A. J., French A. D. and Cranage J. D. (1980) The effect of fluoridation upon the relationship between caries experience and social class in 5-year-old children in Newcastle and Northumberland. *Br. Dent. J.* **149**, 163–167.

Dean H. T., Arnold F. A. and Elvove E. (1942) Domestic water and dental caries V. Additional studies of the relation of fluoride domestic waters to dental caries experience in 4425 white children aged 12 to 14 years of 13 cities in 4 states. *Public Health Rep. (Wash.)* **57**, 1155–1179.

Dean H. T., Jay P., Arnold F. A. jun., McClure F. J. and Elvove E. (1939) Domestic water and dental caries, including certain epidemiological aspects of oral *L. acidophilus*. *Public Health Rep.* **54**, 862–888.

Denby G. C. and Hollis M. J. (1966) The effect of fluoridation on a dental public health programme. *N.Z. Dent. J.* **62**, 32–36.

Gillody C. J., Heinz H. W. and Eastman P. W. (1954) A dental caries and fluoride study of 19 Nebraska cities. *J. Neb. Dent. Assoc.* **31**, 3–13.

Jackson D. (1974) Personal communication.

Jackson D., Goward P. E. and Morrell G. V. (1980) Fluoridation in Leeds. *Br. Dent. J.* **149**, 231–234.

Jackson D., Gravely J. F. and Pinkham I. O. (1975) Fluoridation in Cumbria. *Br. Dent. J.* **139**, 319–322.

Jackson D., James P. M. C. and Wolfe W. B. (1975) Fluoridation in Anglesey. *Br. Dent. J.* **138**, 165–171.

Künzel W. (1976) Trinkwasserfluoridierung Karl-Marx-Stadt XIII. *Stomat. DDR* **26**, 458–465.

Lewis F. D. and Leatherwood E. C. (1959) Effect of natural fluorides on caries incidence in three Georgia cites. *Public Health Rep. (Wash.)* **74**, 127–131.

Murray J. J. (1969a) Caries experience of five-year-old children from fluoride and non-fluoride communities. *Br. Dent. J.* **126**, 352–354.

Murray J. J. (1969b) Caries experience of 15-year-old children from fluoride and non-fluoride communities. *Br. Dent. J.* **127**, 128–131.

Murray J. J. and Atkinson K. (1971) Caries experience of West Hartlepool children aged 2–18 years. *Dent. Pract. Dent. Rec.* **21**, 387–388.

Nevitt G. A., Diefenbach V. and Presnell C. E. (1953) Missouri's fluoride and dental caries study. *J. Mo. Dent. Assoc.* **33**, 10–26.

Rock W. P., Gordon P. H. and Bradnock G. (1981) Dental caries experience in Birmingham and Wolverhampton school children following the fluoridation of Birmingham water in 1964. *Br. Dent. J.* **150**, 61–66.

Rugg-Gunn A. J., Carmichael C. L., French A. D. and Furness J. A. (1977) Fluoridation in Newcastle and Northumberland: A clinical study of 5 -year-old children. *Br. Dent. J.* **142**, 359–402.

Rugg-Gunn A. J., Nicholas K. E., Potts A., Cranage J. D., Carmichael C. L. and French A. D. (1981) Caries experience of 5 year old children living in four communities in N.E. England receiving differing water fluoride levels. *Br. Dent. J.* **150**, 9–12.

Tank G. and Storvick C. A. (1964) Caries experience of children 1–6 years old in two Oregon communities (Corvallis and Albany). 1. Effects of fluoride on caries experience and eruption of teeth. *J. Am. Dent. Assoc.* **69**, 749–757.

Weaver R. (1944) Fluorosis and dental caries on Tyneside. *Br. Dent. J.* **76**, 29–40.

Whittle J. G. and Downer M. C. (1979) Dental health and treatment needs of Birmingham and Salford schoolchildren. *Br. Dent. J.* **147**, 67–71.

Winter G. B., Rule D. C., Mailer G. P., James P. M. C. and Gordon P. H. (1971) The prevalence of dental caries in pre-schoolchildren aged 1–4 years. *Br. Dent. J.* **130**, 271–277.

CHAPTER 3

WATER FLUORIDATION AND ADULT DENTAL HEALTH

Although many studies have shown conclusively that water fluoridation is effective in reducing caries in the permanent teeth of children, some doubts have been raised as to whether the observed reductions are due to a delay in the onset of clinical dental caries in the permanent dentition, or whether water fluoridation is having a truly long-term caries-preventive effect. The best way of resolving this problem is to carry out studies on adults continuously resident in fluoride and non-fluoride areas.

Deatherage (1943) made a study of the dental health in 2026 white national service selectees (mainly aged 21–28 years) living in 91 Illinois communities, with public water supplies varying in fluoride content. The communities were graded according to the content of the drinking water as follows:

F = 0·0–0·1 ppm—Fluoride-free areas
F = 0·9 ppm—Suboptimal fluoride areas
F = 1·0 ppm and over—Fluoride areas

The mean DMF of selectees continuously resident in fluoride areas (F = 1·0 ppm) was 6·21 compared with a mean DMF value of 10·79 for selectees who had lived in fluoride-free areas all their lives.

Weaver (1944) examined 100 mothers attending Maternity and Child Welfare clinics in North Shields (F = 0·25 ppm) and South Shields (F = 1·2–1·8 ppm). Third molar teeth were not assessed because of their varied eruption pattern. The results are presented in *Table* 15.

Weaver concluded that the South Shields mothers initially had a delay of caries experience of about 5 years; this delay was not constant and by 30–34 years caries experience in South Shields was similar to that in North

Table 15. Mean DMF of Mothers in North Shields and South Shields (*Weaver, 1944*)

Age (yrs)	*North Shields* No. examined	Mean DMF	Age (yrs)	*South Shields* No. examined	Mean DMF
20	1	6	20	4	5
20–24	25	11	20–24	32	7
25–29	33	15	25–29	19	9
30–34	22	17	30–34	20	15
35–39	12	18	35–39	16	17
40+	7	19	40+	9	17

45

Shields. The evidence given by Weaver cannot be regarded as conclusive. Apart from the fact that the numbers and selected sample upon which he based his conclusions were too small for adequate analysis, the DMF index cannot be regarded as a true measure of caries experience in adults because of the increasing number of caries-free teeth extracted for periodontal, prosthetic or surgical reasons. The M fraction of the index occupies approximately 85 per cent of the total DMF in Weaver's study: this very high extraction rate would certainly have masked any caries-inhibitory property of fluoride drinking water.

Forrest et al. (1951) examined adults from three high-fluoride areas, South Shields (0·82 ppm F), Colchester (1·45 ppm F) and Slough (0·9 ppm F), and three low-fluoride areas, North Shields (0·07 ppm F), Ipswich (0·3 ppm F) and Reading (0·1 ppm F). To obtain groups of like social status mothers attending antenatal and infant welfare centres were examined. Only those continuously resident in one of the above communities were examined. In all 286 mothers were seen in high-fluoride areas and 296 mothers were seen in low-fluoride areas. An uncorrected DMF index was used: the results are presented in *Table* 16. The authors stated that at each age caries incidence was lower in the high-fluoride areas than in the low-fluoride areas, but that the difference seemed to indicate a delay in onset of dental caries of about 10 years. Even in this study, which was of a highly selected sample, the numbers in the older age groups are too small to allow firm conclusions to be drawn.

Table 16. Caries Experience of Expectant and Nursing Mothers in Low- and High-Fluoride Communities (*Forrest et al., 1951*)

Age (yrs)	No. examined		Mean DMF		% Difference
	Low F	High F	Low F	High F	
20	22	17	12·5	8·5	33
21–25	92	91	16·2	10·0	38
26–30	107	69	19·3	12·5	35
31–35	40	61	21·5	16·2	25
36–40	30	23	22·8	19·0	16
40+	5	7	26·4	22·0	17

Russell and Elvove (1951) also studied the effect of fluoride on dental caries experience in an adult population. Residents in Colorado Springs, Colo. (population 36 789 in 1940) were selected for the investigation, principally because of the long and reliable fluoride history of this town; the water supply contained 2·55 ppm F. Nearby Boulder, Colo. (population 13 000 in 1940) was utilized as a control; in this town there was only a trace of fluoride in the drinking water. Examination lists were based on school census records, birth records, marriage records and city directories. Age limits of 20–44 years were established. When the sample lists were assembled they were found to constitute a random cross-section of all people from the two communities. An attempt was made to examine each listed person; approximately 80 per cent of the actual number of eligible persons agreed to a dental examination. Most of the men were professional or semi-professional workers, business proprietors, skilled craftsmen or students. There were comparatively few unskilled or semi-skilled workers in either group. More than half of the women examined were housewives and the remainder were mostly clerical and sales workers. College graduates constituted a high percentage of each sample—about 40 per cent in Boulder and 20 per cent at Colorado Springs. Both groups had received a high level of dental care and dental hygiene was generally good. For the purpose of this study 'continuous residence' was defined as 'residence unbroken except for periods not exceeding 60 days during the time of development and eruption of the permanent teeth; thereafter more than half the life had to be spent in the respective community'. The results of this study are recorded in *Table* 17. Russell and Elvove concluded that total rates for DMF permanent teeth were about 60 per cent lower in Colorado Springs than in Boulder for each age group. Caries inhibition apparently continued undiminished up to at least 44 years. Boulder residents had lost three to four times as many teeth from dental caries as had those of Colorado Springs.

Table 17. Mean Number of DMF Teeth, together with its Standard Deviation (SD), in Adults from Boulder and Colorado Springs (excluding Third Molars) (*Russell and Elvove, 1951*)

Age (yrs)	Male	Female	Both	Mean DMF	± SD
Boulder					
20–24	22	29	51	14·0	4·9
25–29	26	15	41	16·5	5·5
30–34	17	12	29	18·3	5·2
35–39	8	14	22	21·8	5·1
40–44	6	6	12	21·7	6·0
20 +	79	76	155	17·2	
Colorado Springs					
20–24	36	36	72	5·4	5·1
25–29	61	40	101	6·5	5·0
30–34	55	27	82	7·1	4·9
35–39	51	24	75	9·2	7·0
40–44	36	19	55	10·3	6·4
20 +	239	146	385	7·5	

In a further article concerned with the same study Russell (1953) assessed the inhibition of approximal caries in adults with lifelong fluoride exposure. He comments that studies of approximal caries in children are complicated by variation in the time risk factor for individual tooth types. This difficulty is minimized when adults are considered, but unfortunately progressive tooth loss in adults prevents the true pattern of surface attack from being determined. Because of this the most desirable age group to study is the oldest in which tooth loss has been minimal. Russell concluded that the optimal age was 35 years and proceeded to group all adults up to this age: there were 68 such persons at Boulder and 183 at Colorado Springs. The mean age of the Boulder group was 29·0 years and of the Colorado group 29·6 years. The mean number of missing teeth was 2·2 and 0·6 respectively; the corresponding mean DMF values were 16·8 and 6·6. In this investigation, approximal tooth areas were used as the unit of estimation. For example, an approximal area was made up of the distal surface of the maxillary first molar and the mesial surface of the maxillary second molars. The results were expressed as a percentage of approximal site areas at risk which were decayed, missing or filled, because of dental caries. In Colorado Springs the prevalence of DMF approximal site areas affected was 61–100 per cent lower than in Boulder.

Englander and Wallace (1962) stated that there was a need to compare the dental caries experience of a large sample of adults who had continuously resided in a city having approximately 1 ppm F in its domestic water with that of a similar sample of adults in a nearby city who had consumed water low in fluoride. The communities they chose for study were Aurora, Illinois (F = 1·2 ppm), and Rockford, Illinois (fluoride-free). The main purpose of the Englander and Wallace study concerned the effect of fluoride on periodontal disease and hence only persons with at least 10 natural teeth present were examined. In each city local workers telephoned mature residents and asked them to volunteer for examination. Newspapers, television and radio were used to solicit cooperation of all persons who met the residential criteria. A careful review of information received by telephone showed that of all persons over 20 years old contacted, 14 per cent were edentulous in Rockford and less than 2 per cent were edentulous in Aurora. No edentulous persons, or those with fewer than 10 natural teeth, were asked to report for examination. This population was therefore highly selected. A total of 896 continuous residents in Aurora and 935 residents in Rockford were examined. Women constituted 61 per cent of the sample in Aurora and 63 per cent of the sample in Rockford. The number in each age group, and the DMF values, for Aurora and for Rockford, are given in *Table* 18. The authors state that dental caries experience was significantly less for Aurora residents than for residents of Rockford. The mean DMF for Aurora was approximately 10 compared with approximately 17 for residents of Rockford. Overall reduction in DMF teeth for Aurorans over residents of Rockford was 40 per cent approximately, in comparison with the reduction of approximately 60 per cent found by Russell. Englander and Wallace suggested that failure to duplicate Russell's reduction was probably due to various factors, such as the elimination of people with fewer than 10 natural teeth, differences in examination techniques, and the

Table 18. Mean DMF Values against Age for Residents in Aurora (1·2 ppm F) and Rockford (no F) (*After Englander and Wallace, 1962*)

Age group	*Aurora* No. in group	Mean DMF	*Rockford* No. in group	Mean DMF
18–19	162	6·05	120	11·27
20–29	188	8·78	223	16·92
30–39	255	11·03	342	17·65
40–49	205	12·41	191	18·00
50–59	86	12·58	59	13·34
All ages	896	10·13	935	16·78

inclusion of persons over 45 years of age. In Rockford the mean DMF value in the 50–59-year age group (13·34) was much lower than that for younger age groups, and this suggests that the persons examined in the oldest age groups belonged to a biased sample. From the figures in the 50–59-year age group the mean DMF values for Aurora (12·58) and Rockford (13·34) are very similar.

Between individuals of similar age, the extent of dental disease varies over a wide range. Because of this, population estimates must be based on large numbers of people. This requirement is easily met in child studies because schoolchildren are effectively a captive population. This does not apply to adults, and hence adult studies are far more difficult to carry out. It is almost impossible to obtain a perfect sample of adult residents within any community for the purposes of dental study. Bulman et al. (1968) attempted to obtain a random sample of adults in Salisbury and Darlington by taking a sample of adults whose names were selected at random from the electoral registers of the two areas. In the end only 68 per cent of those interviewed in Salisbury and 79 per cent of those interviewed in Darlington were examined. A similar level of cooperation was obtained in the Adult Dental Health Survey of England and Wales (Gray et al., 1970) where 77 per cent of selected samples were examined and interviewed. These studies, however, were not of continuous residents. It would be impossible to ascertain the total pool of continuous residents within a community unless each resident was contacted. Even then, not all the continuous residents would give permission for a dental examination to be carried out. This is a very real problem of dental health studies in fluoride and non-fluoride areas, where it is essential to examine continuous residents.

In 1968–1969 4774 adults from Hartlepool and York were examined to try to measure in greater detail the long-term effect of fluoride in drinking water (Murray, 1971a). The County Borough of Hartlepool, population 100 000, is situated in the south-east corner of County Durham, some 8 miles north of the River Tees. Domestic water is supplied to Hartlepool by the Hartlepool Water Company, founded in 1841; it is a private company and its pipelines are not connected to any of the surrounding local authority water boards. The fluoride concentration in the drinking water is 1·5–2·0 ppm.

The City of York was used as a control town. Domestic water is supplied to the City of York by the York Water Company, which obtains its water from the River Ouse. The fluoride content of the water varies between the limits of 0·15 ppm and 0·28 ppm, depending on whether or not the river is in spate. The mean fluoride concentration is 0·2 ppm. The population of York is 105 000, very similar to that of Hartlepool. The socioeconomic status of active males in the two towns is very similar (1961 Census). Furthermore, caries experience of 5-year-old and 15-year-old York children was found to be very similar to that of the 'national average' for non-fluoride towns in England (Murray, 1968), suggesting that the pattern of caries experience in York was probably very similar to that of other low-fluoride towns. It was for these reasons that York was chosen as a control town.

In order to determine the full effect of fluoride drinking water on the dental structures, it is necessary to examine people who have been born and lived virtually all their lives in a fluoride area. The following definition of 'continuous residence' was adopted: a person who had been born in Hartlepool, had lived all his/her school life in the town (except for holidays) and had been away from the town during his/her life for no more than 6 years. This meant that all those people termed 'continuous residents' had been exposed to fluoride drinking water during birth and childhood and had spent nearly all, if not all, of their adult life in the town. The definition was sufficiently flexible to allow people attending colleges, or working in other areas for short periods, or those who had done military service, to be included in the sample.

In order to obtain a sample of Hartlepool adults, large establishments were approached and asked to cooperate in the study. The aims of the project were discussed with the management and representatives of the workers in order to obtain as much cooperation as possible. Once approval had been given, a letter was sent to each person in the factory or establishment explaining the reason for the survey and asking for his/her cooperation. Subsequently arrangements were made for those people who had been born in Hartlepool, and who had agreed to a dental examination, to be seen in the place of work. Thirteen establishments, including all sections of Hartlepool Council, were visited in order to obtain as representative a sample of Hartlepool adults as possible. The number of Hartlepool adults examined in each quinquennial age group is recorded in *Table* 19.

Although the sample of people examined cannot be called a true random sample of Hartlepool adults, it included people from all the major places of work in Hartlepool and spanned the whole social scale: directors,

Table 19. Number of Adults examined in each Age Group in Hartlepool and York

| | | Hartlepool | | | York | |
Age	Male	Female	Total	Male	Female	Total
15–19	141	450	591	61	102	163
20–24	132	298	430	149	158	307
25–29	107	75	182	199	76	275
30–34	102	77	179	186	56	242
35–39	100	77	177	188	83	271
40–44	86	77	163	225	106	331
45–49	83	80	163	270	123	393
50–54	48	51	99	167	86	253
55–59	55	49	104	185	65	250
60 +	34	13	47	132	22	154

professional people, white-collar workers, skilled, semi-skilled and unskilled workers. The percentage of people in each social class in the sample examined is recorded in *Table* 20; 80 per cent of the people examined were in social classes III and IV. It is therefore felt that every effort was made to achieve as representative as possible a sample of Hartlepool adults, concomitant with examining large numbers of people, and bearing in mind the fact that many people, particularly in the older age groups, were excluded from the study because they did not fulfil the criteria for 'continuous residence'.

Table 20. Social Class of Adults examined in Hartlepool and York

| | Hartlepool | | York | |
Class	No.	Per cent	No.	Per cent
I	3	0·1	14	0·5
II	202	9·5	371	14·0
III	899	42·1	1337	50·7
IV	805	37·7	797	30·2
V	226	10·6	120	4·6

A similar procedure to that used in Hartlepool was adopted in York to obtain a population sample of a low-fluoride area. Three large establishments agreed to cooperate in this study. The purpose of the survey was explained to representatives of the management and employees in each case. After approval had been given, a letter was sent to each person in the place of work asking for his/her cooperation in the study. Three people who had lived for a time in Hartlepool and one person who was born in Colchester and lived in Mersea (all high-fluoride areas) were excluded from the results.

The number of York adults examined in each quinquennial age group is recorded in *Table* 19 and the number of people in each social group is recorded in *Table* 20. As in Hartlepool, the people examined spanned the whole social scale. The percentage of adults in social classes I, II and III who were examined was slightly higher in York than in Hartlepool and the percentage of adults in social classes IV and V who were examined was slightly lower in York than in Hartlepool. However, in both communities approximately 80 per cent of adults examined were in social classes III and IV, so that overall, the fluoride sample and the non-fluoride sample were fairly well balanced with respect to social class. The mean DMF values for all people examined, including edentulous persons, is shown in *Fig.* 12.

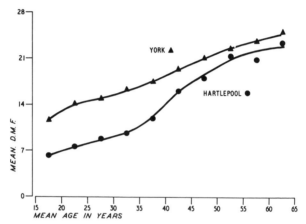

Fig. 12. Mean DMF values in adults from Hartlepool and York, including edentulous persons. (From Murray, 1971a.) (*Reproduced by courtesy of the Editor, 'British Dental Journal'.*)

Unfortunately, the DMF index is not an accurate measure of caries experience in adults because of the increasing number of caries-free teeth which are extracted (for periodontal and prosthetic reasons) as age advances. In order to try to measure the full caries inhibitory effect of fluoride in the drinking water, it is essential to try to measure more accurately caries experience in an adult population in fluoride and non-fluoride areas. Russell and Elvove (1951) attempted to compensate for the inaccuracy of the DMF index in adults by recording the primary reasons for extraction based upon a history of signs and symptoms. Apart from the fact that subjective evidence of this nature is unreliable, a tooth removed for any reason other than caries may have suffered caries attack also. Unless reliable life records are available, an accurate assessment of the cumulative incidence of dental caries over a wide age range would seem to be impossible.

Three different approaches were made in the Hartlepool–York study to try to overcome this problem. Firstly, it can be argued that the greatest error in the DMF index when used in adults is the inclusion of edentulous people in the DMF count, because it is these people who will have had the greatest proportion of caries-free teeth extracted in order to wear full dentures. On the other hand, those people who want to keep their teeth will have had relatively few caries-free teeth extracted and thus a more accurate measure of caries experience would be to calculate the observed DMF (DM_0F) in dentate persons (*Fig.* 13). Comparing *Figs.* 12 and 13 it will be seen that, using the latter index, the difference between the communities is much more clear cut.

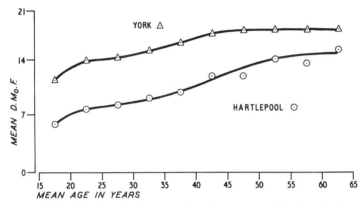

Fig. 13. Mean DMF values in adults from Hartlepool and York, excluding edentulous persons. (From Murray, 1971a.) (*Reproduced by courtesy of the Editor, 'British Dental Journal'.*)

A second approach is to use the method put forward by Jackson (1961) who suggested that if, by a sampling survey, the percentage number of extracted teeth which were carious was known for any specific community, it would appear reasonable to apply correction factors to the M fraction of the DMF value at each age group, in order to obtain a more accurate measurement of caries experience in an adult population. This procedure was adopted in order to obtain 'correction factors' for the Hartlepool–York data.

All 7 dental practitioners in Hartlepool and 19 of the dental practitioners in York agreed to cooperate in the study by collecting teeth extracted in their surgeries, over a specified period of time. Ten polythene bottles marked according to the quinquennial age groups used in the study (15–19 years, 20–24 years and so on) were supplied to each practitioner. In Hartlepool only those teeth extracted from people who had been born and lived most of their lives in Hartlepool were collected. This part of the study extended from March 1968 to April 1969 in York and from January 1968 to September 1969 in Hartlepool. The teeth were separated according to age and type and examined for dental caries. A probe was used if caries was not obvious to the naked eye. All filled teeth were presumed to have been carious. In all 7933 extracted teeth were collected in York and 2958 teeth were collected in Hartlepool. The correction factors for each tooth type and the corrected DMF values (DM_cF) for the total population (including the edentulous) were calculated (Murray, 1971b).

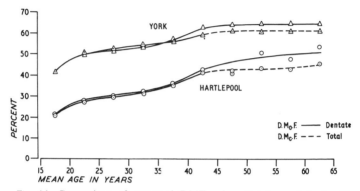

Fig. 14. Comparison of corrected DMF values (total population) with observed values. (From Murray, 1971b.) (*Reproduced by courtesy of the Editor, 'British Dental Journal'.*)

The DM_cF values at any year age group can only be an approximation of true caries experience in the whole population. As a check on the validity of the correction factors, the DM_cF values for the total population were compared with the DM_oF values for the dentate population in each community (*Fig.* 14). (The dentate population includes only those people with at least one natural tooth.) The DM_cF values (total population) were effectively identical with the DM_oF values (dentate population) up to the age of 45 years in both communities. Thereafter the DM_oF (dentate) values were slightly higher than the DM_cF (general) values; this is to be expected because even in a dentate population one would imagine that a small proportion of caries-free teeth would have to be extracted for periodontal, prosthetic or surgical reasons. Overall, it is considered that the DM_cF values give a good estimate of caries experience in the population throughout the whole age range in Hartlepool and York. The ceiling DM_cF value in Hartlepool was 45·6 per cent and in York it was 61·0 per cent; this means that the maximum DMF in Hartlepool was 25 per cent lower than it was in York.

Unfortunately, the DMF index gives no indication of the number of surfaces affected by caries. Thus the third approach is to ignore missing teeth altogether and not attempt to apply correction factors or assume that a missing tooth should be counted as 3 or 5 surfaces. Instead the number of decayed or filled surfaces in teeth present in the mouth can be measured and this method gives perhaps the most accurate measure of the extent of caries in adults in different communities. Data using this method have been reported (Jackson et al., 1973). Three types of tooth sites were considered: smooth-surface sites (mesial, distal and buccal cervical), occlusal surfaces and pit sites. The increment in caries was virtually nil in persons aged 45 years and above. Thus in this age group permanent differences between Hartlepool and York can be observed. In persons aged 45 years and above 36 678 specified sites in the York population were examined; of these 7182 or approximately 20 per cent were carious. In Hartlepool 17 422 specified sites were examined and of these 1909 or approximately 11 per cent were carious. Thus in dentate persons aged 45 years and above the number of carious sites was 44 per cent lower in Hartlepool than it was in York. Data for the number of DF sites in standing teeth in 10-year age groups for the two communities are recorded diagrammatically in *Fig.* 15. Taking this information as a whole, it can be stated that fluoride in drinking water does not have a merely short-term delaying effect on the appearance of dental caries, but has substantial lifelong caries-preventive effects.

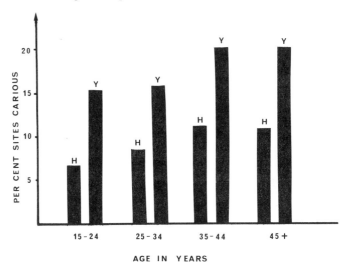

Fig. 15. The percentage number of decayed/filled sites in teeth present in the mouths of Hartlepool and York adults. (From Murray, 1974.) (*Reproduced by courtesy of the Editor, 'Community Health'.*)

REFERENCES

Bulman J. S., Slack G. L., Richards N. D. and Wilcocks A. J. (1968) A survey of the dental health and attitudes towards dentistry in two communities. Part 2, Dental data. *Br. Dent. J.* **124**, 549–554.

Deatherage C. F. (1943) Fluoride domestic waters and dental caries experience in 2026 white Illinois selective service men. *J. Dent. Res.* **22**, 129–137.

Englander H. R. and Wallace D. A. (1962) Effects of naturally fluoridated water on dental caries in adults. *Public Health Rep.* **77**, 887–893.

Forrest J. R., Parfitt G. J. and Bransby E. R. (1951) The incidence of dental caries among adults and young children in three high and three low fluoride areas in England. *Monthly Bull. Minist. Health* **10** 104–111.

Gray P. G., Todd J. E., Slack G. L. and Bulman J. S. (1970) *Adult Dental Health in England and Wales in 1968.* Government Social Survey. London, HMSO, Department of Health and Social Security.

Jackson D. (1961) An epidemiological study of dental caries prevalence in adults. *Arch. Oral Biol.* **6**, 80–93.

Jackson D., Murray J. J. and Fairpo C. G. (1973) Lifelong benefits of fluoride in drinking water. *Br. Dent. J.* **134**, 419–422.

Murray J. J. (1968) M.Ch.D. Thesis. University of Leeds.

Murray J. J. (1971a) Adult dental health in fluoride and non-fluoride areas. *Br. Dent J.* **131**, 391–395.

Murray J. J. (1971b) Adult dental health in fluoride and non-fluoride areas. Part 2. Caries experience in each tooth type. *Br. Dent. J.* **131**, 437–442.

Murray J. J. (1974) Water fluoridation: a choice for the community. *Community Health* **6**, 75–83.

Russell A. L. (1953) The inhibition of approximal caries in adults with lifelong fluoride exposure. *J. Dent. Res.* **32**, 138–143.

Russell A. L. and Elvove E. (1951) Domestic water and dental caries, VII. A study of the fluoride dental caries relationship in an adult population. *Public Health Rep.* **66**, 1389–1401.

Weaver R. (1944) Fluorine and dental caries: further investigations on Tyneside and in Sunderland. *Br. Dent. J.* **77**, 185–193.

CHAPTER 4

COMMUNITY FLUORIDATION SCHEMES
THROUGHOUT THE WORLD

Reductions in dental caries observed in the communities which were the first to fluoridate have been reported and reviewed extensively (Adler, 1970; Backer Dirks, 1974). Following the early favourable reports, many other communities decided to fluoridate their public water supplies so that by 1978 approximately 155 million people worldwide were consuming fluoridated water, in addition to the 40 million or so people receiving naturally fluoride-rich water supplies (Backer Dirks et al., 1978). Dental health has been monitored in many of these communities, and findings of surveys in artificially fluoridated areas will be reviewed here, since such information is not readily available because reports are frequently written and published in the language of the country concerned (*Table* 21). This review has been confined to those studies reporting standard caries indices (i.e. deft, DMFT); information on reduction in dental care cost is not so internationally comparable and will be discussed separately on page 252.

THE AMERICAS

The world's first artificial fluoridation plant began at Grand Rapids, USA, in 1945. By 1977, 49 per cent (105·3 million) of Americans on piped-water supply received fluoridated water. The US authorities have also been most conscientious in monitoring its effectiveness. The classic Grand Rapids–Muskegon (Arnold et al., 1962), Newburgh–Kingston (Ast et al., 1956) and Evanston–Oak Park (Blayney and Hill, 1967) studies are well known. Fluoridation has been monitored in at least 103 other communities, although some of these reports have only appeared as press articles and many are published in state health department reports and newsletters. It is inevitable, as the effectiveness of fluoridation has been demonstrated repeatedly in the USA, that results of fresh surveys will be published less frequently. This review is therefore incomplete as far as the USA is concerned, but is believed to be more comprehensive for countries outside the USA.

In Central America, most of Puerto Rico is fluoridated and in 1961 fluoridation reached 93 per cent of the population on piped supply or 63 per cent of the total population (Guzman, 1961).

Canada has a long history of fluoridation, beginning in Brantford in 1945; by 1970, fluoridation was reaching 6·6 million Canadians. The

Table 21. Results of Surveys into the Effectiveness of Public Water Fluoridation Schemes throughout the World

Country	Fluoridated community	Reference	Year fluoridation began	Year of study	Age of subjects (yrs)	Caries index	Non-fluoridated community caries experience	Per cent caries reduction
USA	Grand Rapids	Arnold et al. (1956)	1945	1951	5	deft	5·3	57
	Grand Rapids	Arnold et al. (1962)	1945	1960	15	DMFT	12·4	50
	Newburgh	Ast et al. (1956)	1945	1955	6–9	DMFT	2·3	58
	Marshall	Taylor and Bertram (1965)	1945	1956	10	DMFT	4·3	67
	Sheboygan	Schreiber (1966)	1946	1950	5	dmft	4·8	45
	Evanston	Blayney and Hill (1967)	1946	1961	14	DMFT	11·7	49
	Lewiston	Young (1958)	1947	1957	10	DMFT	7·0	79
	Oshkosh	Steele (1977)	1948	1975	14	DMFT	9·1	50
	Charlotte	Szwejda (1962)	1949	1961	6	deft	5·3	51
	Charlotte	Szwejda (1962)	1949	1961	11	DMFT	3·3	57
	Antigo	Lemke et al. (1970)	1949–1960	1966	5–6	deft	5·3	53
	Newark	Musselman (1957)	1950	1955	6	DMFT	1·1	82
	New Britain	Erlenbach and Tracy (1961)	1950	1961	10	DMFT	3·9	48
	Milan	Trithart and Denney (1956)	1951	1956	6	deft	6·9	42
	Louisville	Gernert (1958)	1951	1956	6	deft	6·0	46
	Athens	Chrietzberg and Lewis (1958)	1951	1957	6	DMFT	1·2	85
	Iowa	Iowa State DOH (1960)	1951	1958	5	deft	5·1	44
	Tuscaloosa	Klymko (1959)	1951	1959	6	deft	5·6	52
	Tuscaloosa	Klymko (1959)	1951	1959	8	DMFT	2·3	73
	Fort Wayne	Mollenkopf (1963)	1951	1962	10	DMFT	3·7	50
	Columbus	Trubman (1965)	1951	1962	10	DMFT	3·3	47
	Grand Junction	Reger et al. (1963)	1951	1962	6	deft	5·3	50

Location	Reference		Year		Index		%
Grand Junction	Reger et al. (1963)	1951	12	1962	DMFT	5·9	68
Norway	Garcelon (1956)	1952	7	1955	DMFT	2·1	71
Antioch	Stadt et al. (1960)	1952	5	1957	deft	4·1	42
Orangeburg	Bunch (1959)	1952	6	1958	deft	5·5	47
Orangeburg	Bunch (1964)	1952	10	1963	DMFT	3·3	41
Maryland	Russell and White (1961)	1952	5	1959	deft	2·8	65
Maryland	Russell and White (1961)	1952	7	1959	DMFT	1·1	77
Baltimore	McCauley et al. (1961)	1952	6	1960	DMFT	1·2	68
Easton	Sogaro (1964)	1952	5	1962	deft	5·0	71
Easton	Sogaro (1964)	1952	10	1962	DMFT	3·6	53
Amery	Arra and Lemke (1964)	1952	9	1962	DMFT	3·8	29
Roundup	Anon. (1962)	1952	10	1962	DMFT	4·0	60
Washington, DC	Ostrow (1963)	1952	10	1962	DMFT	2·2	37
Cleveland, Tenn.	Holmes (1963)	1952	11	1963	DMFT	7·6	63
Hagerstown	Leonard (1963)	1952	11	1963	DMFT	4·2	62
Rush City	Jordan (1964)	1952	10	1964	DMFT	5·0	50
Providence	Yacovone and Parente (1974)	1952	13	1972	DMFT	8·4	63
Richmond	Crooks and Konikoff (1972)	1952	13	1972	DMFT	7·2	50
Monmouth	Ross et al. (1960)	1953	6	1959	DMFT	0·8	50
Milwaukee	Schultz (1969)	1953	5	1959	deft	3·6	35
Milwaukee	Schultz (1969)	1953	10	1965	DMFT	3·6	56
Boseman	Snyder (1964)	1953	10	1964	DMFT	5·0	50
Mystic-Stonington	Erlenbach (1964)	1953	11	1964	DMFT	4·4	35
Corvallis	Tank and Storvick (1964)	1953	5	c. 1962	deft	6·0	45
Puerto Rico	Guzman (1961)	1953	6	1958	DMFT	1·2	66
Salem	Anon (1971)	1953	12	1971	DMFT	6·9	67
Philadelphia	Bronstein (1969)	1954	5	1967	deft	3·2	50
Philadelphia	Gordon (1975)	1954	15	1969–1970	DMFT	9·3	52

Table 21 (cont.)

Country	Fluoridated community	Reference	Year fluoridation began	Year of study	Age of subjects (yrs)	Caries index	Non-fluoridated community caries experience	Per cent caries reduction
	St Louis	Smith and Paquin (1962)	1955	1961	7	DMFT	0·8	50
	Kingsport	Bryan and Smith (1966)	1955	1965	10	DMFT	3·9	62
	Albert Lea	Jordan (1970)	1955	1969	6	deft	5·7	42
	Albert Lea	Jordan (1970)	1955	1969	12	DMFT	6·2	53
	Cleveland	Healy (1963)	1956	1962	5–6	deft	3·4	62
	Lebanon	Fishman and Collier (1965)	1956	1964	6	deft	5·4	47
	Lebanon	Fishman and Collier (1965)	1956	1964	8	DMFT	2·4	68
	Chicago	Weinstein (1972)	1956	1972	14	DMFT	11·6	51
	Fayette	Moncrief (1970)	1957	1969	10	DMFT	5·1	63
	Mobile	Russell (1965)	1958	1965	6	deft	5·6	32
	Mobile	Russell (1965)	1958	1965	7	DMFT	2·0	72
	Silver Bay	Jordan et al. (1969)	1958	1968	5	deft	4·6	46
	Silver Bay	Jordan et al. (1969)	1958	1968	10	DMFT	3·6	45
	Kalamazoo	Margolis et al. (1975)	<1964	1974	4–6	deft	2·4	47
	Kalamazoo	Margolis et al. (1975)	<1964	1974	7–10	DMFT	1·6	36
	Asheville	Dudney et al. (1977)	1965	1976	6	dft	3·6	20
	Asheville	Dudney et al. (1977)	1965	1976	10	DMFT	3·3	59
	Winona	Flaven (1977)	1965	1976	5	deft	4·0	74
	Winona	Flaven (1977)	1965	1976	10	DMFT	3·4	57
	Cudahy	Doherty and Krippene (1972)	1966	1971	5	deft	3·9	56
	New Haven	Konick (1979)	1967	1977	10	DMFT	3·5	51

Country	Location	Reference			Age	Index		%
Canada	Brantford	Brown et al. (1960)	1945	1959	12–14	DMFT	7·5	57
	Brandon	Connor and Harwood (1963)	1955	1962	6–8	deft	6·5	41
	Brandon	Connor and Harwood (1963)	1955	1962	6–8	DMFT	2·0	74
	Toronto	Lewis (1976)	1963	1975	5	deft	3·9	56
	Toronto	Lewis (1976)	1963	1975	11	DMFT	3·6	35
	Prince George	Hann (1968)	1955	1968	12–14	DMFT	11·2	60
Brazil	Campinas	Viegas and Viegas (1974)	1962	1972	5	deft	5·5	68
	Campinas	Viegas and Viegas (1974)	1962	1972	10	DMFT	5·1	55
Columbia	San Pedro	Mejia et al. (1976)	1965	1972	8	DMFT	3·8	78
UK	Anglesey	DHSS (1969)	1955	1965	5	deft	4·8	40
	Anglesey	Jackson et al. (1975)	1956	1974	15	DMFT	11·4	44
	Watford	DHSS (1969)	1956	1967	5	deft	2·8	43
	Watford	DHSS (1969)	1956	1967	10	DMFT	3·1	35
	Kilmarnock	DHSS (1969)	1956	1961	5	deft	6·9	42
	Balsall Heath	Beal and James (1971)	1964	1970	5	deft	5·2	62
	Northfield	Beal and James (1971)	1964	1970	5	deft	4·9	50
	Birmingham	Whittle and Downer (1979)	1964	1977	5	deft	3·6	54
	Birmingham	Whittle and Downer (1979)	1964	1977	12	DMFT	4·0	45
	Leeds	Jackson et al. (1980)	1968	1979	5	deft	3·3	62
	Cumbria	Jackson et al. (1975)	1969	1975	5	deft	4·4	46
	Newcastle upon Tyne	Rugg-Gunn et al. (1977)	1969	1975	5	deft	6·1	57
	Northumberland	Rugg-Gunn et al. (1977)	1969	1975	5	deft	6·1	67
Ireland	Dublin	O'Hickey (1976)	1964	1969	5	deft	5·8	65
	Cork	Collins and O'Mullane (1970)	1965	1969	5	deft	6·4	45

Table 21 (cont.)

Country	Fluoridated community	Reference	Year fluoridation began	Year of study	Age of subjects (yrs)	Caries index	Non-fluoridated community caries experience	Per cent caries reduction
Netherlands	Tiel	Kwant et al. (1973)	1953	1969	15	DMFT	13·9	51
Finland	Kuopio	Nordling and Tulikoura (1970)	1959	1968	7	DMFT	3·1	55
Switzerland	Basel	Gülzow and Maeglin (1979)	1962	1977	15	DMFT	7·2	59
DDR	Karl-Marx-Stadt	Künzel (1968)	1959	1966	5	deft	2·9	76
	Karl-Marx-Stadt	Künzel (1976)	1959	1972	12	DMFT	4·1	66
Czechoslovakia	Tabor	Jirásková et al. (1969)	1958	1964	6–7	deft	5·3	36
Poland	Wroclaw	Wigdorowicz-M. et al. (1975)	1967	1972	5	deft	5·5	38
	Wroclaw	Wigdorowicz-M. et al. (1978)	1967	1975	8	DMFT	1·9	42
Romania	Tirgu-Mures	Csögör et al. (1968)	1960	1965	5	deft	3·6	37
	Tirgu-Mures	Csögör et al. (1973)	1960	1971	10	DMFT	3·3	52
USSR	Murmansk	Rybakov et al. (1978)	1966	1976	10	DMFT	3·0	50
	Monchegorsk	Rybakov et al. (1978)	1968	1976	8	DMFT	2·7	54
	Ivan-Frankovsk	Gabovich et al. (1972)	1966	1970	8	DMFT	2·2	55
	Leningrad	Strelyukhina et al. (1976)	1969	1974	5	deft	4·9	29

Country	Place	Reference						
Singapore	Singapore	Wong et al. (1970)	1956	1968	7–9	deft	10·7	31
	Singapore	Wong et al. (1970)	1956	1968	7–9	DMFT	2·9	31
Malaysia	Kluang	Awang (1973)	1966	1973	7	deft	7·2	37
	Kluang	Awang (1973)	1966	1973	7	DMFT	2·3	75
Taiwan	Chung-Hsing	Hsieh et al. (1979)	1972	1978	5	deft	8·5	26
Japan	Yamashina	Minoguchi (1964)	1952	1963	11	DMFT	3·6	33
Australia	Tamworth	Martin and Barnard (1970)	1963	1969	5	deft	5·7	48
	Tamworth	Barnard (1980)	1963	1979	15	DMFT	12·3	78
	Canberra	Carr (1976)	1964	1974	5	deft	5·0	71
	Canberra	Carr (1976)	1964	1974	10	DMFT	4·4	51
	Townville	Videroni et al. (1976)	1965	1975	6	deft	5·3	57
	Townville	Videroni et al. (1976)	1965	1975	10	DMFT	4·8	54
	Kalgoorlie	Medcalf (1975)	1968	1973	6	deft	6·3	40
	Perth	Medcalf (1978)	1968	1977	6	deft	4·4	48
	Perth	Medcalf (1978)	1968	1977	10	DMFT	3·9	51
New Zealand	Hastings	Ludwig (1965)	1954	1964	5	deft	8·4	52
	Hastings	Ludwig (1971)	1954	1970	15	DMFT	16·8	49
	Lower Hutt	Hollis and Knowsley (1970)	1959	1969	5	deft	8·0	47
	Lower Hutt	Hollis and Knowsley (1970)	1959	1969	10	DMFT	6·2	42

Only surveys reporting deft or DMFT data have been included. In studies where results are given for several ages, for deciduous teeth age 5 years was preferred, and age 15 years for permanent teeth.

results of the Brantford–Sarnia–Stratford study are well known (Brown and Poplove, 1965), but caries experience has also been monitored in Brandon (Connor and Harwood, 1963) and Toronto (Lewis, 1976), which fluoridated in 1955 and 1963 respectively. The Toronto survey is one of the best investigations into the effectiveness of water fluoridation as a public health measure, and should serve as a guide to other cities which are operating, or planning to introduce, fluoridation schemes.

Fluoridation is fairly widespread in South America, with 10·3 per cent of the population on piped-water supplies receiving fluoridated water in 1968 (WHO, 1969). The highest proportion occurs in Paraguay (100 per cent), although only one-tenth of the population receives a piped supply. On the other hand, about half the people of Chile are on a piped supply and 56 per cent of these receive fluoridated water. Fluoridation is also wide-spread in Panama and Nicaragua. In Brazil, where 1·5 million people received fluoridated water in 1968, Viegas and Viegas (1974) have studied the effect of 10 years' fluoridation in Campinas City.

EUROPE

In the United Kingdom, fluoridation began in 1955 in three trial areas: Watford, Kilmarnock and Anglesey. Apart from these three areas, the dental aspects of fluoridation have been monitored and substantial caries reductions found in Birmingham, Cumbria, Newcastle, Northumberland and Leeds (*see* pp. 34–37).

In Ireland fluoridation became mandatory in 1960, and by 1975 57 per cent of the population were receiving fluoridated water (O'Hickey, 1976). Because of widespread fluoridation, the choice of control towns has been difficult, but its effectiveness has been assessed in the two largest cities, Cork (Collins and O'Mullane, 1970) and Dublin (O'Hickey, 1976).

In Belgium, the town of Assesse was fluoridated in 1956 with a population of 0·4 million people in 1974, but its effectiveness has not been monitored. A pilot fluoridation scheme began in Kassel–Wahlershausen (West Germany) in 1952, but was later discontinued, so that by 1978 there was no fluoridation in that country; detailed data on the effectiveness of fluoridation in Kassel have not been published although Auermann and Lingelbach (1964) reported a 28 per cent caries reduction. In Norrköping in Sweden, which was fluoridated only from 1952 to 1962, a 52 per cent reduction in caries in 7-year-old children was observed (Quentin and Lingelbach, 1963).

One of the best studies into the effect of water fluoridation was conducted in Holland, where Tiel fluoridated in 1953. Reports on this well-known study provide detailed information on the effect of fluoridation on different teeth and types of tooth surface (Backer Dirks et al., 1961; Kwant et al., 1973). Indeed this study gives almost the only data available on the effect of fluoridation in continuously resident 18-year-olds, showing a 53 per cent reduction, or an absolute difference of 19 cavities per person (Kwant et al., 1974). Fluoridation ceased in Tiel in 1974, at a time when 2·7 million Dutch people (20 per cent of the population) were receiving fluoridated water.

The only Finnish community to fluoridate has been the city of Kuopio, where fluoridation began in 1959 with Jyväskylä as control (Nordling and Tulikoura, 1970). In Switzerland, although the first community to fluoridate was Aigle in 1960, the effects of fluoridation have been studied more thoroughly in Basel (1962) (Gülzow et al., 1978; Gülzow and Maeglin, 1979).

By 1972 10 cities in East Germany (DDR) had fluoridated with planned extension to half the population by the middle 1980s. The effectiveness of this measure has been thoroughly studied in Karl-Marx-Stadt by Künzel (1968, 1976): fluoridation began in 1959 with the city of Plauen as control, until 1971 when Plauen itself fluoridated. Examinations were conducted in alternate years on children 3–18 years of age. Künzel also gives data for each tooth type separately for each age group, confirming that incisor teeth benefit most.

In Hungary, attempts to introduce fluoridation have not been success-ful: it was started in the town of Szolnok in 1962 but abandoned 1 year later. It has been reported that 63 per cent of the population of Bulgaria were drinking fluoridated water in 1974, but no data on its effectiveness could be traced. On the other hand, the effectiveness of water fluoridation in Czechoslovakia, Poland and Romania has been documented. In Czechoslovakia, Tabor has been the main test town, fluoridating in 1958, with Pisek as control. In addition to the 36 per cent caries reduction in Tabor (Jirásková et al., 1969), a small reduction was observed in children in Bialystok after 6 years' fluoridation (Januszko et al., 1977) and a 70 per cent caries reduction in Brünn after 3 years (Auermann and Lingelbach, 1964). By 1972, 36 Czech communities had fluoridated, covering 10 per cent of the population.

Progress in fluoridation has been slower in Poland where, by 1974, 3·7 per cent of the population (1·3 million) were receiving fluoridated water. The effect is being monitored in the city of Wroclaw which commenced fluoridation in 1967 (Wigdorowicz-Makowerowa et al., 1978).

The town of Tirgu-Mures in Romania fluoridated its water supplies in 1960, and in 1972 was the only fluoridated community in that country. From 1962 onwards, caries experience has been monitored in 3- to 14-year-old children (Csögör et al., 1968, 1973), but due to technical difficulties, fluoridation has not been continuous and between 1960 and 1971 operated on only 64 per cent of the total possible number of days.

Fluoridation of public water supplies has advanced rapidly in the USSR since it commenced in Norilsk in 1958. By 1972, 13 million people were receiving fluoridated water in 24 communities, but this had risen to 20 million by 1977. After 7 years of fluoridation, dental caries in Norilsk 7-year-olds had decreased by 43 per cent with an overall reduction in the cost of filling materials in Norilsk of 30 per cent, despite the fact that fluoridation was said to be intermittent (Toth, 1972). Fluoridation began in 1966 in Ivano-Frankovsk with Dolina as control (Gabovich et al., 1972), and in Leningrad in 1969 with surrounding areas as control (Strelyukhina et al., 1976). One of the more comprehensive USSR studies has monitored fluoridation in Murmansk, commencing in 1966, and Monchegorsk, commencing in 1968, in the Arctic regions. This is being undertaken by the Central Research Institute of Stomatology (CRIS), Moscow, in collaboration with the World Health Organisation (Rybakov et al., 1978).

ASIA

By 1975, only one Malaysian state, Johore, had fluoridated its water supplies. Results of dental surveys carried out before and after 7 years of fluoridation in the towns of Johore Bahru and Kluang indicated reductions of 60 and 75 per cent respectively in caries experience (Awang, 1973). Fluoridation began in Singapore in 1956, and by 1958 was extended to the entire water system, which supplied 2 million people in 1970 (Wong et al., 1970). No data on the effectiveness of fluoridation in Hong Kong, where 3·6 million people receive fluoridated water, could be traced.

Fluoridation commenced on an experimental basis in Taiwan in 1972. In the fluoridated village of Chung-Hsing, caries experience in 5-year-olds changed from 6·5 dft in 1971 to 6·3 dft in 1978 after 6 years' fluoridation at 0·6 ppm F. However, caries experience in the control, non-fluoridated village of Tsao-Tun increased from 6·4 dft in 1971 to 8·5 dft in 1978; the increase probably being due to the rise in sugar consumption, a result of increasing economic prosperity.

There is at present no fluoridation in Japan. The only town to fluoridate, Yamashina, began in 1952 but fluoridation has now ceased. The average caries experience for 11-year-old children was 1·53 DMFT in 1952 but this had increased to 2·39 after 11 years' fluoridation. However, caries experience in the control town of Shugakuin increased even more, from 1·36 to 3·59 DMFT over the same time period, in the same age group. Therefore, if the caries experience in the fluoridated and control town in 1963 are compared, a 33 per cent reduction in caries was observed, although this may be an underestimate as caries experience was higher in Yamashina than in Shugakuin before fluoridation (Minoguchi, 1964; Adler, 1970).

AUSTRALASIA

Fluoridation has been widely introduced in Australia, so that by 1971 4·9 million Australians were drinking fluoridated water. One of the first communities to fluoridate was Tamworth, which began in 1963 (Martin and Barnard, 1970; Barnard, 1980), but one of the most thorough investigations into its effectiveness has been conducted in Canberra (Carr, 1976). Areas of Western Australia were fluoridated in 1968 and Medcalf (1971, 1975) reported on its effect upon caries experience in the Kalgoorlie area after 6 years of fluoridation. The city of Townsville, Queensland, fluoridated in 1965; data from 16 neighbouring low-fluoride towns acted as negative control and 4 naturally fluoridated areas as positive control, in a survey in 1975 after 10 years' fluoridation (Videroni et al., 1976).

Hastings was the first New Zealand community to fluoridate and the reports of its effectiveness are well known (Ludwig, 1965, 1971). The very high caries experience found in New Zealand has meant that, in real terms, a larger number of teeth are prevented from becoming carious in Hastings, for a given percentage reduction, than in other communities. For example, the mean DMFT for 15-year-old children in 1954 was 16·8, which fell to 8·5 by 1970, a per cent reduction of 49 per cent or 8·3 teeth less. The corresponding figures for tooth surfaces were 42·5 DMFS in 1954 and 17·4 in 1970, a 59 per cent reduction or the large difference of 25 tooth surfaces, 15 of which were approximal. Gingival surfaces benefited most (87 per cent), approximal surfaces by 73 per cent and occlusal surfaces least (39 per cent). The effect of 10 years' fluoridation in the city of Lower Hutt has been reported (Hollis and Knowsley, 1970). In 1980, 54 per cent of the total population of New Zealand (or 84 per cent of the population on public water supplies) were receiving fluoridated water (Donaldson, 1980).

SUMMARY

Table 21 contains the results of 95 studies, from 20 countries, into the effectiveness of artificial water fluoridation. Fifty-five studies are from the USA and 40 from the remaining 19 countries throughout the world. *Fig.* 16 contains the frequency distributions of the percentage caries reductions observed in the 55 studies reporting data for deciduous teeth and the 73 studies giving results for permanent teeth. The modal percentage caries reduction is 40–50 per cent for deciduous teeth and 50–60 per cent for permanent teeth—this is in agreement with the oft-quoted statement that 'water fluoridation reduces dental decay by half'.

In a few countries (e.g. USA, New Zealand) a very high proportion of the population who receive a public water supply drink optimally fluoridated water. At present, the biggest programme for introducing artificial fluoridation is in progress in Eastern Europe and the USSR. Little information is available for South American countries, but it has been reported that fluoridation programmes are widespread. There is virtually no expansion of fluoridation in Western Europe, largely for political reasons.

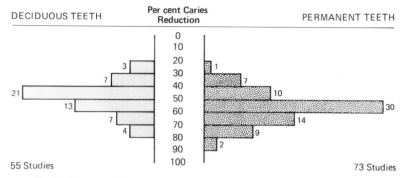

Fig. 16. Per cent caries reductions observed in 95 studies into the effectiveness of artificial fluoridation in 20 countries. Fifty-five studies gave results for the deciduous dentition (dmft) and 73 studies for the permanent dentition (DMFT).

REFERENCES

Adler P. (1970) Fluorides and dental health, In: *Fluorides and Human Health. WHO Monogr. Ser.* No. 59, Geneva, WHO, chap. 9.

Anon. (1962) Dental decay reduced by 60 per cent in Round-up fluoridation program. *Treasure State Health (Montana)* **12**, Oct., 1.

Anon. (1971) Salem dental survey 1971. *J. Oreg. Dent. Assoc.* Sept., **18**, 16–17.

Arnold F. A., Dean H. T., Jay P. and Knutson J. W. (1956) Effect of fluoridated public water supplies on dental caries prevalence. *Public Health Rep.* **71**, 652–658.

Arnold F. A., Likins R. C., Russell A. L. and Scott D. B. (1962) Fifteenth year of Grand Rapids fluoridation study. *J. Am. Dent. Assoc.* **65**, 780–785.

Arra M. C. and Lemke C. (1964) Effects of adjusted fluoridated water on dental caries in school children of Amery, Wis. *J. Am. Dent. Assoc.* **69**, 460–464.

Ast D. B., Smith D. J., Wachs B. and Cantwell K. T. (1956) Newburgh–Kingston caries-fluorine study XIV. Combined clinical and roentgenographic dental findings after ten years of fluoride experience. *J. Am. Dent. Assoc.* **52**, 314–325.

Auermann E. and Lingelbach H. (1964) Status and prospects of fluoridation in Europe. *J. Am. Public Health* **54**, 1545–1550.

Awang A. R. (1973) *Report of the Results of Seven Years of Fluoridation at Kluang, Johore.* Annual Conference of Directors of Medical and Health Services, Malaysia, Kuala Lumpur, Ministry of Health.

Backer Dirks O. (1974) The benefits of water fluoridation. *Caries Res.* **8** (suppl.), 2–15.

Backer Dirks O., Houwink B. and Kwant G. W. (1961) The results of $6\frac{1}{2}$ years of artificial fluoridation of drinking water in the Netherlands. *Arch. Oral Biol.* **5**, 284–300.

Backer Dirks O., Künzel W. and Carlos J. P. (1978) Caries-preventive water fluoridation. *Caries Res.* **12** suppl. 1, 7–14.

Barnard P. D. (1980) Fluoridation in Tamworth after 15 years. *Dent. Outlook* **6**, 46–47.

68

Beal J. F. and James P. M. C. (1971) Dental caries prevalence in 5-year-old children following five and a half years of water fluoridation in Birmingham. *Br. Dent. J.* **130**, 284–288.

Blayney J. R. and Hill I. N. (1967) Fluorine and dental health. *J. Am. Dent. Assoc.* **74**, 233–302.

Bronstein E. (1969) A survey of caries-experience among the pre-school children of Philadelphia. *J. Public Health Dent.* **29**, 24–26.

Brown H. K., McLaren H. R. and Poplove M. (1960) The Brantford–Sarnia–Stratford fluoridation caries study—1959 report. *J. Can. Dent. Assoc.* **26**, 131–142.

Brown H. K. and Poplove M. (1965) The Brantford–Sarnia–Stratford fluoridation caries study. Final survey 1963. *J. Can. Dent. Assoc.* **31**, 505–511.

Bryan E. T. and Smith C. E. (1966) The results of ten years of continuous fluoridation in Kingsport, Tennessee. *J. Tenn. State Dent. Assoc.* **46**, 30–34.

Bunch G. A. (1959) Post-fluoridation dental survey. *S. Carolina Dent. J.* **17**, 3–17.

Bunch G. A. (1964) Results of ten year post-fluoridation survey. *S. Carolina Dent. J.* **22**, 7–11.

Carr L. M. (1976) Fluoridation in Canberra. Part III. Dental caries after ten years. *Aust. Dent. J.* **21**, 440–444.

Chrietzberg J. E. and Lewis F. D. (1958) An evaluation of caries prevalence after five years of fluoridation. *J. Am. Dent. Assoc.* **56**, 192–193.

Collins C. K. and O'Mullane D. M. (1970) Dental caries experience in Cork city schoolchildren aged 4–11 years after $4\frac{1}{2}$ years of fluoridation. *J. Irish Dent. Assoc.* **16**, 130–134.

Connor R. A. and Harwood W. R. (1963) Dental effects of water fluoridation in Brandon, Manitoba: second report. *J. Can. Dent. Assoc.* **29**, 716–722.

Crooks E. L. W. and Konikoff A. B. (1972) A twenty-year study of the effectiveness of fluoride in the Richmond water supply. *Virginia Dent. J.* **49**, 24–26.

Csögör L., Guzner N. and Cristoloveanu R. (1968) Prophylaxis of dental decay in the town of Tirgu Mures by fluoridation of the drinking water. *Stomatol. (Buch.)* **15**, 33–38.

Csögör L., Guzner N., Cristoloveanu R. and Shapira M. (1973) Prophylaxie de la carie dentaire par fluorisation de l'eau potable dans la ville de Tirgu-Mures. *Rev. Port. Estomatol. Cir. Maxilofac.* **14**, 89–98.

Department of Health and Social Security (1969) *The Fluoridation Studies in the United Kingdom and the Results Achieved After Eleven years.* Report No. 122. London, HMSO.

Doherty J. M. and Krippene B. (1972) Fluoridation in Cudahy—five-year evaluation. *J. Wis. State Dent. Soc.* Aug., 247–249.

Donaldson E. W. (1980) New Zealand—fluoridation. *Br. Dent. J.* **148**, 80.

Dudney G. G., Rozier R. G., Less M. F. and Hughes J. T. (1977) Ten years of fluoridation in Asheville, North Carolina. *N. Carolina Dent. J.* **60**, 11–16.

Erlenbach F. M. (1964) Mystic-Stonington dental survey. *Conn. Health Bull.* **78**, 231–234.

Erlenbach F. M. and Tracy E. T. (1961) Tenth year of New Britain, Connecticut, fluoride study. *Conn. Health Bull.* **75**, 371–382.

Fishman S. R. and Collier D. R. (1965) Eight years fluoridation—Lebanon, Tenn. *J. Tenn. State Dent. Assoc.* **45**, 48–57.

Flaven B. M. (1977) *Benefits of Eleven Years of Fluoridated Water—the Winona Report*. Minneapolis, Minnesota Department of Health, Feb. 1977.

Gabovich R. D., Dmitrochenko A. S. and Stepanenko G. A. (1972) The effect of fluoridation of water in Ivano-Frankovsk on dental caries in the population. *Stomatol. (Mosk.)* **51**, 14–17.

Garcelon A. H. (1956) Fluoridation of water supply; the Norway, Maine study. *New Engl. J. Med.* **254**, 1072–1077.

Gernert E. B. (1958) Five year report on fluoridation in Louisville, Kentucky. *J. Kentucky Dent. Assoc.* July 1958, 29–32.

Gordon J. J. (1975) *Fluoridation in Philadelphia*. Report to Mr. J. Small, USPHS, Bethesda, Feb. 1975.

Gülzow H.-J., Kränzlin H. and Maeglin B. (1978) Ist der Kariesrückgang nach Trinkwasser fluoridierung in Basel auf eine Verzögerung in Zahndurchbruch zurückzuführen? *Schweiz. Monatsschr. Zahnheilkd.* **88**, 1192–1200.

Gülzow H.-J. and Maeglin B. (1979) Kariesstatistische Ergebnisse nach 15 jähriger Trinkwasser-fluoridierung. *Dtsch. Zahnärzl. Z.* **34**, 118–123.

Guzman R. M. (1961) Status of fluoridation in Puerto Rico. *J. Am. Waterwks Assoc.* **53**, 141–145.

Hann H. J. (1968) *The Dental Benefits of Water Fluoridation; 1968 Prince George Report*. Prince George, British Columbia, Prince George and District Dental Society and the Northern Interior Health Unit, Oct. 1968.

Healy T. F. (1963) *Study of the Effects of Fluoride on Teeth of Children in Cleveland Public Schools*. Cleveland, Ohio, Cleveland Public Schools.

Hollis M. J. and Knowsley P. C. (1970) Ten years of fluoridation in Lower Hutt. *N.Z. Dent. J.* **66**, 235–238.

Holmes C. B. (1963) Eleven year fluoridation evaluation on dental health status and practice. *J. Tenn. State Dent. Assoc.* **43**, 223–233.

Hsieh C.-C., Guo M.-K. and Hong Y.-C. (1979) Effect of water fluoridation on prevalence of dental caries in Chung-Hsing New Village after six years. *J. Formosan Med. Assoc.* **78**, 168–176.

Iowa State Department of Health (1960) *Controlled Fluoridation in Public Water Supplies. Iowa New Series* No. 1822 (Jan. 15) and No. 1850 (Nov. 5). State University of Iowa.

Jackson D., Gravely J. F. and Pinkham I. O. (1975) Fluoridation in Cumbria; a clinical study. *Br. Dent. J.* **139**, 319–322.

Jackson D., James P. M. C. and Wolfe W. B. (1975) Fluoridation in Anglesey; a clinical study. *Br. Dent. J.* **138**, 165–171.

Jackson D., Goward P. E. and Morrell G. V. (1980) Fluoridation in Leeds; a clinical survey of 5-year-old children. *Br. Dent. J.* **149**, 231–234.

Januszko T., Komenda W., Dobrowolski J., Smorczewska B., Szymaniak E., Zalewska E. and Kisiel A. (1977) Evaluation of effectiveness of drinking water fluoridation for prevention of dental caries in children of elementary schools in the city of Bialystok. *Czas. Stomat.* **30**, 555–560.

Jirásková M. et al. (1969) Water fluoration in Czechoslovakia. *V. Csek. Stomatol.* **69**, 129–138.

Jordan W. A. (1964) The Rush City report—ten years of fluoridated water. *Minn. Dept Health Rep.* **832**, July 1964.

Jordan W. A. (1970). Fluoridated water benefits continue; Albert Lea's 1969 dental survey. *North-West Dent.* **49**, 77–80.

Jordan W. A., Pugnier V. A. and McKee D. P. (1969) Silver Bay reports, following ten years of fluoridated water. *North-West Dent.* **48**, 7–10.

Klymko M. B. (1959) The effect of artificial water fluoridation on the teeth of Tuscaloosa school children. *J. Ala. Dent. Assoc.* **43**, 5–9.

Konick L. (1979) Dental health survey of New Haven schoolchildren after ten years of fluoridation. *Conn. Health Bull.* **93**, 32–40.

Künzel W. (1968) Results and prospects of water fluoridation in the German Democratic Republic. *Caries Res.* **2**, 172–179.

Künzel W. (1976) *Trinkwasserfluoridierung als Kollektive Kariesvorbeugende Massnahme*, 2nd ed. Berlin, VEB Verlag Volk und Gesundheit Berlin.

Kwant G. W., Groenveld A., Pot T. J. and Purdell Lewis D. (1974) Fluoride-toeveeging aan het drinkwater v; Een vergelijking van de gebitsgezondheid van 17- en 18-jarigen in Culemborg en Tiel. *Ned. Tijdschr. v. Tandheelkd.* **81**, 251–261.

Kwant G. W., Houwink B., Backer Dirks O., Groeneveld A. and Pot T. J. (1973) Artificial fluoridation of drinking water in the Netherlands; results of the Tiel–Culemborg experiment after $16\frac{1}{2}$ years. *Neth. Dent. J.* **80**, suppl. 9, 6–27.

Lemke C. W., Doherty J. M. and Arra M. C. (1970) Controlled fluoridation; the dental effects of discontinuation in Antigo, Wisconsin. *J. Am. Dent. Assoc.* **80**, 782–786.

Leonard R. C. (1963) Fluoridation in Maryland. *Md. State Dept. Health Month. Bull.* **35** (5), 1–4.

Lewis D. W. (1976) *An Evaluation of the Dental Effects of Water Fluoridation, City of Toronto 1963–1975*. Toronto, City Hall, Department of Public Health.

Ludwig T. G. (1965) The Hastings fluoridation project V—Dental effects between 1954 and 1964. *N.Z. Dent. J.* **61**, 175–179.

Ludwig T. G. (1971) The Hastings fluoridation project VI—Dental effects between 1954 and 1970. *N.Z. Dent. J.* **67**, 155–160.

McCauley H. G., Frazier T. M. and Rivas L. P. (1961) Dental caries in Baltimore schoolchildren after seven years of fluoridation of the public water supply. Baltimore Bureau of Statistics. *Q. Statist. Rep.* **13**, 14–21.

Margolis F. J., Reames H. R., Freshman E., McCauley J. C. and McLaffrey H. (1975) Fluoride—ten-year prospective study of deciduous and permanent dentition. *Am. J. Dis. Child.* **129**, 794–800.

Martin N. D. and Barnard P. D. (1970) Tamworth dental survey results 1963, 1969. *Dental Outlook* **23**, 6–7.

Medcalf G. W. (1971) First permanent molars of six-year-old children after two and a half years of fluoridation in Western Australia. *Aust. Dent. J.* **16**, 252–254.

Medcalf G. W. (1975) Six years of fluoridation on the goldfields of Western Australia. *Aust. Dent. J.* **20**, 170–173.

Medcalf G. W. (1978) Ten years of fluoridation in Perth, Western Australia. *Aust. Dent. J.* **23**, 474–476.

Mejia D. R., Espinal F., Velez H. and Aguirre S. M. (1976) Use of fluoridated salt in four Columbian communities VIII. *Bol. Sanit. Panam.* **80**, 205–219.

Ministry of Health, Scottish Office, Ministry of Housing and Local Government (1962) *The Conduct of the Fluoridation Studies in the United Kingdom and the Results Achieved After Five Years*. Report No. 105. London, HMSO.

Minoguchi G. (1964) Eleventh year of fluoridation study at Yamashina in Kyoto and some problem about the fluoridation of waterworks in Japan. *Bull. Stomatol. Kyoto Univ.* **4**, 45–124.

Mollenkopf J. (1963) Benefits of fluoridation apparent in Fort Wayne. *Ind. St. Board Health Month. Bull.* Feb. 1963, 6–8.

Moncrief E. W. (1970) Results of eleven years of fluoridation in Fayette Alabama. *J. Ala. Dent. Assoc.* **54**, 18–25.

Musselman P. (1957) Report on dental findings in Newark, Delaware children after five years of fluoridation. *J. Am. Dent. Assoc.* **54**, 783–785.

Nordling H. and Tulikoura I. (1970) Results of the fluoridation of drinking water in Kuopio. *Suom. Hammaslääk.* **17**, 517–524.

O'Hickey S. (1976) Water fluoridation and dental caries in Ireland: background, introduction and development. *J. Irish Dent. Assoc.* **22**, 61–66.

Ostrow A. H. (1963) *Ten Year Fluoridation Report.* Report of the Washington Dept. Public Health, Bureau of Dental Health, March 18, 1963.

Quentin K.-E. and Lingelbach H. (1963) Trinkwasserfluoridierung in Europa. In: Hardwick J. L., Dustin J. P. and Held H. R. (eds), *Advances in Fluorine Research and Dental Caries Prevention.* Oxford, Pergamon, pp. 23–32.

Reger R. H., Dunn M. M. and Downs R. A. (1963) *The effects of 10 years of fluoridation on the teeth of school-age continuous residents of Grand Junction 1951–1962.* Denver, Colo., Colorado Department of Health, Appendix, pp. 4–11.

Ross M. R., Hecht S. J. and Gleeson J. C. (1960) Results of five years of fluoridation in 21 Monmouth County municipalities. *J. New J. State Dent. Soc.* **31**, 14–16.

Rugg-Gunn A. J., Carmichael C. L., French A. D. and Furness J. A. (1977) Fluoridation in Newcastle and Northumberland; a clinical study of 5-year-old children. *Br. Dent. J.* **142**, 395–402.

Russell A. L. and White C. L. (1961) Dental caries in Maryland and children after seven years of fluoridation. *Public Health Rep.* **76**, 1087–1093.

Russell D. L. (1965) Dental caries rate of Mobile County school children; comparison of children in areas supplied by fluoridated and non-fluoridated communal water supplies. *Ala. J. Med. Sci.* **2**, 381–388.

Rybakov A. I., Pakhomov G. N., Kuklin G. S. and Alimsky A. V. (1978) A decade of experience in drinking water fluoridation and dynamics of caries among schoolchildren in the European part of the USSR beyond the Arctic Circle. Personal communication, World Health Organisation.

Schreiber M. F. (1966) Sheboygan led fluoridation 'war' on tooth decay. Wis. State Board of Health, *Fluoridation News* **3**(2), 1.

Schultz W. E. (1969) Results of the city of Milwaukee dental surveys 1950, 1959, 1965. *J. Wis. St. Dent. Soc.* **45**, 195–198.

Smith J. E. and Paquin O. (1962) The effect of five and one-half years of water fluoridation on the continuous resident child population of St. Louis, Missouri. *J. Missouri Dent. Assoc.* **42**(7), 10–16.

Snyder J. R. (1964) Benefits of fluoridation in Boseman. Montana State Board of Health, *Treasure State Health* **13**(11), 4.

Sogaro L. H. (1964) Phillipsburg, N. J.–Easton, Pa. fluoridation study. *J. Am. Dent. Assoc.* **69**, 295–299.

Stadt Z. M., Blum H. L., Barney E. E. and Fletcher E. (1960) Contra Costa County fluoridation reports. *J. Cal. State Dent. Assoc.* and *Nevada State Dent. Assoc.* Apr., 109–113.

Steele A. (1977) Oshkosh School dental survey indicates decay decline. Wis. Dept. of Health and Social Services *Fluoridation News* **13**(1), 3.

Strelyukhina T. F., Belova T. A., Belyaevskaya L. A. and Gromova E. M. (1976) Influence of water fluoridation on dental caries experience among schoolchildren in Leningrad. *Stomatol. (Mosk.)* **8**, 66–69.

Szwejda L. (1962) Eleven years of fluoridation in Charlotte, N. Carolina. *Dent. Soc. J.* **45**, 107–113.

Tank G. and Storvick C. A. (1964) Caries experience of children one to six years old in two Oregon communities. *J. Am. Dent. Assoc.* **69**, 750–757.

Taylor E. and Bertram F. P. (1965) Marshall Study credit is due; discussion of the tabular data from the ten-year Marshall, Texas dental fluoridation study. *Texas Dent. J.* Feb., 30–31.

Toth K. (1972) The methods and results of caries prevention with fluorides in Hungary and in Eastern European countries. *Rev. Belge Med. Dent.* **27**, 521–527.

Trithart A. H. and Denney R. P. (1956) Study of caries experience rates of 6-yr-old children of Milan, Tenn. after 5 yrs of fluoridation. *J. Tenn. State Dent. Assoc.* **36**, 156–159.

Trubman A. (1965) Dental caries in Mississippi children; comparison of a fluoride with non-fluoride towns. *J. Miss. Dent. Assoc.* **21**, 19–23.

Videroni W., Sternberg G. S. and Davies G. N. (1976) Effect on caries experience of lifetime residents after 10 years of fluoridation in Townsville, Australia. *Community Dent. Oral Epidemiol.* **4**, 248–253.

Viegas Y. and Viegas A. R. (1974) Data analysis of the prevalence of dental caries in Campinas city (S. Paulo, Brazil) after ten years of water fluoridation. *Rev. Saude Publica* **8**, 399–409.

Weinstein H. N. (1972) Effectiveness of fluoridation. *Chicago Board of Health Newsletter* **12**, 1–2.

Whittle J. G. and Downer M. C. (1979) Dental health and treatment needs of Birmingham and Salford schoolchildren. *Br. Dent. J.* **147**, 67–71.

Wigdorowicz-Makowerowa N., Plonka B. and Dadun-Sek A. (1975) Evaluation of water fluoridation effectiveness in children in Wroclaw during 5 years. *Czas. Stomatol.* **28**, 253–259.

Wigdorowicz-Makowerowa N., Dadun-Sek A. and Plonka B. (1978) Comparison of effectiveness of water fluoridation during 5 and 8 years in Wroclaw. *Czas. Stomatol.* **31**, 817–823.

Wong M. Q., Goh S. W. and Oon. C. H. (1970) A ten-year study of fluoridation of water in Singapore. *Dent. J. Malaysia Singapore* **10**, 20–40.

World Health Organisation (1969) *Status of Water Fluoridation in the Americas.* Document No. HP/DH/2. Dental Health Section, Department of Health Services and the Department of Engineering and Environmental Sciences, Pan American Health Organisation, Regional Office of WHO, 1969.

Yacovone J. A. and Parente A. M. (1974) Twenty years of community water fluoridation: the prevalence of dental caries among Providence, R. I. schoolchildren. *R. I. Dent. J.* June, 3–18.

Young W. O. (1958) Fluorides and dental caries in Idaho V; ten years of fluoridation in Lewiston. *Idaho State Dent. Assoc. Newsletter* Feb. 1958.

CHAPTER 5

OTHER METHODS OF SYSTEMIC ADMINISTRATION OF FLUORIDE

Although the importance of fluoride in the prevention of dental caries in the first half of this century principally concerned fluoride in public water supplies, other vehicles for fluoride have been recommended for almost as long a time. Tablets containing calcium fluoride were recommended for 'the strengthening of teeth' in the last century, as was bone meal, which makes one suspect that, in those early days, calcium was considered to be of at least equal importance to fluoride.

Initially it was thought that, to be effective, the fluoride had to be ingested, absorbed into the body and laid down in the forming tooth enamel. This undoubtedly occurs and has come to be known as the 'systemic' method of fluoride administration. Since enamel formation is completed (except for third molars) by about the age of 12 years, fluoride administration was thought to be only effective up to this age. However, in the 1940s workers in America suggested that it might be possible to increase the amount of fluoride in tooth enamel by applying solutions of fluoride to the enamel after the teeth had erupted into the mouth. This was named the 'topical' method of fluoride administration. There are, therefore, two ways of increasing the concentration of fluoride in enamel; the systemic method while teeth are forming, and the topical method after they erupt although, as will be seen later, the division between these two methods is not so clear cut as was first thought.

SYSTEMIC ADMINISTRATION

Water fluoridation is the most natural of all the methods of giving fluoride since many millions of people already drink the optimum amount of fluoride without any adjustment to their water supply (Chapter 4). It is also the most cost-effective method (Chapter 16). Because piped-water supplies are not universal and, where they are available, many communities have not agreed to implement public water fluoridation, alternatives have been considered. As has been mentioned earlier, fluoride-containing tablets have been available for many years throughout the world. Fifty million fluoride tablets were sold in the UK in 1980. For younger children drops have sometimes been preferred to tablets. Recently, in the USA, fluoridation of school water supplies has been investigated as an alternative to fluoridation of the public water system. Because daily intake of salt in man varies less than for many other foods, the addition of fluoride (not to be confused with iodide) to salt has been investigated in Europe and South America. Milk has also been considered as a vehicle for fluoride with the alternative of fluoride-containing fruit juices in warmer climates. The addition of fluoride to flour and even to sugar has been suggested (there are good theoretical reasons for choosing sugar), but because intake of these foods varies widely they have not been investigated further.

TOPICAL ADMINISTRATION

The application of concentrated fluoride solutions (around 1 per cent F) to erupted teeth has been investigated since 1940. This has come to be known as 'clinical topical fluoride administration' because it is most commonly carried out by qualified personnel in a dental chair, although application is sometimes made by other ancillary personnel, or by the children themselves under supervision. The fluoride can be applied in water solutions or in gels, in varnishes or incorporated in prophylactic pastes. Their action is purely topical and they should not be swallowed.

A mouthwash is a second type of vehicle; the fluoride concentration being 0·1 per cent F or less. Again, the action of mouthwashes is topical and in general they should not be swallowed, although, to complicate matters, a few are especially formulated for rinsing and swallowing.

From the public's point of view the best-known vehicle for fluoride is toothpaste (or dentifrice as it is known in the USA). The fluoride concentration is almost invariably around 0·1 per cent F. Ninety-five per cent of all toothpastes sold in the UK in 1978 contained fluoride and the price of a non-fluoride and fluoride toothpaste is now the same.

Apart from the above three types of vehicle for topical administration of fluoride, many of those developed primarily for systemic administration also have a topical action while they are in the mouth. Nearly half the effect of water fluoridation is reported to come from its topical action in the mouth, despite a very low concentration of fluoride (Backer Dirks, 1967). In proportion, the topical effect of school water fluoridation is likely to be even greater, and tablets are now especially made to dissolve slowly in the mouth, rather than to be swallowed whole or crushed with food as was previously advised, to give a greater topical effect. Although there is a lack of information on the subject, the topical action of fluoride in salt and milk is likely to be slight; fluoridated fruit juice might, in theory, have a slightly greater topical effect because of the greater availability of fluoride.

Topical methods of fluoride administration are discussed later in this book; the remainder of this chapter will include descriptions of school water fluoridation, salt and milk fluoridation, while fluoride tablets and drops will be considered in a separate chapter.

SCHOOL WATER FLUORIDATION

Two advantages of water fluoridation are that, first, no effort is required by the recipients and, second, that the cost per person is low. However, the cost per person increases as the size of the population served by each fluoridation plant decreases. It was of interest, therefore, to see whether fluoridation of a school's water supply was effective and economical. Unlike other school-based preventive programmes (e.g. F tablets and mouthrinses), no action is required by the children. As yet, school water fluoridation has been tested only in the USA where 40 million people live in areas without community water supplies and many rural schools are supplied by their own well. By the end of 1976 125 000 children attending 400 schools in 13 states in the USA were benefiting from school fluoridation programmes (Jenny and Heifetz, 1978).

The first investigation began in 1954 in the Virgin Islands with fluoridation of the water supply at 2 schools at a level of 2·3 ppm F. Because one of the schools was altered and enlarged during the study, and operation of the machinery was intermittent and eventually broke down, the study cannot be considered satisfactory. In 1962, 7–13-year-old children in the school receiving the more consistent supply of fluoridated water (for 8 years) were examined, together with children of similar age in other schools in the same district. The children attending the fluoridated school had about 22 per cent less DMFT than the control children, at least indicating that school water fluoridation might be beneficial (Horowitz et al., 1965).

Since then three major studies, each planned to last 12 years, have been undertaken in mainland USA. The first two, in Pike County, Kentucky, and Elk Lake, Pennsylvania, began in 1958, while the third in Seagrove, North Carolina, began in 1968 with final examinations planned for 1980. In Elk Lake, the final examinations (after 12 years) took place in 1970, but this was not possible in Pike County where the organization at the 2 test schools changed and school fluoridation ceased after the 8-year follow-up examination in 1966.

In the Pike County schools, water was fluoridated at 3·0 ppm (or 3·3 times the optimum level for public water supplies in the same area), while in the Elk Lake schools the water fluoride level was 5 ppm (or 4·5 times the optimum public water supply level). These levels were chosen because children consume part of their daily water intake at school and only attend school for a maximum of about 200 days per year. In addition, children do not enter school before 6 years, an age when incisor teeth can be considered to be no longer at risk of developing mottled enamel. Since no objectionable mottling was observed in any teeth in the children attending the Pike County and Elk Lake schools, a higher fluoride level (6·3 ppm or 7 times the optimal community water fluoride level) was tested in the third American study in Seagrove. In all three of these studies children in the test schools were examined before fluoridation of the school's water supply began, and the results of these baseline examinations then served as control data for comparison with the results of the surveys after 4, 8 and 12 years' school fluoridation.

Interim results after 8 years of school fluoridation in Pike County and Elk Lake (Horowitz et al., 1968) showed that children who had continually attended schools in the two study areas had very similar reductions in DMFT of about 33 and 35 per cent respectively, compared with similarly aged children who attended these schools before fluoridation began.

Results after 8 years' school fluoridation in Elk Lake (5·0 ppm F) and Seagrove (6·3 ppm F) are given in *Table* 22. It can be seen that children of

Table 22. Mean DMF Surface Scores by Age at Baseline and after 8 Years of Fluoridated Water at School (*Heifetz et al., 1978*)

	1968 (*Baseline*)		1976		*Difference in mean DMFS*	% *Difference from baseline*
Age	No. of children	Mean DMFS	No. of children	Mean DMFS		
Seagrove, NC (6·3 ppm F)						
Total		9·34*		5·63*	−3·71	−39·7
6	27	1·07	38	0·71	−0·36	−33·6
7	76	2·29	96	1·40	−0·89	−39·0
8	79	3·86	68	2·06	−1·80	−46·7
9	89	5·69	80	3·28	−2·42	−42·4
10	78	7·91	96	6·04	−1·87	−23·6
11	90	10·26	74	6·93	−3·33	−32·4
12	77	14·23	82	7·10	−7·13	−50·1
13	63	15·21	72	9·22	−5·99	−39·4
14	51	21·82	40	12·68	−9·15	−41·9
Elk Lake, Pa (5·0 ppm F)						
Total		9·86*		6·42*	−3·44	−34·9
6	91	1·00	109	0·35	−0·65	−65·0
7	84	2·77	106	1·30	−1·47	−53·1
8	64	4·33	98	2·44	−1·89	−43·7
9	85	5·92	114	4·31	−1·61	−27·2
10	81	7·72	79	6·01	−1·71	−22·2
11	123	10·15	103	7·25	−2·90	−28·6
12	90	15·73	90	9·93	−5·80	−36·9
13	114	18·12	88	10·53	−7·59	−41·9
14	85	20·81	93	14·16	−6·65	−32·0

*Adjusted to combined baseline age distribution of both schools.

all ages in the range 6–14 years appeared to benefit and that, on average, the reduction was marginally higher in Seagrove (39·7 per cent) for all ages compared with Elk Lake (34·9 per cent); the difference between the two studies in tooth surfaces prevented was about 0·25 DMFS for all years combined. Although the per cent reductions were high in younger children the actual number of DMF surfaces prevented was much higher in the older children (up to 9 surfaces prevented per child). None of the 130 children who had been exposed to 6·3 ppm F for 8 years in Seagrove showed any definite signs of fluorosis in their canines, premolars and second molars, teeth which were still calcifying during their school years (Heifetz et al., 1978).

In all three studies it was observed that the relative effectiveness of fluoridation was twice as great on the late erupting teeth (canines, premolars and second molars) than on the early erupting teeth (incisors and first molars). This may be because the late erupting teeth received both a systemic and topical exposure to fluoride, while the early erupting teeth received only a topical exposure, although difference in length of time exposed to the cariogenic challenge in the mouth may be an additional explanation (Horowitz, 1973). Likewise the overall percentage reduction increased in Elk Lake from about 22 per cent after 4 years, to 35 per cent after 8 years, to 39 per cent after 12 years, as the proportion of teeth receiving both systemic and topical effect increased. As is commonly found in fluoride trials, caries protection was greatest on the approximal tooth surfaces. The number of teeth extracted fell from 80 to 28 per 100 children in Elk Lake between 1958 and 1970 (Horowitz, 1973).

In summary, fluoridation of school water supplies is technically feasible, results in a substantial reduction in caries experience in school-children and the cost of this public health measure is low (about US $1·5 per person per year) (Horowitz and Heifetz, 1979). In the opinion of Heifetz et al. (1978), from the results so far, the slightly bigger benefit achieved with 6·3 ppm F is not sufficiently greater than that observed with 5 ppm F to warrant the higher fluoride level, and they therefore re-commend school fluoridation at the lower level of 5 ppm F, or 4·5 times the optimum level of fluoridation of community water supplies in that locality.

FLUORIDATED SALT

As a dietary vehicle for ensuring adequate ingestion of fluoride, domestic salt comes second to drinking water; salt's enrichment with iodide already provides an effective means of preventing goitre. Indeed it was a medical practitioner concerned with the prevention of goitre in Switzerland who, over 30 years ago, pioneered the addition of fluoride to salt as a caries-preventive measure (Wespi, 1948, 1950). Fluoridated salt has been on sale in Switzerland since 1955, and by 1967 three-quarters of domestic salt sold in Switzerland was fluoridated at 90 mg F/kg salt (or 90 ppm F). However, it was soon accepted that the original estimates of salt intake, upon which calculations of fluoride concentrations in salt were based, were too high and the ingestion of fluoride too low. In more recent investigations the level of fluoride has been raised to 200, 250 and 350 mg F/kg salt, with enhanced effectiveness. Toth (1976, 1980) has suggested that the urinary fluoride concentration is the most accurate guide for estimating fluoride intake in communities using fluoridated salt. From these results he concluded that, in Hungary, 250 mg F/kg provide too low a fluoride intake compared with optimally fluoridated water, and he is therefore currently testing 350 mg F/kg salt.

Despite the widespread use of fluoridated salt in Switzerland, its effectiveness is not easily measured since, in many Swiss communities, other preventive programmes (e.g. fluoride brushing; *see* Chapter 16) have been introduced in addition to fluoridated salt. However, Marthaler et al. (1977, 1978) concluded that the caries-preventive effectiveness of 250 mg F/kg salt used in the Swiss canton of Vaud was greater than the 25 per cent or so reduction observed following the addition of 90 mg F/kg in other Swiss cantons (Marthaler and Schenardi, 1962).

Toth (1976) reported the effectiveness of 250 mg F/kg salt fluoridation in Hungary after 8 years' use. The results (*Table* 23) indicated a reduction

Table 23. Caries Experience (deft) for 6-year-old Children living in Test and Control Communities in Hungary after 8 Years' Salt Fluoridation (at 250 mg F/kg) (*Toth, 1976*)

	Experimental	Control
1966	6·8	8·6
1974	4·1	9·2
Difference	−2·7 (−39·5%)	+0·6 (+7·1%)

of 39 per cent in deft in 6-year-old children in the test community, while caries experience increased by 7 per cent in the control community children over the same period. Although there was an imbalance in caries experience between the two communities at the start of the experiment in 1966, this alone could not explain the differences observed in 1974. After 10 years' exposure to salt fluoridation, Toth (1979) observed that 5- to 6-year-olds in the same test community had 2·8 deft, compared with 6·0 deft in the control community, and 1·4 deft in children of the same age living in an area with fluoridated water. These 10-year results indicated that a substantial caries reduction occurred after the introduction of salt fluoridation, but this was less than occurred with water fluoridation. No results are yet available from the studies testing 350 mg F/kg salt in Hungary.

In 1964, a well-planned study was initiated in four Colombian communities (Mejia et al., 1976). In the village of Montebello, sodium fluoride was added to domestic salt (at 200 mg F/kg), while in Armenia calcium fluoride was added to domestic salt (at 200 mg F/kg), in San Pedro drinking water was fluoridated (at 1 ppm F) and Don Matias remained as the control community. At the end of the project, after 8 years, reductions in caries prevalence and experience in 8-year-old children were large in the three communities receiving fluoride in salt or water, although a small reduction was also observed in the control town (*Table* 24). When all children aged 6–14 years were included in the data analyses, the reduction in DMFT between 1964 and 1972 was 50 per cent in Montebello (NaF in salt), 48 per cent in Armenia (CaF_2 in salt), 60 per cent in San Pedro (water F) and 5 per cent in the control town Don Matias. Analysis of urine samples throughout the year revealed that fluoride excretion was similar in the two fluoridated salt communities, but excretion levels in the salt communities were 20 per cent lower than those recorded in the fluoridated water town.

Table 24. Caries Experience (DMFT) for 8-year-old Children living in Three Test Communities and One Control Community in Colombia, South America, after 8 Years (*Mejia et al., 1976*)

	NaF salt	CaF$_2$ salt	Water F	Control
1964	3·7	3·8	3·8	4·3
1972	1·4	1·1	0·8	3·8
Difference	2·3 (61%)	2·7 (72%)	3·0 (78%)	0·5 (13%)

Encouraging results were also reported after the addition of NaF to domestic salt in a closed children's institution in Pamplona, Spain (Vines, 1971). Because of the high estimated salt intake, particularly in their special salt bread, the fluoride level was only 112 mg F/kg salt but, after 4 years, reductions in caries experience were observed in all ages in the range 8–13 years.

During the 20 years' experience of large-scale production of fluoridated salt in Switzerland, technical problems have been overcome. When sodium fluoride was first added to domestic salt, separation tended to occur, but this problem was solved by the addition of tricalcium phosphate (Restrepo, 1967). The proportion of the fluoride in salt which is absorbed into the body has not been established: Alanen and Pohto (1977) suggested, from in vitro experiments, that this was not likely to be greater than 50–60 per cent of the fluoride consumed. However, because of the difficulties of accurately estimating salt intake, measurement of urinary fluoride output would seem to be the preferred method for establishing the optimum level of fluoride in domestic salt (Toth, 1979). Data would appear to indicate (Toth, 1976, 1979) that, in Hungary at least, 350 mg F/kg is likely to be close to the optimum fluoride concentration in domestic salt. Substantial reductions in caries experience observed in teeth exposed only post-eruptively to fluoridated salt (Marthaler et al., 1978) appear to indicate that, surprisingly, a topical as well as a systemic action occurs.

In summary, the caries-preventive effectiveness of fluoridated salt is substantial, although it appears to be slightly less than that observed with fluoridated water. This view is based on a comparatively small number of studies (compared with the data on water fluoridation) which have lasted for a maximum of 10 years. From urinary analyses data, it is probable that doses tested so far (up to 250 mg F/kg) are suboptimal and the results of trials of higher doses are awaited with interest to see whether the effectiveness approaches that achieved by water fluoridation. Salt appears to be a safe vehicle for fluoride administration (Mühlemann, 1967; Ruzicka et al., 1976). Salt fluoridation uses only 3 per cent of the quantity of fluoride required for water fluoridation (Toth, 1978), but it has the same advantage that no personal effort is needed by the public.

FLUORIDATED MILK AND FRUIT JUICES

Both bovine and human milk contain low levels of fluoride—about 0·03 ppm F (Ericsson and Ribelius, 1971). Because milk is recommended as a good food for infants and children, it was considered, over 20 years ago, to be a suitable vehicle for supplementing children's fluoride intake in areas with fluoride-deficient water supplies. Ericsson (1958) showed that fluoride was absorbed in the gut just as readily from milk as from water, refuting the suggestion that the high calcium content of milk would render the fluoride unavailable. However, the binding of added fluoride to calcium or protein might reduce the topical fluoride effect in the mouth compared with fluoride in water (Duff, 1981).

Despite its potential promise, only three studies have been reported. Although all three studies indicated that the addition of fluoride to milk might have a caries-preventive effect, the first two studies can be criticized in certain respects. The study of Rusoff et al. (1962) involved 171 children aged 6–9 years from 2 schools in Louisiana, USA. Children from one school received a half-pint of homogenized milk daily, fortified with 2·2 mg NaF (yielding 1 mg F). The fluoride was added in the form of 0·5 ml NaF solution to each half-pint before sealing. During the summer vacation parents of children in the study group were given bottles of aqueous sodium fluoride solution so that 8 drops could be added to their 8 oz glass of milk per day. Children in the control group received homogenized milk without fluoride. This pilot study lasted $3\frac{1}{2}$ years, when 65 children aged 9–12 years remained in the fluoride group and 64 children of similar age in the control group. Unfortunately the two groups were not well balanced with respect to first-molar caries experience at the beginning of the experiment. The DMFT in second molars and first and second premolars, after $3\frac{1}{2}$ years' consumption of fluoridated milk, was 0·34 in the fluoride group and 1·70 in the control group. A difference was still apparent 18 months after cessation of the experiment. However, because of the considerable divergence in caries attack on first molars between groups before the study and the small size of the groups, the lower caries rate in the experimental children must be viewed with caution. The data indicated that some of the effect was likely to be topical.

Ziegler (1962) reported his attempts to introduce fluoridated milk in Winterthur, Switzerland. At first, a sealed plastic bottle of 0·22 per cent sodium fluoride solution was made available to the public in pharmacies against a prescription. Each parent then added 1 ml of this fluoride solution to 1 litre of milk to produce 1 ppm F fluoridated milk. Thus the amount of fluoride ingested depended on the amount of milk consumed— a half-litre of milk contained 0·5 mg F. In 1955, school milk was fluoridated at the central dairy in Winterthur; initially 0·2 mg F was placed in 200 ml milk, but this was increased to 0·5 mg in 1961. A little later, the size of milk bottles was increased to 250 ml, which contained 0·625 mg F. The results of clinical surveys indicated that dental caries was lower in children who had consumed the fluoridated milk for 6 years, compared with control children (Wirz and Ziegler, 1964, quoted in WHO, 1970).

Davis (1975) has reported that clinical studies of fluoridated milk have been conducted in Germany and Japan, but as yet no details of these studies are available. In a recent publication, Stephen et al. (1981) reported that consumption of 200 ml of milk containing 1·5 mg F each school day for 4 years reduced the occurrence of caries in first permanent molars in Glaswegian primary schoolchildren by 34 per cent. The 49 test children had a mean of 1·7 DMFT (first permanent molars) at the age of 9 years, compared with 2·4 DMFT in the 59 control children who also drank 200 ml of milk each school day but with no added fluoride. The difference of 0·7 teeth between the groups was statistically significant ($P < 0.01$).

In warm climates, fluoridated fruit juices may be a practical alternative to fluoridated milk. Gedalia et al. (1981) have recently reported a 28 per cent reduction in DMFS increment in 6–9-year-old Israeli children who consumed 1 mg F in 100 ml of pure orange juice ($\equiv$10 ppm F) each school day for 3 years. The 111 test-group children developed 2·5 DMFS over 3 years compared with 3·5 DMFS in the 111 control children who had no beverage. However, interpretation of the results was complicated by the observation that a third group of similarly aged children, who consumed 100 ml of orange juice with no added fluoride, developed 2·9 DMFS over the 3-year period. It would appear, therefore, that the fluoride per se might have been responsible for only part of the difference between the fluoride drink group and the no-drink group.

Since absorption of fluoride from water and milk would appear to be about equal, it is likely that their systemic caries-preventive effect would be similar. Fluoridated milk has been shown to have a topical caries-preventive effect in rats (Poulsen et al., 1976) and possibly in humans (Rusoff et al., 1962), although Rugg-Gunn et al. (1976) did not find an increase in plaque fluoride after children had consumed milk containing

5 ppm F, and Gedalia et al. (1981) reported no increase in enamel fluoride in children who consumed 100 ml of 10 ppm F fruit juice for 3 years. Kempler et al. (1977) have reported that, in hamsters, acidulated fluoride beverages have a greater caries-preventive effect than a neutral fluoride beverage. Although this suggests that low pH fruit drinks may be a better vehicle for fluoride than milk (at a neutral pH), these findings await confirmation from comparative human clinical trials, since acidulated fluoride mouthrinses have not been shown to be superior to neutral fluoride mouthrinses in preventing caries in human subjects (*see* Chapter 11).

In summary, although milk and fruit juices are possible vehicles for fluoride, clinical data are limited. In addition, the intake of milk varies widely and methods previously tested have required parental or school effort. It would, therefore, seem that salt fluoridation would appear to be a more promising alternative to water fluoridation in areas unable to implement the latter.

REFERENCES

Alanen E. and Pohto P. (1977) Non-ionized fluoride in fluoridated domestic salt solution. *Proc. Finn. Dent. Soc.* **73**, 225–227.

Backer Dirks O. (1967) The relation between the fluoridation of water and dental caries experience. *Int. Dent. J.* **17**, 582–605.

Davis J. G. (1975) Fluoridised milk for children, part 2. *Dairy Industries* **40**, 48–51.

Duff E. J. (1981) Total and ionic fluoride in milk. *Caries Res.* **15**, 406–408.

Ericsson Y. (1958) The state of fluorine in milk. *Acta Odont. Scand.* **16**, 51–77.

Ericsson Y. and Ribelius U. (1971) Wide variations of fluoride supply to infants and their effect. *Caries Res.* **5**, 78–88.

Gedalia I., Galon H., Rennert A., Biderco I. and Mohr I. (1981) Effect of fluoridated citrus beverage on dental caries and on fluoride concentration in the surface enamel of children's teeth. *Caries Res.* **15**, 103–108.

Heifetz S. B., Horowitz H. S. and Driscoll W. S. (1978) Effect of school water fluoridation on dental caries: results in Seagrove, NC, after eight years. *J. Am. Dent. Assoc.* **97**, 193–196.

Horowitz H. S. (1973) School fluoridation for the prevention of dental caries. *Int. Dent. J.* **23**, 346–353.

Horowitz H. S. and Heifetz S. B. (1979) Methods for assessing the cost-effectiveness of caries preventive agents and procedures. *Int. Dent. J.* **29**, 106–117.

Horowitz H. S., Law F. E. and Pritzker T. (1965) Effect of school water fluoridation on dental caries, St. Thomas, V.I. *Publ. Hlth Rep.* **80**, 382–388.

Horowitz H. S. et al. (1968) School fluoridation studies in Elk Lake, Pennsylvania, and Pike County, Kentucky—results after eight years. *Am. J. Public Health* **50**, 2240–2250.

Jenny J. and Heifetz S. B. (1978) Prevention update. *Dental Hygiene* **52**, 187–194.

Kempler D., Anaise J., Westreich V. and Gedalia I. (1977) Caries rate in hamsters given non-acidulated and acidulated tea. *J. Dent. Res.* **56**, 89.

Marthaler T. M. and Schenardi C. (1962) Inhibition of caries in children after $5\frac{1}{2}$ years use of fluoridated table salt. *Helv. Odont. Acta* **6**, 1–6.

Marthaler T. M., de Crousaz Ph., Meyer R., Regolati B. and Robert A. (1977) Fréquence globale de la carie dentaire dans le canton de Vaud, après passage de la fluoruration par comprimés à la fluoruration du sel alimentaire. *Schweiz. Monatsschr. Zahnheilkd.* **87**, 147–158.

Marthaler T. M., Mejia R., Toth K. and Vines J. J. (1978) Caries-preventive salt fluoridation. *Caries Res.* **12**, suppl. 1, 15–21.

Mejia D. R., Espinal F., Velez H. and Aguirre S. M. (1976) Use of fluoridated salt in four Colombian communities VIII. Results achieved from 1964 to 1972. *Bol. Sanit. Panam.* **80**, 205–219.

Mühlemann H. R. (1967) Fluoridated domestic salt; a discussion of dosage. *Int. Dent. J.* **17**, 10–17.

Poulsen S., Larsen M. J. and Larson R. H. (1976) Effect of fluoridated milk and water on enamel fluoride content and dental caries in the rat. *Caries Res.* **10**, 227–233.

Restrepo D. (1967) Salt fluoridation: an alternate measure to water fluoridation. *Int. Dent. J.* **17**, 4–9.

Rugg-Gunn A. J., Edgar W. M., Jenkins G. N. and Cockburn M. A. (1976) Plaque F and plaque acid production in children drinking milk fluoridated to 1 and 5 ppm F. *J. Dent. Res.* **55**, D143 (abstr.).

Rusoff L. L., Konikoff B. S., Frye J. B., Johnston J. E. and Frye W. W. (1962) Fluoride addition to milk and its effect on dental caries in school children. *Am. J. Clin. Nutr.* **11**, 94–107.

Ruzicka J. A., Mrklas L. and Rokytova K. (1976) The influence of salt intake on the incorporation of fluoride into mouse bone. *Caries Res.* **10**, 386–389.

Stephen K. W., Boyle I. T., Campbell D., McNee S., Fyffe J. A., Jenkins A. S. and Boyle P. (1981) A 4-year double blind fluoridated school milk study in a vitamin-D deficient area. *Br. Dent. J.* **151**, 287–292.

Toth K. (1976) A study of 8 years domestic salt fluoridation for prevention of caries. *Community Dent. Oral Epidemiol.* **4**, 106–110.

Toth K. (1978) Some economic aspects of domestic salt fluoridation *Caries Res.* **12**, 110 (abstr.).

Toth K. (1979) 10 years of domestic salt fluoridation in Hungary. *Caries Res.* **13**, 101 (abstr.).

Toth K. (1980) Factors influencing the urinary fluoride level in subjects drinking low fluoride water. *Caries Res.* **14**, 168 (abstr.).

Vines J. J. (1971) Fluorprofilaxis de la caries dental a traves de la sal fluorurada. *Revta Clin. Esp.* **120**, 319–334.

Wespi H. J. (1948) Gedanke zur Frage der optimalen Ernährung in der Schwangerschaft. Salz and Brot als Träger zusätzlicher Nahrungsstoffe. *Schweiz. Med. Wochenschr.* **78**, 153–155.

Wespi H. J. (1950) Fluoriertes Kochsalz zur Cariesprophylaxe. *Schweiz. Med. Wochenschr.* **80**, 561–564.

World Health Organisation (1970) *Fluorides and Human Health. WHO Monogr. Ser.* No. 59, Geneva, WHO.

Ziegler E. (1962) Milk fluoridation. *Bull. Schweiz. Akad. Med. Wiss.* 18.

CHAPTER 6

FLUORIDE TABLETS AND DROPS

EFFECTIVENESS IN CARIES PREVENTION

About 55 reports on the effectiveness of fluoride tablets or drops have appeared in the literature, although some of these are difficult to interpret because of the small size of the test group, the short experimental period or inadequate reporting. The remaining investigations fall into two groups: first, those where the fluoride supplements were given daily at home and were started before school age, and second, those where tablets have been distributed in school, on school days only, usually without additional supplementations during holidays or before school age. The effectiveness of the use of fluoride tablets at home is very much harder to investigate because it is difficult to choose a comparable control group and there is frequently a marked fall-off cooperation; these difficulties do not usually arise in school-based trials. An excellent review of the effectiveness of fluoride tablets is given by Driscoll (1974), and *Tables* 25 and 26 are based on his report, but with additional recent data.

Deciduous Teeth

Summaries of 20 trials into the effect of fluoride tablets on the deciduous dentition are given in *Table* 25. Twelve were conducted in Europe, 5 in the USA and 3 in Australia. Sodium fluoride was used in all but one study (although the compound was not stated in one further study), sometimes in combination with vitamins.

The initial age of the subjects and the length of time the tablets were taken varied considerably, making it difficult to draw conclusions on effectiveness accurately. Nevertheless it would appear that a caries-preventive effect was consistently observed (about 50–80 per cent reduction) in studies where the initial age was 2 years or younger. In the three studies in which no effect was found, the children were initially aged 3 years or older. In a more thorough analysis of effectiveness in relation to the age at which ingestion of tablets began, Granath et al. (1978) suggested that while buccolingual surfaces may benefit if the commencement age is over 2 years, the effect on approximal surfaces is very much less if the commencement age is 2 years or over. This suggests that the topical effect is greater on the more exposed buccolingual surfaces than on the less accessible approximal surfaces.

The study of Hennon et al. (1977) is the only clinical trial of fluoride tablets conducted in an area with an almost optimal water fluoride level

Table 25. Caries-preventive Effects of Fluoride Tablets/Drops on Deciduous Teeth (*Based on Driscoll, 1974 and Binder et al., 1978*)

Study	F compound	Daily dosage (mg)	Initial age of subjects (yrs)	No. of subjects in F group	Duration of F intake (yrs)	Caries reduction (%) deft	Caries reduction (%) defs	Statistical significance
Arnold et al. (1960)	NaF	0·5–1	Birth–6	121	1–12	'Comparable to water F'		NR
Pollak (1960)[5]	NaF+V	1	3	100	2	80		NR
	NaF+V	1	4	111	2	20		NR
Ziemnowicz-Glowaka (1960)[5]	NaF	0·8	3	139	2		26	S
Lutomska and Kominska (1962)[5]	NaF	0·6	3–4	154	2	'No significant effect'		NR
Kamocka et al. (1964)[5]	NaF	0·75[1]	3	64	3	0		NS
	NaF	0·75[1]	4	79	3	0		NS
Leonhardt (1965)[5]	NaF+V	1+	3	Not known	2	38		NR
	NaF+V	1+	4	Not known	2	30		NR
Hennon et al. (1966, 1967, 1970)	NaF+V	0·5–1	Birth–5½	85	3		63	S
	NaF+V	0·5–1	Birth–5½	54	4		68	S
	NaF+V	0·5–1	Birth–5½	60	5		66	S
Margolis et al. (1975)	NaF+V	0·5–1	Birth	149	4–6	76		S
	NaF+V	0·5–1	4	77	0–2	29		NS
Hoskova (1968)	NaF	0·25–1	Prenatal	78	4	93		S
	NaF	0·25–1	Birth–1	151	4	54		S
Kailis et al. (1968)	NaF	?	Prenatal	50	4–6	82		S
	NaF	?	Birth	92	4–6	56		S

Study	Compound	Conc.	Age administration started	No. of children	Age at examination	% reduction	% reduction	Significance
Stolte (1968)[5]	?	1	3	130	3	11		NR
Prichard (1969)	NaF	?	Prenatal	176	6–8	70		S
	NaF	?	Birth	282	6–8	40		S
Hamberg (1971)	NaF+V (drops)	0·5	Birth	342	3	57		NR
	NaF+V (drops)	0·5	Birth	342	6	49		NR
Kraemer (1971)[5]	CaF_2	1	4	170	2	22		NR
	CaF_2	1	5	82	2	18		NR
Schützmannsky (1971)	NaF	1	Prenatal	100	<1	13		S
	NaF	0·25–1	Prenatal	100	9	30		S
	NaF	0·25–1	Birth	100	9	14		S
Aasenden and Peebles (1974)	NaF+V[2]	0·5–1	Birth	87	8–11		78	S
Fanning et al. (1975)	NaF	0·5–1	<1	581	5	33		NR
Andersson and Grahnen (1976)	NaF	0·25–0·5	1	127	5[3]	31		S
Hennon et al. (1977)[4]	NaF+V	0·5–1	<1	44	5		47	S
	NaF+V	0·5	<1	47	5		37	S
Granath et al. (1978)	NaF	0·25–0·5	<2	48	2–4		46 BL	NS
							51 AP	S
	NaF	0·25–0·5	2–3	123	1–2		33 BL	NS
							−1 AP	NS

V. Vitamins; S, Statistically significant; NS, statistically non-significant; NR, No statistical test reported; BL, Buccolingual; AP, Approximal surfaces.

[1] Tablets given only on school days.

[2] A NaF + V combination was given up to 3 years of age. Beyond this age, some children received NaF + V, while others received only NaF.

[3] Aged 8–10 at examination.

[4] In F area (0·6–0·8 ppm F).

[5] Quoted by Driscoll (1974).

Table 26. Caries-preventive Effects of Fluoride Tablets on Permanent Teeth (*Based on Driscoll, 1974 and Binder et al., 1978*)

Study	F compound	Daily dosage (mg)	Initial age of subjects (yrs)	No. of subjects in F group	Duration of F intake (yrs)	Caries reduction (%) DMFT	DMFS	Statistical significance
Stones et al. (1949)	NaF	1·5	6–14	125	2	0		NS
Bibby et al. (1955)	NaF	1	5–14	133	1		Nil	NR
	NaF	1	5–14	119	1		Tentative finding: 'possible'	NR
Niendenthal (1957)[4]	NaF	1[1]	6–7	251	3	22		NR
Wrzodek (1959)[4]	NaF	1[1]	6–9	8381	3	21		NR
	NaF	1[1]	6–9	13 585	4	22		NR
Arnold et al. (1960)	NaF	0·5–1	Birth–6	121	1–15	'Comparable to water F'		NR
Krusic (1960)[4]	CaF$_2$	Not known	8–15	480	1–3	70		NR
Pollak (1960)[4]	NaF+V	1	6–7	300	2	38		NR
Ziemnowicz-Glowaka (1960)[4]	NaF	0·8[1]	3–6	704	2		33	S
	NaF	0·8[1]	5–6	204	3		28	S
Jez (1962)[4]	CaF$_2$	Not known	7–11	7200	2½	0		NR
Krychalska-Karwan and Laskowa (1963)[4]	NaF	Not known	Grammar school	134	4		5	NR
Minoguchi et al. (1963)	NaF+V	0·25	Birth–6	75	6	36		NR
Grissom et al. (1964)	NaF	1[1]	6–11	178	2		34	S
Kamocka et al. (1964)[4]	NaF	0·75[1]	3	64	3	17		NS
	NaF	0·75[1]	4	79	3	60		S
Leonhardt (1964)	NaF	1	6	398	4	32		NR
	NaF	1	7	429	3	25		NR
Hippchen (1965)[4]	Not known	1	6	500	3	32		NR
Schützmannsky (1965)	NaF	0·75[1]	6	580	4		25	NR
	NaF	0·75[1]	6	197	6		27	NR

Study	Agent	Dose[1]	Age (years)	Number	Years	Reduction (%)	Reduction (%)	
Berner et al (1967)	NaF	0·5-1[1]	5-7	105	3		84 (except 1st molar) 33 (1st molar)	NR
De Paola and Lax (1968)	NaF	1[1]	7-9	158	4	16		NR
	NaF	1[1]	7-9	160	6	20		NR
	NaF	1[1]	7-9	109	7	24		NR
	APF	1[1]	6-8	130	2		23	S
Girardi-Vogt (1968)[4]	NaF	1	6	Not known	3	31		NR
Stolte (1968)[4]	Not known	1	3	150	3	69		NR
Marthaler (1969)	NaF	0·5-1[1]	7	450	1-8	36	47	S
Hamberg (1971)	NaF+V	0·5	Birth	342	7	70		NR
Schützmannsky (1971)	NaF	1	Prenatal	100	<1	6		NS
	NaF	0·25-1	Prenatal	100	9	43		S
	NaF	0·25-1	Birth	100	9	39		S
Aasenden et al. (1972)	APF	1[1]	8-11	109	3		30	S
	NaF	1[1]	8-11	114	3		27	S
Plasschaert and Konig (1974)	NaF	1	7	208	2		38	S
Aasenden and Peebles (1974)	NaF+V[2]	0·5-1	Birth	100	8-11		80	S
Binder (1974)	NaF	0·25-1	Birth-14	3084	8-14	43		S
Margolis et al. (1975)	NaF+V	0·5-1	Birth	56	7-10	58		S
	NaF+V	0·5-1	4	31	3-6	14		NS
Andersson and Grahnén (1976)	NaF	0·25-0·5	1	127	5[3]		40	S
Stephen and Campbell (1978)	NaF	1[1]	5½	54	3		81	S
Driscoll et al. (1978)	APF	1[1]	6-7	150	6		28	S
	APF	2[1]	6-7	135	6		29	S

V, Vitamins; S, Statistically significant; NS, Statistically non-significant; NR, No statistical test reported.
[1] Tablets given only on school days.
[2] A NaF+V combination was given up to 3 years of age. Beyond this age, some children received NaF+V, while others received only NaF.
[3] Aged 8-12 at examination
[4] Quoted by Driscoll (1974).

(0·6–0·8 ppm F), although the observations of Glenn (1979) were on children living in a fluoridated community. A substantial preventive effect was observed by Hennon et al. in the children taking fluoride tablets, in addition to the benefit that could be expected to be derived from living in an area with a moderate water fluoride level. In their study one group of children received 0·5 mg F from birth throughout the 5-year trial period while another group received 0·5 mg F up to 3 years of age and 1 mg for the remaining 2 years. The effect was slightly greater (47 per cent reduction compared with 37 per cent) in the latter group.

Permanent Teeth

Summaries of investigations into the effectiveness of fluoride tablets in preventing caries in the permanent dentition are given in *Table* 26; again, most of the studies are European. The initial age of the subjects and the duration of fluoride tablet intake varied widely. In only four of the studies (Hamberg, 1971; Schützmannsky, 1971; Aasenden and Peebles, 1974; Margolis et al., 1975) were fluoride tablets taken from birth for at least 7 years. Reductions ranged from 39 per cent in Schützmannsky's trial to 80 per cent in the trial of Aasenden and Peebles. In the trial of Margolis et al., the children who started taking fluoride tablets at birth showed a 58 per cent reduction in DFT compared with only a 14 per cent reduction in the group of children who started at the age of 4 years, suggesting the importance of ingestion in the first few years of life, before the permanent teeth erupted.

In the four studies conducted in school (initial age 6–7 years) and lasting at least 5 years, the following reductions in caries have been reported: 27 per cent (Schützmannsky, 1965), 20–24 per cent (Berner et al., 1967), 36 per cent (Marthaler, 1969) and 28–29 per cent (Driscoll et al., 1978). The only study conducted in the UK was by Stephen and Campbell (1978), where an 81 per cent reduction was reported after a 3-year trial in Glasgow children initially aged $5\frac{1}{2}$ years.

Prenatal

Six trials have investigated the effectiveness of the ingestion of prenatal fluoride tablets, although results of only four of these are given in *Tables* 25 and 26, because in the remaining two (Feltman and Kosel, 1961; Glenn, 1979) insufficient data were reported. In all these trials (*Tables* 25 and 26) the per cent caries reduction was greater in the children whose mothers received fluoride tablets in pregnancy. But in spite of the apparent greater benefit of prenatal fluoride, Hoskova (1968) concluded that fluoride administration should begin as soon after birth as possible, attributing the greater benefit to better home conditions in the prenatal group. Feltman and Kosel (1961) compared the caries experience of 672 children who had received (1) only prenatal supplements (162 children), (2) pre- and post-natal supplements (228 children) and (3) only postnatal tablets from varying ages (282 children). Prenatal fluoride appeared to confer benefit additional to that derived from postnatal fluoride exposure. The trial of Schützmannsky (1971) was better reported and also had three groups: a prenatal fluoride-only group, a pre- and postnatal group (for 9 years) and a postnatal-only group (also for 9 years). The reductions for deciduous teeth were 13 per cent, 30 per cent and 14 per cent respectively (*Table* 25) and 6 per cent, 43 per cent and 39 per cent respectively for permanent teeth (*Table* 26), suggesting that a small benefit may be derived from prenatal fluoride ingestion, particularly in the deciduous dentition.

Glenn (1979) reported caries prevalence in children attending a private practice who had received prenatal fluoride supplements in addition to receiving an optimum water fluoride level; data on the use of postnatal fluoride tablets or drops were not given. Nineteen of the 24 children aged 5–17 years who received prenatal supplements were caries-free.

Although it would seem likely that ingestion of fluoride tablets by gravid women may reduce the caries experience of their offspring, the benefits are likely to be limited to the deciduous dentition and may be of insufficient magnitude to warrant administration. Because of this, authorities in some countries (e.g. UK, USA) do not recommend prenatal fluoride administration.

Fluoride–Vitamin Combination

From the results of the studies listed in *Tables* 25 and 26 it would seem that the effectiveness of fluoride tablets/drops is neither enhanced nor reduced by their combination with vitamins. There would seem, therefore, little advantage in these combinations and they are not at present marketed in the UK.

Type of Fluoride Compound

The results of the three trials testing CaF_2 compounds are very variable (0–70 per cent reduction); all were short-term trials. The impressive result of Krusic (1960) is surprising since the insolubility of CaF_2 would obviate the likelihood of a topical effect compared with NaF, and a systemic effect would be very unlikely to occur in this short trial in 8–15-year-old children.

From the three trials in which APF compounds were used, the effectiveness would appear to be no greater than that observed in the larger number of NaF trials. APF tablets are considerably more expensive than NaF tablets (Driscoll et al., 1978), and the greater salivary flow caused by the low pH of the APF tablets is likely to reduce the concentration of fluoride around the teeth and hasten its clearance from the mouth. It would appear that to ensure high and long-lasting salivary F levels, tablets should contain NaF rather than APF, disintegrate slowly in the mouth without being sucked, and possess as little flavour as possible, so long as the tablets are acceptable to children (McCall et al., 1981).

Dosage and Effectiveness

Hennon et al. (1977) have conducted the only study in which the effect of varying the daily dosage level has been investigated in deciduous teeth. One group of children received 0·5 mg F from soon after birth onwards, while a second group received 0·5 mg F up to 3 years of age and 1 mg F after the age of 3 years. The effect was slightly greater in the latter group (47 per cent reduction compared with 37 per cent reduction) after 5 years but the difference between these two test groups was not statistically significant and not observed consistently at all ages. The authors attribute this lack of difference partly to the fact that the subjects lived in an area with moderate (0·6–0·8 ppm F) water fluoride levels.

Driscoll et al. (1974, 1977, 1978) conducted a carefully controlled trial in which subjects, initially aged $6\frac{1}{2}$ years, were randomly divided into 2 test groups and 1 control group. One test group chewed and swallowed 1 tablet (containing 1 mg F as APF) while the second group chewed and swallowed 2 such tablets, taking the first in morning school and the second in afternoon school. After 6 years there was no difference in the preventive effect between the groups of children taking 1 or 2 tablets (28 per cent and 29 per cent reduction respectively). The caries-preventive effect did not diminish, in either of the test groups, $1\frac{1}{2}$ years after the tablet programme ended (Driscoll et al., 1979).

SUMMARY OF EFFECTIVENESS OF FLUORIDE TABLETS AND DROPS

From the results of published trials (*Tables* 25 and 26) it would seem that there is no doubt that the use of fluoride tablets or drops is effective in preventing dental caries in both the deciduous and permanent dentitions. The effectiveness would seem to be greater the earlier the child begins to take the fluoride supplement—from 40 to 80 per cent reduction being expected in both deciduous and permanent dentitions if supplementation is commenced before 2 years of age. For school-based schemes the effectiveness would appear to be lower and more variable (30–80 per cent reduction). NaF would appear to be the compound of choice, but the data are insufficient to judge whether the size of the daily dose influences effectiveness.

Results of the home-based trials have to be interpreted with caution, for the attitude to dental health of the mothers who gave their children supplements from birth is likely to be more favourable than mothers who began supplementation later or who formed the control group. This problem has been investigated in the following three studies. Although Andersson and Grahnén (1976) observed that the per cent caries reduction recorded after use of fluoride tablets was not affected by differences in social class between the test and control group, in a more thorough study Granath et al. (1978) found that two factors—diet and oral hygiene—were important in interpreting such clinical trials. They found that 4-year-old children who had taken fluoride tablets for at least 2 years had 69 per cent less approximal caries and 57 per cent less buccal and lingual caries than children who had not taken tablets. However, when the variables of diet and oral hygiene were kept constant in the analyses, these caries reductions were reduced to 51 per cent and 46 per cent respectively. Tijmistra et al. (1978) found that the difference in caries experience of 15-year-old children who had or had not taken fluoride tablets fell from 15 per cent to 3 per cent when the data were standardized on diet, oral hygiene and father's occupation.

It has to be admitted that daily administration of tablets at home from birth (or prenatally) requires a very high level of parental motivation, and campaigns to get parents to give their children fluoride supplements have not been successful in the UK. Smyth and Withnell (1974) reported that when parents of 3500 pre-school children in Gloucestershire were asked to give their children fluoride tablets, only 759 (22 per cent) entered the scheme and only 70 of these (2 per cent of those originally invited) were still giving tablets at the end of 9 months, despite widespread publicity and subsidy of the cost of the tablets. Silver (1974) found that only 6 per cent of 3-year-olds in Hertfordshire were consuming fluoride tablets despite their widespread recommendation and availability. The acceptability of school-based tablet programmes would appear to be much better (Driscoll et al., 1977; Poulsen et al., 1981).

DISCUSSION OF THE DOSAGE OF FLUORIDE TABLETS AND DROPS

At least 18 different dosage régimes for fluoride tablets and drops have been published (Rugg–Gunn, 1980). These range from the high dosage level recommended before 1976 in Australia of 0·5 mg F daily from birth to 12 months and 1·0 mg F from 1 year onwards (McEniery and Davies, 1979), to the low dosage level in Denmark since 1978 of 0·25 mg F from 6 to 24 months and 0·5 mg F from 2 years onwards (Thylstrup et al., 1979). In the UK the most widely advocated dosage regime has been 0·5 mg F from birth to 2 years and 1 mg F from 2 years onwards (Silverstone, 1973; Murray, 1976). In recent years there has been a trend to reduce the dosage of daily fluoride supplements in Australia, the USA and in Scandinavia.

In the UK Dowell and Joyston-Bechal (1981) have recently recommended 0·25 mg F from birth to 2 years, 0·5 mg F from 2 to 4 years and 1·0 mg F over 4 years. Most regimes give sliding scales of dosages depending upon water fluoride levels (*Table* 27). Since there is considerable disagreement between countries on the recommended dosage levels it is pertinent to discuss the reasons for changes in dosage schedules.

Table 27. Fluoride Supplements—Age-related Dosages (mg F/day)
(*Dowell and Joyston-Bechal, 1981*)

Age	Concentration of fluoride in drinking water (ppm F)		
	<0·3	0·3–0·7	>0·7
2 wks to 2 yrs	0·25	0	0
2–4 yrs	0·50	0·25	0
4–16 yrs	1·00	0·50	0

The objective of any systemic fluoride administration is to obtain the maximum caries-preventive effect with a low risk of unacceptable enamel mottling. As far as water fluoridation is concerned this is achieved, in temperate climates, where drinking water contains 1 ppm F. In the past, fluoride tablet dosages have been calculated in an attempt to duplicate the fluoride intake which occurs in people receiving optimally fluoridated drinking water. However, the situation where a dosage of fluoride is given at a particular time in a day is physiologically different from water fluoridation where fluoride is taken throughout the day, and both the effectiveness of fluoride tablets and the risk of mottling have to be considered separately from water fluoridation.

The relative effectiveness of different dosage levels of fluoride tablets has already been discussed. It must be pointed out that many currently recommended dosage levels have not been tested in clinical trials but, of those which have been tested, there is little indication that higher dosages result in a greater caries-preventive effect.

The Problem of Mottling

The only fluoride tablet trial to report the occurrence of dental fluorosis is that by Aasenden and Peebles (1974) in which children received 0·5 mg F from birth to 3 years and 1 mg F from 3 years onwards. Fourteen per cent of the children developed moderate fluorosis and a further 19 per cent mild fluorosis in permanent teeth. However, in a follow-up study (Aasenden and Peebles, 1978), the proportion of children with dental fluorosis had fallen, possibly due to 'continuous mineralization or to abrasion'. It has been reported that mild fluorosis has been seen in children of dentists and doctors in Switzerland (Driscoll, 1974) and in Australia (McEniery and Davies, 1979). On the other hand, in a trial using the same fluoride tablet dosage as Aasenden and Peebles, Margolis et al. (1975) recorded an absence of fluorosis. Hennon et al (1977) observed some fluorosis in children receiving fluoride tablets in an area with moderate (0·6–0·8 ppm) water fluoride levels, although in no case was the fluorosis aesthetically unacceptable.

Despite these equivocal findings, authorities in the USA have reduced their recommended fluoride tablet dosage levels. The main reason for this is that infants fed on formula milk manufactured in areas with, and made up with, fluoridated water may be receiving adequate levels of fluoride from this source alone (Wei et al., 1977). In addition, baby foods manufactured in fluoride areas may have high F levels (Tinanoff and Mueller, 1978). It is also argued that the use of fluoride-containing toothpastes is now widespread and that a significant amount is likely to be ingested by young children, although it should be noted that an increase in mottling has not been observed in the USA where nearly all toothpastes have contained fluoride for over 15 years.

The influence of these likely increases in fluoride intake in infants and young children on the prevalence of unacceptable fluorosis remains speculative. Nevertheless, because on present evidence the caries-preventive effect may not be greatly reduced by reducing tablet dosage levels, adoption of the American Council on Dental Therapeutics dosage schedule (Driscoll and Horowitz, 1978) would seem a sensible compromise in the UK. In this schedule 0·25 mg F is given between birth and 2 years, 0·50 mg F between 2 and 3 years and 1 mg F for children 3 years of age and older.

Some authorities, because they consider that an increase in fluoride tablet dosage is likely to lead to greater caries prevention, recommend higher dosages for special groups (such as the medically or mentally handicapped). Some flexibility, therefore, in the dosage of fluoride tablets prescribed should be accepted.

REFERENCES

Aasenden R. and Peebles T. C. (1974) Effects of fluoride supplementation from birth on human deciduous and permanent teeth. *Arch. Oral Biol.* **19**, 321–326.

Aasenden R. and Peebles T. C. (1978) Effects of fluoride supplementation from birth on dental caries and fluorosis in teen-aged children. *Arch. Oral Biol.* **23**, 111–115.

Aasenden R., De Paola P. F. and Brudevold F. (1972) Effects of daily rinsing and ingestion of fluoride solutions upon dental caries and enamel fluoride. *Arch. Oral Biol.* **17**, 1705–1714.

Andersson R. and Grahnén H. (1976) Fluoride tablets in pre-school age—effect on primary and permanent teeth. *Swed. Dent. J.* **69**, 137–143.

Arnold F. A., McClure F. J. and White C. L. (1960) Sodium fluoride tablets for children. *Dent. Prog.* **1**, 8–12.

Berner L., Fernex E. and Held A. J. (1967) Study on the anticarious effect of sodium fluoride tablets (Zymafluor). Results recorded in the course of 13 years of observation. *Schweiz. Monatsschr. Zahnheilkd.* **77**, 528–539.

Bibby G. G., Wilkins E. and Witol E. (1955) A preliminary study of the effects of fluoride lozenges and pills on dental caries. *O. Surg. O. Med. O. Pathol.* **8**, 213–216.

Binder K. (1974) In: Davies G. N., *Cost and Benefit of Fluoride in the Prevention of Dental Caries. WHO Offset Publication* No. 9 Geneva, WHO, p. 64, *Table* 23.

Binder K., Driscoll W. S. and Schützmannsky G. (1978) Caries-preventive fluoride tablet programs. *Caries Res.* **12**, suppl. 1, 22–30.

De Paola P. F. and Lax M. (1968) The caries-inhibiting effect of acidulated phosphate-fluoride chewable tablets: a two-year double-blind study. *J. Am. Dent. Assoc.* **76**, 554–557.

Dowell T. B. and Joyston-Bechal S. (1981) Fluoride supplements—age related dosages. *Br. Dent. J.* **150**, 273–275.

Driscoll W. S. (1974) The use of fluoride tablets for the prevention of dental caries. In: Forrester D. J. and Schulz E. M. (eds.), *International Workshop on Fluorides and Dental Caries Prevention.* Baltimore, University of Maryland, pp. 25–111.

Driscoll W. S. and Horowitz H. S. (1978) A discussion of optimal dosage for dietary fluoride supplementation. *J. Am. Dent. Assoc.* **96**, 1050–1053.

Driscoll W. S., Heifetz S. B. and Brunelle J. A. (1979) Treatment and post-treatment effects of chewable fluoride tablets on dental caries: findings after $7\frac{1}{2}$ years. *J. Am. Dent. Assoc.* **99**, 817–821.

Driscoll W. S., Heifetz S. B. and Korts D. C. (1974) Effect of acidulated phosphate-fluoride chewable tablets on dental caries in school children: results after 30 months. *J. Am. Dent. Assoc.* **89**, 115–120.

Driscoll W. S., Heifetz S. B. and Korts D. C. (1978) Effect of chewable fluoride tablets on dental caries in schoolchildren: results after six years of use. *J. Am. Dent. Assoc.* **97**, 820–824.

Driscoll W. S., Heifetz S. B., Korts D. C., Meyers R. J. and Horowitz H. S. (1977) Effect of acidulated phosphate-fluoride chewable tablets in schoolchildren: results after 55 months. *J. Am. Dent. Assoc.* **94**, 537–543.

Fanning E. A., Cellier K. M. and Leadbeater M. M. (1975) South Australian kindergarten children: fluoride tablet supplements and dental caries. *Aust. Dent. J.* **20**, 7–9.

Feltman R. and Kosel G. (1961) Prenatal and postnatal ingestion of fluorides—fourteen years of investigation—final report. *J. Dent. Med.* **16**, 190–198.

Girardi-Vogt J. (1968) *Results of Fluoridation in Darmstadt.* Dissertation. Frankfurt, Germany, Johan Wolfgang Goethe University, p. 127.

Glenn F. B. (1979) Immunity conveyed by sodium-fluoride supplement during pregnancy: part II. *J. Dent. Child.* **46**, 17–24.

Granath L.-E., Rootzen H., Liljegren E., Holst K. and Kohler L. (1978) Variation in caries prevalence related to combinations of dietary and oral hygiene habits and chewing fluoride tablets in 4-year-old children. *Caries Res.* **12**, 83–92.

Grissom D. K., Dudenbostel R. E., Cassel W. J. and Murray R. T. (1964) A comparative study of systemic sodium fluoride and topical stannous fluoride applications in preventive dentistry. *J. Dent. Child.* **31**, 314–322.

Hamberg L. (1971) Controlled trial of fluoride in vitamin drops for prevention of caries in children. *Lancet* **1**, 441–442.

Hennon D. K., Stookey G. K. and Beiswanger B. B. (1977) Fluoride–vitamin supplements: effects on dental caries and fluorosis when used in areas with suboptimum fluoride in the water supply. *J. Am. Dent. Assoc.* **95**, 965–971.

Hennon D. K., Stookey G. K. and Muhler J. C. (1966) The clinical anti-cariogenic effectiveness of supplementary fluoride-vitamin preparations. Results at the end of three years. *J. Dent. Child.* **33**, 3–12.

Hennon D. K., Stookey G. K. and Muhler J. C. (1967) The clinical anti-cariogenic effectiveness of supplementary fluoride-vitamin preparations. Results at the end of four years. *J. Dent. Child.* **34**, 439–443.

Hennon D. K., Stookey G. K. and Muhler J. C. (1970) The clinical anti-cariogenic effectiveness of supplementary fluoride-vitamin preparations. Results at the end of five and a half years. *J. Pharmacol. Ther. Dent.* **1**, 1–6.

Hippchen P. (1965) Caries prevention with fluorides in Düsseldorf children. *Zahnaerztl. Mitt.* **55**, 897–898.

Hoskova M. (1968) Fluoride tablets in the prevention of tooth decay. *Cesk. Pediatr.* **23**, 438–441.

Jez M. (1962) Izledki mnozicne fluorizacije zobovja solske mladine. *Zobozdrav. Vest.* **17**, 113–118.

Kailis D. G., Taylor S. R., Davis G. B., Bartlett L. G., Fitzgerald D. J., Grose I. J. and Newton P. D. (1968) Fluoride and caries: Observations on the effects of prenatal and postnatal fluoride on some Perth pre-school children. *Med. J. Aust.* **11**, 1037–1040.

Kamocka D., Sebastyanska Z. and Spychalska M. (1964) The effect of administration of 'Fluodar' tablets on the appearance of caries in children of pre-school age in Szczecin. *Czas. Stomatol.* **17**, 299–303.

Kraemer O. (1971) *Results of Two Years of Dental Caries Prophylaxis by Oral Administration of Fluoride in Bonn Kindergartens.* Dissertation. Bonn, West Germany, Rheinische Friedrich Wilhelm University.

Krusic V. (1960) Our tests in fluoridation with the calcium fluoride 'Fluokalcia' (CaF_2). *Zobozdrav. Vest.* **15**, 27–31.

Krychalska-Karwan Z. and Laskowa L. (1963) Use of fluoride tablets in Polish children. *Czas. Stomatol.* **16**, 201–205.

Leonhardt H. (1964) Results of fluorine tablet applications in Salzburg school children. In: Hardwick J. L., Dustin J. P. and Held H. R. (eds), *Advances in Fluorine Research and Dental Caries Prevention,* Vol. 2. Oxford, Pergamon, pp. 49–56.

Leonhardt H. (1965) Mulgatum and Mulgatum-Fluoratum in preschool children. *Therapie der Gegenwart* **104**, 118–133.

Lutomska K. and Kominska D. (1962) Effect of fluoride tablets. *Czas. Stomatol.* **15**, 493–501.

McCall D., Stephen K. W. and McNee S. G. (1981) Fluoride tablets and salivary fluoride levels. *Caries Res.* **15**, 98–102.

McEniery M. and Davies G. N. (1979) Brisbane dental survey 1977: a comparative study of caries experience of children in Brisbane, Australia over a 20 year period. *Community Dent. Oral Epidemiol.* **7**, 42–50.

Margolis F. J., Reames H. R., Freshman E., Macauley J. C. and Mehaffey H. (1975) Fluoride—ten year prospective study of deciduous and permanent dentition. *Am. J. Dis. Child.* **129**, 794–800.

Marthaler T. M. (1969) Caries-inhibiting effect of fluoride tablets. *Helv. Odontol. Acta* **13**, 1–13.

Minoguchi G., Ono T. and Tamai S. (1963) Prophylactic application of fluoride for dental caries in Japan. *Int. Dent. J.* **13**, 510–515.

Murray J. J. (1976) *Fluorides in Caries Prevention*, Ist ed. Bristol, Wright.

Niedenthal A. (1957) Caries prophylaxis with sodium fluoride tablets in Offenbach school children. *Zahnaerztl. Mitt.* **45**, 576–587.

Plasschaert A. J. M. and Konig K. G. (1974) The effect of information and motivation towards dental health and of fluoride tablets on caries in school children: 1. Increment over the initial 2-year experimental period. *Int. Dent. J.* **24**, 50–65.

Pollak H. (1960) Caries prophylaxis with Mulgatum F. Result of an investigation over a period of two years in Nordheim-Westphalia. *Dtsch. Zahnaerzteble.* **14**, 363–365.

Poulsen S., Gradegaard E. and Mortensen B. (1981) Cariostatic effect of daily use of a fluoride-containing lozenge compared to fortnightly rinses with 0.2% sodium fluoride. *Caries Res.* **15**, 236–242.

Prichard J. L. (1969) The prenatal and postnatal effects of fluoride supplements on West Australian school children, aged 6, 7 and 8, Perth, 1967. *Aust. Dent. J.* **14**, 335–338.

Rugg-Gunn A. J. (1980) *Published Dosage Regimes for Dietary Fluoride Supplementations*. Evidence to British Dental Association Dental Health Committee, Feb. 1980.

Schützmannsky G. (1965) Further results of our tablet fluoridation in Halle. *Dtsch. Stomatol.* **15**, 107–114.

Schützmannsky G. (1971) Fluorine tablet application in pregnant females. *Dtsch. Stomatol.* **21**, 122–129.

Silver D. H. (1974) The prevalence of dental caries in 3-year-old children. *Br. Dent. J.* **137**, 123–128.

Silverstone L. M. (1973) Preventive dentistry: systemic fluoride part 2. *Dental Update* **1**, 101–105.

Smyth J. F. A. and Withnell A. (1974) Daily fluoride tablets. *Health Soc. Sci. J.* **84**, 419–423.

Stephen K. W. and Campbell D. (1978) Caries reduction and cost benefit after 3 years of sucking fluoride tablets daily at school. *Br. Dent. J.* **144**, 202–206.

Stolte G. (1968) Results of three years of caries prophylaxis by oral fluoride application in Solingen kindergartens. *Zahnaerztl. Mitt.* **58**, 380–382.

Stones H. H., Lawton F. E., Bransby E. R. and Hartley H. O. (1949) The effect of topical applications of potassium fluoride and of the ingestion of tablets containing sodium fluoride on the incidence of dental caries. *Br. Dent. J.* **86**, 264–271.

Thylstrup A., Fejerskov O., Brunn C. and Kann J. (1979) Enamel changes and dental caries in 7-year-old children given fluoride tablets from shortly after birth. *Caries Res.* **13**, 265–276.

Tijmistra T., Brinkman-Engels M. and Groeneveld A. (1978) Effect of socioeconomic factors on the observed caries reduction after fluoride tablet and fluoride toothpaste consumption. *Community Dent. Oral Epidemiol.* **6**, 227–230.

Tinanoff N. and Mueller B. (1978) Fluoride content in milk and formula for infants. *J. Dent. Child.* **45**, 53–55.

Wei S. H. Y., Wefel J. S. and Parkins F. M. (1977). Fluoride supplements for infants and preschool children. *J. Prev. Dent.* **4**, 28–32.

Wrzodek G. (1959) Does the prevention of caries by means of fluorine tablets promise success? *Zahnaerztl. Mitt.* **47**, 1–5.

Ziemnowicz-Glowaka W. (1960) Prevention of caries by means of 'Fluodar' tablets. *Czas. Stomatol.* **13**, 719–728.

CHAPTER 7

FLUORIDE TOOTHPASTES AND
DENTAL CARIES

Investigations into the effectiveness of adding fluoride to toothpaste have been carried out since 1945, and cover a wide range of active ingredients in various chemical combinations. There have probably been more reports in the literature on the caries-inhibitory property of fluoride in toothpaste than on any other aspect of topical fluoride therapy. Fluoride compounds which have been tested for caries-inhibitory properties when incorporated into a toothpaste include: sodium fluoride, acidulated phosphate fluoride, stannous fluoride, sodium monofluorophosphate and amine fluoride.

In Britain, a dramatic change in the use of a fluoride toothpaste took place in the 1970s, largely as a result of decisions made by manufacturers to improve their product. Before 1970 less than 10 per cent of branded toothpastes contained fluoride; now over 96 per cent of all toothpaste sold contains fluoride (*Fig.* 17). In 1975 the British Dental Association endorsed a number of fluoride toothpastes which, on the basis of clinical trials, had been shown to be effective in reducing dental decay. Pastes receiving this 'seal of approval' were Colgate, Crest, Macleans and Signal 2. However, following attempts to involve the British Dental

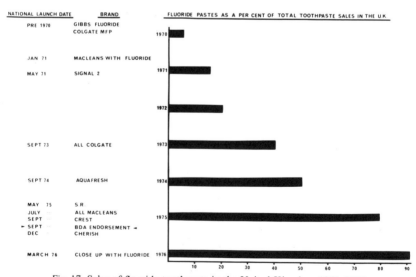

Fig. 17. Sales of fluoride toothpaste in the United Kingdom 1970–1976.

Association (BDA) in competing claims within the dentifrice industry, the BDA has now withdrawn its endorsement, on the grounds that its objective of bringing the advantages of fluoride toothpaste to the notice of the public has been largely achieved (*BDA News*, 1981).

TOOTHPASTES CONTAINING SODIUM FLUORIDE
(*Table* 28)

Sodium fluoride was the first fluoride compound to be incorporated in a conventional toothpaste as the active agent. A 2-year study investigating the unsupervised use of such a paste was published by Bibby in 1945. The active ingredient was 0·1 per cent sodium fluoride but the nature of the abrasive system was not published. It seems reasonable to assume it was of a type used in conventional toothpastes commercially available at that time, probably calcium carbonate. Bibby found no significant reduction in caries increment for the test group using the sodium fluoride paste, in comparison to the use of a placebo paste by a control group. The significance of the study is doubtful in view of the small numbers in the groups, and the wide age range of the study participants. Winkler et al. (1953), in spite of changing the test formulation, found no significant benefit for supervised use of a 0·15 per cent sodium fluoride paste for 18 months.

Investigations testing the unsupervised use of a paste containing 0·2 per cent sodium fluoride were published introducing alternative abrasive systems. Muhler et al. (1955b) investigated a combination of 0·2 per cent sodium fluoride and heat-treated calcium orthophosphate, finding a reduction in caries increment of only 0·3 of a surface for the test group over the 12-month study period. The reduction was neither clinically nor statistically significant.

Kyes et al. (1961), using a combination of 0·2 per cent sodium fluoride and 2 per cent sodium N-lauroyl sarcosinate, explored the possibility of using an insoluble sodium metaphosphate abrasive system, but found no significant clinical benefit. Brudevold and Chilton (1966) investigated relative caries-preventive effects for several toothpaste formulas covering a range of active ingredients, including 0·22 per cent sodium fluoride— dicalcium phosphate formula. Two years of unsupervised use gave no statistically significant caries reduction in the test group compared to a control group using a placebo. Thus the early studies tended to suggest that sodium fluoride did not have a caries-preventive effect when incorporated in a toothpaste.

However, in 1961 Ericsson investigated the compatibility of fluoride compounds with conventional constituents of toothpaste and reported that the abrasive systems of calcium carbonate and phosphate inactivate the sodium fluoride by formation of calcium fluoride. He recommended

Table 28. Clinical Trials of Sodium Fluoride Dentifrices

Investigators	% NaF + Abrasive		Unsupervised (U) or supervised (S) use	Duration of trial	No. of carious surfaces saved per year	Reduction in carious surface increment (%)	Level of statistical significance
Bibby (1945)	0·1	CaCO$_3$	S	2 years	—	—	—
Winkler et al.	0·1	CaCO$_3$	U	2 years	—	—	—
(1953)	0·15	CaCO$_3$	S	18 months	—	—	—
Muhler et al. (1955b)	0·22	Heat-treated Ca ortho-phosphate	U	1 year	—	—	—
Kyes et al. (1961)	0·2	IMP + 5% anhydrous DCP	U	1 year	—	—	—
Torell and Ericsson (1965)	0·24	NaHCO$_3$	U	2 years	1-2	—	0·01
Brudevold and Chilton (1966)	0·22 0·22	IMP Sec. Ca phosphate	U	2 years	—	—	0·01
Peterson and Williamson (1968)	0·22	IMP	U	2 years	0·6	14	0·05
Koch (1967a)	0·22	Acrylic	S	3 years	3·2	40–48	0·001
Koch (1967b)	0·22	Acrylic	U	2 years	2·1	38	0·01

Reference	F (%)	Abrasive	Exam	Duration	Control	% reduction	'Test significantly better than control'
Weisenstein and Zacherl (1972)	0·22	CaPP	U	21 months	0·7	25	0·05
Zacherl (1972a)	0·22	CaPP	U	20 months	1·1	28	0·05
Reed (1973)	0·055	CaPP	U	2 years	0·15	7·5	
	0·11	CaPP	U	2 years	0·2	8·5	
	0·22	CaPP	U	2 years	0·4	20·0	0·05
Forsman (1974)	0·05	SiO₂	U	2 years	0·2*	10–17*	NS
					0·8†	5–48†	NS
Stookey and Beiswanger (1975)	0·22	CaPP	U	27 months	0·8	25	0·05
Gerdin (1975)	0·22 (NaF)	Acrylic	S	2 years			
	0·24 (KF)	Acrylic	S				
Reed and King (1975)	0·22	CaPP	U	2 years	0·65	30	0·05
Edlund and Koch (1977)	0·22	SiO₂	S	3 years	0·8	23**	0·05
Ennever et al. (1980)	0·22	CaPP	U	28 months	0·60	37	0·05
	0·22	CaPP			0·53	34	0·05
Zacherl (1981)	0·24 (pH 10)	SiO₂	U	3 years	0·82 (0·35‡)	41 23‡	0·05
Beiswanger and Gish (1981)	0·24	SiO₂	U	3 years	(0·22†)	15‡	0·05

IMP, Insoluble metaphosphate; DCP, Dicalcium phosphate.
* Clinical examination.
† Radiographic examination.
** Versus MFP positive control. Placebo not included.
‡ Against SnF₂ positive control.

103

sodium bicarbonate as a compatible abrasive system for sodium fluoride. Subsequently a clinical investigation by Torell and Ericsson (1965) tested the unsupervised use of 0·2 per cent sodium fluoride–sodium bicarbonate formulation and found a cumulative caries reduction of one surface per child for 2 years for the study group.

The clinical value of the abrasive property of a toothpaste is a controversial question. In 1967 Koch published results of a study testing a toothpaste formulation containing 0·22 per cent sodium fluoride, but without a conventional inorganic abrasive. He substituted acrylic particles which are low in abrasivity but allow a maximum of free ionized fluoride, his assumption being that in relation to oral cleanliness, the thoroughness with which one brushes is more relevant than the physical composition of the abrasive. The paste was tested for 3 years of once-a-day brushing at school under supervision. Study participants and their immediate families were supplied with non-fluoridated paste to use at home, to eliminate the possible use of commercial fluoride pastes during the study period. The comparability of the groups initially was good, and the number of reversals of diagnoses recorded was small, and comparable for test and control groups. The cumulative reduction in new carious surfaces for the test groups represented a saving of 7 surfaces per child for the younger group and a saving of 10 surfaces for the older age group. The observed caries reductions in the test groups, as compared to the control groups, were highly significant ($P < 0.001$). The inhibitory effect was sustained over the study period, and increased in magnitude with successive years, until, in the third year, the reduction in new carious surfaces for the test groups was of the order of 50–58 per cent ($P < 0.001$). There was no statistical significance in the difference in caries increments observed between the sexes. The largest relative reduction was noted for the buccal surfaces.

When this trial ended in 1966, a follow-up was organized for 57 children in the younger age study group, to attempt to evaluate the long-term prophylactic effect of 3 years' daily supervised tooth-brushing with a fluoride paste. For the 2-year period immediately after the study had finished there was a 13 per cent reduction in caries increment for the group who had used the fluoride paste, relative to the control group (Koch, 1970). The reduction in 2 years of 1–2 surfaces per child for the test group was not statistically significant and indicated little long-term practical protection attributable to 3 years' use of a sodium fluoride paste, once regular use of the paste had ceased. This is one of the very few studies reported in the literature which attempts to evaluate whether there is any long-term benefit achieved with use of a fluoride paste. The results of this study suggest that any caries-inhibitory effect of fluoride toothpastes is reliant on regular and sustained applications.

Two recent trials (Beiswanger and Gish, 1981; Zacherl, 1981) have reported that a new 0·243 per cent sodium fluoride–silica abrasive toothpaste (yielding 1000 ppm F) was superior to a 0·4 per cent stannous fluoride–calcium pyrophosphate toothpaste, also yielding 1000 ppm F and marketed as Crest. It has been suggested that the new formulation maintains a higher fluoride ion concentration and allows a greater uptake of fluoride into the outer layers of enamel (Cilley and Haberman, 1981; Mobley and Tepe, 1981).

TOOTHPASTES CONTAINING ACIDULATED PHOSPHATE FLUORIDE (*Table* 29)

In search of a more potent fluoride agent for caries prevention, it was postulated that the effectiveness of a topical agent was directly related to its ability to deposit fluoride as fluorapatite in enamel. Brudevold et al. (1963), while investigating topical applications of fluoride in solution, showed large amounts of fluoride were deposited from high concentrations at a low pH. Unfortunately calcium fluoride was formed in addition to fluorapatite, and was not retained in the enamel as it was soluble in saliva at neutral pH, and washed away within a few hours (Brudevold et al., 1967).

Grøn and Brudevold (1967) postulated a hypothesis that failure to achieve significant results with original neutral sodium fluoride formulations was related not only to the chemical nature of the abrasive but also to the pH values of the formulations. Reports of successful trials of topical acidulated phosphate fluoride solutions encouraged attempts to incorporate this active ingredient into a toothpaste. Brudevold and Chilton (1966) and Peterson and Williamson (1968) published investigations of 2 years' unsupervised use of a formula containing 0·22 per cent sodium fluoride acidulated with 1·5 per cent soluble orthophosphate. The abrasive system used was insoluble sodium metaphosphate which Ericsson (1961) had found did not reduce the amount of available fluoride in sodium fluoride solutions. In both trials the control group did not use a true placebo but a commercially available fluoride-free dentifrice. Caries-reduction effects observed in the test groups were of a similar order (a saving of 1–2 surfaces for each child for the 2-year period). The reduction effects observed in the test group were statistically significant ($P < 0·01$).

Slack et al. (1971) conducted a 3-year trial of normal home use of the same paste in 11–12-year-olds. Again, a commercially available fluoride-free toothpaste was used for a control paste, while a second control group carried on with normal toothbrushing habits and pastes. No significant difference was found in caries increment for groups using the acidulated phosphate fluoride formulation compared with those for the two control groups over the 3-year period. From the results of these trials, it was not possible to establish whether insoluble metaphosphate was indeed a more

Table 29. Clinical Trials of Acidulated Phosphate Fluoride Dentifrices

Investigators	Active ingredient (%conc.)	Abrasive system	pH	Duration (yrs)	Age	Use	Statistically significant reductions surfaces		
							saved	% redn	P
Brudevold and Chilton (1966)	0·22% NaF + 1·5% soluble orthophosphate	IMP	4·8–5·3	2	11–17	U	1–2	*	0·01
Peterson and Williamson (1968)		IMP	4·8–5·3	2	9–15	U	1	*	*
Slack et al. (1971)		IMP	*	3	11–12	U	—	—	—
Zacherl (1972b)	0·22% NaF	Calc. pyro.	5·5	$1\frac{2}{3}$	7–14	U	—	—	—

U. Unsupervised use.   * Information not given in paper.

106

suitable abrasive system in combination with fluoride as the study lacked a true control paste.

A combination of 0·22 per cent acidulated phosphate fluoride and calcium pyrophosphate was investigated by Zacherl (1972b). After unsupervised home use of the test paste for 20 months there was no significant reduction in caries increment observed in the test group compared to similar use of a placebo dentifrice by the control group. The use of a potentially incompatible abrasive system (established by in vitro experiments by Ericsson (1961)) and the wide range in age of the study participants could have served to reduce the significance of Zacherl's results. The majority of study participants were known to have regularly used naturally fluoridated well water (F level of 0·8–1·5 ppm), which could have reduced the magnitude of the observed differences between test and control groups.

The clinical value of using acidulated sodium fluoride as an active agent in fluoride toothpastes has not been conclusively established in these published studies. The only investigation using a calcium pyrophosphate abrasive system did not establish any efficacy of this combination. While inadequacy of study design could have clouded the results, the abrasive system may well have been responsible for reduced activity of the paste. In the trials using an insoluble sodium metaphosphate abrasive system, the paste used by the control group was a commercially available fluoride-free paste. The reductions observed in caries increments for test groups could have been attributable to the fluoride ion activity per se, but whether the effect of the paste was enhanced by acidulation remains unestablished from these clinical trials. The magnitude of the clinical reductions observed using the same test formula were of a similar order, that is 1–2 surfaces per child for 2 years. A further point for consideration is the possible effect of regular and sustained use of commercially available fluoride toothpastes by participants before the start of any particular trial. While it is known that 33 per cent of the participants in the Brudevold–Chilton study were previous users of fluoride toothpastes, similar information is not available for the Peterson and Williamson study. Slack et al. (1971) reported that 10 per cent of the participants had previously used a fluoride paste, but felt that this would have no significant reflection on the results. As very few studies have investigated the duration and magnitude of benefit from routine use of a fluoride paste, the magnitude of this effect on the observed results is not known.

TOOTHPASTES CONTAINING STANNOUS FLUORIDE (*Table* 30)

Following the initial negative results achieved in clinical trials testing the efficacy of sodium fluoride as an active toothpaste ingredient, attention

Table 30. Clinical Trials of Stannous Fluoride Dentifrices

Investigators	% SnF_2 + Abrasive	Unsupervised (U) or supervised (S) use	Duration of trial	No. of carious surfaces saved per year	Reduction in carious surface increment (%)	Level of statistical significance
Muhler et al. (1955a)	0·4	CaPP	U	1 year	1·48	49	0·0001
Muhler et al. (1955b)	0·4	CaPP	U	1 year	0·87	36	0·013
Muhler and Radike (1957) (Adults)	0·4	CaPP	U	2 years	0·84	34	0·005
Jordan and Peterson (1959)	0·4	CaPP	U S	2 years 2 years	0·28 0·46	13 21	NS 0·01
Muhler (1961)	0·4	CaPP	U	3 years	0·6	63*	0·0001
Kyes et al. (1961) (Adults)	0·4	CaPP	U	2 years	0·18	8	NS
Bixler and Muhler (1962)	0·4	CaPP	U	8 months	1·8	45	0·006
Muhler (1962a)	0·4	CaPP	U	3 years	0·41	22	0·0062
Muhler (1962b)	0·4	CaPP	S	2 years	1·2	46	—
Finn and Jamison (1963)	0·4	CaPP	S	2 years	No true placebo	No true placebo	—
Slack and Martin (1964)	0·4	IMP	U	Planned 3–4 years	Trial not completed		—
Gish and Muhler (1965)	0·4	CaPP	U	1 year	1·67–3·46	71**	0·00001
Torell and Ericsson (1965)	0·4	CaPP	U	2 years	1·16	22	0·01
Bixler and Muhler (1966)	0·4	CaPP	U	3 years	0·58 0·97	37† 58**	0·00001 0·00001

Reference		Abrasive	U/S	Duration	Value		
Brudevold and Chilton (1966)	0·4	IMP	U	2 years	1·08	25	0·05
	0·4	CaPP		2 years	0·2	4	NS
Halikis (1966)	0·4	IMP	U	15 months	1·04	27	0·07
Horowitz et al. (1966)	0·4	CaPP	U	3 years	0·33	17	0·01
	0·4	CaPP	S	3 years	0·42	21	0·01
	0·4	CaPP	S	2 years	N/A	36	0·05
Thomas and Jamison (1966)	0·4	IMP				37	
Jackson and Sutcliffe (1967)	0·4	CaPP	U	3 years	0·32	12	NS
James and Anderson (1967)	0·4	CaPP	U	3 years	1·22	29	
Muhler et al. (1967) (Adults)	0·4	CaPP	U	30 months	1·0	64**	0·001
Naylor and Emslie (1967)	0·4	IMP	U	3 years	0·49	14·5	0·001
Slack et al. (1967a)	0·4	CaPP	U	3 years	0·2	7	NS
Slack et al. (1967b)	0·4	IMP, SiO$_2$	U	3 years	0·0 Clinical	0	NS
					0·3 Radiological	28	0·01
Fanning et al. (1968)	0·4	IMP	U	2 years	1·28	21	0·001
Frankl and Alman (1968)	0·4	CaPP	U	3 years	—	No true placebo	NS
Mergele (1968a)	0·4	IMP	S	2 years	0·3	10	0·05
Mergele (1968b) (Water F 1·0 ppm)	0·4	CaPP	U	3 years	0·25	13	NS
Scola and Ostrom (1968) (Adults)	0·4	CaPP	U	2 years	1·13	42†	0·001
					1·35	48**	0·001
Muhler (1970)	0·4	CaPP	U	1 year	1·18	29	0·05

Table 30 (cont.)

Investigators	% SnF_2 + Abrasive	Unsupervised (U) or supervised (S) use	Duration of trial	No. of carious surfaces saved per year	Reduction in carious surface increment (%)	Level of statistical significance
Zacherl and McPhail (1970)	0·4	CaPP	U	30 months	1·0–0·76	40–44	0·05
Gish and Muhler (1971) (F water area)	0·4	CaPP	U	5 years	0·38	29	0·00078
Slack et al. (1971)	0·4	CaPP	U	3 years	0·76	18	0·01
Zacherl (1972a)	0·4	IMP	U	3 years	1·0	24	0·01
Zacherl (1972b)	0·4	CaPP	U	20 months	1·1	28	0·05
Zacherl (1973)	0·4	CaPP	U	2 years	0·94	22	0·00037
Zacherl (1973)	0·4	CaPP	U	2 years	0·75	30	0·05
Beiswanger et al. (1978)	0·4	CaPP	U	2 years	No placebo	No placebo*	0·05
Fogels et al. (1979)	0·4	SiO$_2$	U	3 years	0·41	15	0·01
	0·4	CaPP	U	3 years	0·40	15	0·01
Ringelberg et al. (1979)	0·4	CaPP	U	30 months	0·44	18	NS
Lu et al. (1980) (Adults)	0·4	CaPP	U	1 year (continuing)	0·23	33	0·05
Zacherl (1981)	0·4	CaPP	U	3 years	0·44	23	0·05

*Combined with topical F.
†Combined with prophylactic F.
**Combined with prophylactic + topical F.

was turned to other soluble fluorides for possible caries inhibitory action. Muhler and his associates at Indiana University, USA, having used stannous fluoride as a topical agent, decided to incorporate this compound into a toothpaste, which was manufactured and marketed under licence with the name of 'Crest' in the USA in 1955.

In formulating a stannous fluoride toothpaste compounded in a watery base, attention had to be paid to the known chemical reactivity and instability of stannous fluoride; in solution, tin and fluoride ions are lost by hydrolysis and oxidation (Hefferen et al., 1966). If the pH is raised, stannous hydroxide is precipitated and a strong stannous fluoride complex is formed (Torell et al., 1958). The conventional abrasive systems of dentifrices at the time were based on calcium salts. However, the chemical affinity of calcium ions for ionic fluoride in solution results in the formation of relatively insoluble calcium fluoride, although the formation of tin fluoride complexes may minimize this change (Torell et al., 1958). Different formulations were tried out by Muhler and his co-workers; the final formulation produced contained 0·4 per cent stannous fluoride and 1 per cent stannous pyrophosphate, in combination with a calcium pyrophosphate abrasive system, formed by treating calcium orthophosphate.

The initial trials began in 1955 and tested a stannous fluoride toothpaste, without the stannous pyrophosphate. The control toothpaste used was of the same composition, but without the active ingredient, and of a pH close to neutrality. Three trials by Muhler and his associates studied the effectiveness of normal home use of this formulation, two of the trials studying children aged 5–15 years for 1 year (Muhler et al., 1955a, b) and a third involving young adults aged 17–36 years (Muhler and Radike, 1957) for 2 years. Reductions in the increment of caries observed in the groups using the test dentifrice for 1 year (compared with the control group) were of the order of 1–1·5 surfaces per child for the study period. The first trial published gave no indication of measures taken to ensure examiner reliability at the examinations and this is reflected in the number of reversals of diagnoses published. For the final examination, the number of reversals for the test group was two and a half times the number recorded for the control group, and these reversals were included in the results. In the second trial there was a loss of two-thirds of the subjects from the groups during the study period, and although there was comparability between the groups at baseline with respect to initial caries experience, there was a lack of this balance at times of re-examination.

The succeeding trials tested a modified formula, containing 1 per cent stannous pyrophosphate, and corresponded to the marketed formula of Crest. Spannous pyrophosphate was added in an attempt to maintain the level of the stannous ion, the hypothesis being that the anti-caries action of fluoride would be augmented by relatively insoluble precipitates formed in enamel by the cation. Subsequent in vitro tests have failed to validate this (Brudevold et al., 1967). The evidence now is that there is no cation effect and fluoride is the effective component.

The new formulation was first investigated by Jordan and Peterson (1959). Supervised brushing once a day with the test dentifrice for 2 years, as well as normal home use of the same, resulted in a reduction in caries increment of one surface in 2 years. Another group of the same age (8–11 years) showed no significant reduction in caries increment for normal home use of the test paste. When brushing was supervised three times a day for 10 months, a caries reduction of one surface per child was observed for the study period. The numbers in the groups were small, and trying to relate the results of this special study with the measure of supervision used to potential reduction benefits in a general population would be unrealistic. Muhler (1960), in a 2-year trial of normal home use of the test dentifrice, observed a reduction benefit of 1·5 surfaces in children aged 6–18 years. The initial effect was maintained with time, the test group showing a relatively stable increment of new DMF surfaces, which was lower than that for the control. The only report of a study of 3 years' duration (Muhler, 1962) observed a reduction of 2 surfaces per child for 3 years of home use of the stannous fluoride dentifrice.

The original stannous fluoride–calcium pyrophosphate Crest formulation has been tested and marketed in many countries, including the USA, Great Britain, Canada and Australia. A summary of over 40 clinical trials is given in *Table* 30, and all have recorded a reduction in caries increment of 1–49 per cent.

In 1964 the Crest formulation was recognized as a therapeutic toothpaste by the Council of Dental Therapeutics of the American Dental Association, and was accorded Grade A status. A number of reports referred to the increased staining observed in test groups brushing with a stannous fluoride dentifrice, compared with controls.

Although the stannous fluoride formulation, marketed as Crest, has been subjected to clinical trials for 25 years, it has now been replaced by a sodium fluoride–silica formulation, marketed as Crest Plus.

TOOTHPASTES CONTAINING SODIUM MONOFLUOROPHOSPHATE (*Table* 31)

Animal experiments (Zipkin and McClure, 1951) and clinical investigations of topically applied solutions containing sodium monofluorophosphate (Hawes et al., 1954; Goaz et al., 1966) established a caries-inhibitory effect attributable to this agent. In vitro investigations by Ericsson (1963), Grøn et al. (1971) and Ingram (1972) have all estimated the uptake of fluoride by intact enamel surfaces to be less from a monofluorophosphate solution than from one of sodium fluoride. At present there are two schools of thought explaining the caries-inhibitory mechanism of the

Table 31. Clinical Trials of Sodium Monofluorophosphate Dentifrices

Investigators	% MFP + Abrasive	Unsupervised (U) or supervised (S) use	Duration of trial	No. of carious surfaces saved per year	Reduction in carious surface increment (%)	Level of statistical significance
Finn and Jamison (1963)	0·76	IMP	S	2 years	0·6	26	0·001
Goaz et al. (1963)	6·0	Solution	S	14 months	0·7	39	0·002
Torell and Ericsson (1965)	0·76	CaCO₃	S	2 years	0·7	25	0·001
Naylor and Emslie (1967)	0·76	DCP +CaCO₃	U	3 years	0·6	18	0·001
Frankl and Alman (1968)	0·76	IMP	U	3 years	0·6	8	0·05
Fanning et al. (1968)	0·70	IMP	U	2 years	1·2	20	0·001
Mergele (1968a) (Houston)	0·76	IMP	U	3 years	0·3	17	0·05
Mergele (1968b) (Austin)	0·76	IMP	S	22 months	0·6	20	0·001
Møller et al. (1968)	0·76	IMP +DCP	U	30 months	1·0	19	0·001
Kinkel and Stolte (1968)	0·76	IMP +silica	U	2 years	—	33	—
Thomas and Jamison (1970)	0·76	IMP	S	2 years	0·7	34	0·05
Zacherl (1972a)	0·76	Ca pyrophosphate	U	20 months	0·9	23	0·05
Kinkel and Raich (1972)			—	2 years	0·7	30·53	0·001
Hargreaves and Chester (1973)	2·0	Al₂O₃	U	3 years	1·1	23	0·01
Lind et al. (1974)	2·0	Al₂O₃	U	3 years	0·9	38	0·001

Table 31 (*cont.*)

Investigators	% *MFP* + Abrasive		Unsupervised (U) or supervised (S) use	Duration of trial	No. of carious surfaces saved per year	Reduction in carious surface increment (%)	Level of statistical significance
Andlaw and Tucker (1975)	0·76	Al₂O₃	U	3 years	0·6	19	0·001
Downer et al. (1976)	0·76	IMP +APF topical applications	S	3 years	0·8	31	0·001
Peterson et al. (1975)	0·76	CaCO₃	S	31 months	0·2	23	0·05
Mainwaring and Naylor (1978)	0·76	IMP	U	3 years	0·6	17	0·01
Shiere (1976)	0·76	CaCO₃	S	2 years	0·7	23	0·05
Edlund and Koch (1977)	0·76	CaPO₄ +CaCO₃	S	3 years	0·7	No placebo group; NaF : SiO₂-containing dentifrice significantly better	
James et al. (1977)	2·0	Al₂O₃	U	3 years	1·2	30	0·01
Howat et al. (1978)	0·76	Silica gel	S	3 years	0·7	26	0·05
Glass and Shiere (1978)	0·76	CaCO₃	U	3 years	0·7	28	0·01
Naylor and Glass (1979)	0·76+ 0·13% CaGP	CaCO₃	U	3 years	0·9	25	0·01
Hodge et al. (1980)	0·76 +0·1% NaF	Al₂O₃	S	3 years	0·6	22	0·05
Hodge et al. (1980)	0·76 +0·1% NaF		S	3 years	0·65	24	0·01
Murray and Shaw (1980)	0·76	Al₂O₃ (Low abrasivity)	U	3 years	0·6	34	0·001
Murray and Shaw (1980)	0·76	Al₂O₃ (Normal	U	3 years	0·5	27	0·001

monofluorophosphate ion. One explanation is that it is essentially a fluoride effect (Ericsson, 1963; Grøn et al., 1971), but the mechanism of fluoride ion release is disputed between these investigators. Ericsson postulates that the monofluorophosphate is deposited in the crystallite lattice and, in subsequent intracrystallite transposition of the deposited monofluorophosphate and apatite hydroxyl groups, fluoride is released and replaces the hydroxyl group in the lattice to form fluorapatite. Grøn et al. (1971) feel the fluoride ion is released at the solution-crystal interface and is deposited on fluorapatite in the enamel by exchange with the hydroxyl groups in the crystal lattice. Both investigators found that the fluoride ion was also released to the oral environment in significant amounts from monofluorophosphate by hydrolysis due to enzymatic action in plaque and saliva. On the other hand, Ingram (1972) has suggested that the anti-cariogenic activity of this compound is a specific monofluorophosphate effect, the MFP ion being incorporated and remaining intact in the crystal lattice by exchange with the phosphate group in the enamel, and as such, the mechanism was less pH dependent than the fluoride reaction with enamel.

In vitro investigations by Erisson (1961) found no reduction in free fluoride ion activity when sodium monofluorophosphate was combined with abrasives of chalk and insoluble metaphosphate (IMP) which had previously been reported to be a mechanically suitable abrasive for a dentifrice system (Van Huysen and Boyd, 1952). The loss of available fluoride from combinations with silica powder and pumice was very small. However, the loss with calcium pyrophosphate was considerable. Ericsson advised the use of sodium lauroyl sulphate as a compatible detergent for sodium monofluorophosphate, and a binder of carboxymethyl cellulose. In these investigations Ericsson found no marked increase in fluoride uptake by intact enamel with reduction in pH, thus making it easier to formulate an actual paste in relation to the slightly alkaline and highly buffered properties of saliva.

Over 20 trials of toothpastes containing sodium monofluorophosphate (usually in a concentration of 0·8 per cent, yielding 1000 ppm F) have been reported and are summarized in *Table* 31. A variety of abrasives have been used; for example, chalk and 2 per cent aerosil (Torell and Ericsson, 1968), insoluble metaphosphate (Finn and Jamison, 1968; Frankl and Alman, 1968), insoluble metaphosphate with anhydrous dicalcium phosphate and 1 per cent hydrated alumina (Møller et al., 1968), dicalcium phosphate dihydrate and chalk (Naylor and Emslie, 1967) and alumina (Hargreaves and Chester, 1973).

Hargreaves and Chester (1973) undertook clinical trials in which they investigated the effect of increasing the concentration of the sodium monofluorophosphate to 2 per cent, the highest fluoride concentration in a toothpaste to date, the assumption being that if the mechanism of effect was that stated by Ingram (1972), by increasing the concentration of monofluorophosphate and using a phosphate-free abrasive system, this would enhance exchange of the monofluorophosphate ions in solution with phosphate in the crystal structure, and help to minimize the inhibitory effect produced by the natural level of phosphate ions present in saliva. The trial investigated 3 years' home use of the paste in three groups of children, aged 5, 8 and 11 years. Home visitors were used to visit each home every 5 weeks to motivate children and families, and maintain interest in the trial. The reductions in caries increments for the test groups relative to the control groups using a placebo paste varied from 1 to 3 surfaces per child over the 3-year period. The observed caries-inhibitory effect did not differ markedly from that observed in studies testing toothpastes containing lower concentrations of monofluorophosphate. The greatest reduction effect was noted on smooth surfaces but worthwhile reductions were recorded in a number of locations where one would expect pit and fissure caries, for example buccal surfaces of the first permanent molars. Similar findings were reported by James et al. (1977).

Hargreaves et al. (1974) re-examined 221 children one year after the termination of their study. It was reported that a statistically significant difference in DMF increment between active and placebo groups still remained. This suggests that 'carry-over protection', for those children who used the sodium monofluorophosphate toothpaste, continued for at least 1 year after withdrawal of the paste.

Lind et al. (1974) carried out a trial in an optimum fluoride area, using a toothpaste of identical formula to that tested by Hargreaves and Chester (1973). After 3 years 1167 children (83 per cent of the original sample) remained in the study. The children were aged 7–12 years initially. The total DMFS increment (clinical and bitewing radiograph scores combined) for the 3-year period was 1·7 surfaces lower in the group receiving the fluoride toothpaste than in the group using the placebo paste (3·71 surfaces as against 5·43 surfaces), a reduction of 32 per cent.

The effectiveness of the fluoride toothpastes in the study by Lind et al. (1974) in natural fluoride areas appears to be very similar to that found by Hargreaves and Chester (1973) and James et al. (1977) using similar toothpastes in low-fluoride areas.

The effect of the varying abrasiveness of toothpaste containing 0·76 MFP has been reported (Murray and Shaw, 1980). Three toothpastes were used in the trial; one MFP toothpaste with low abrasivity (relative dentine abrasivity (RDA) 60), and MFP dentifrice of normal abrasivity (RDA 110) as positive control, and a placebo non-fluoride low-abrasivity toothpaste (RDA 60).

The children who used the test dentifrices containing 0·8 per cent monofluorophosphate had a lower mean caries incidence than those using the placebo paste without any fluoride additive. The lowest mean caries incidence over the 3-year period was in children who were allocated the low-abrasive fluoride paste. Caries increments for all DMF indices for boys and girls seen by both examiners were consistently lower in this group when compared with the other two groups, but statistical analysis indicated that the difference in caries-inhibitory properties between the fluoride paste with reduced abrasivity and that with conventional abrasivity was not significant. When both groups using the monofluorophosphate pastes were compared with children using the placebo dentifrice, the differences in caries increments were statistically significant.

The reports of two studies state that children using a monofluorophosphate dentifrice exhibited significantly less staining than those using a stannous fluoride paste (Naylor and Emslie, 1967; Fanning et al., 1968). This lack of staining associated with use of a monofluorophosphate paste may confer some advantage in acceptability over one containing stannous fluoride. In 1969 a monofluorophosphate dentifrice was recognized by the Council on Dental Therapeutics of the American Dental Association as an accepted dental remedy and was given Grade A status.

A number of agents have been added to MFP toothpastes in an attempt to increase their caries inhibitory effect. Naylor and Glass (1979) detected a consistent, though statistically non-significant trend towards lower caries increment in the group using a toothpaste containing both sodium monofluorophosphate and calcium glycerophosphate. Recently a dentifrice containing both sodium monofluorophosphate and sodium fluoride (1450 ppm F) has been tested (Hodge et al., 1980) and marketed as newly formulated Colgate Dental Cream. It was concluded that the addition of 0·1 per cent sodium fluoride appeared to enhance the effectiveness of a dentifrice containing 0·76 per cent sodium monofluorophosphate. This effect was apparent if the abrasive system was either alumina or dicalcium phosphate. However, in this trial the differences between the positive control (0·76 NaMFP, original Colgate) and the negative (non-fluoride) control were smaller than expected—13·8 per cent in the DMFT index ($P < 0·05$) and 6·6 per cent (non-significant) in the DFS index.

TOOTHPASTES CONTAINING AMINE FLUORIDE (*Table* 32)

The protection afforded enamel from acid decalcification by aliphatic monoamines in in vitro experiments (Irwin et al., 1957) led König and Mühlemann (1961) to test the hypothesis that the detergent action of these organic compounds could be combined with the action of fluoride to give an increased measure of protection to hard tooth structures. In vitro studies with amine fluorides showed some amine fluoride compounds to be superior to inorganic fluorides in reducing enamel solubility (Mühlemann et al., 1957). It was reported by Mühlemann (1967) that amine fluorides were superior to inorganic fluorides in the measure of their caries prevention due to a number of factors. Amine fluorides exhibited a pronounced affinity for enamel, enhancing fluoride uptake by the enamel when used at low concentrations (as in toothpaste). They exhibited a direct anti-enzymatic effect on microbial activity in the plaque by means of the organic moiety of the amine fluoride (Hermann and Mühlemann, 1958; Capozzi et al., 1967). In vitro tests established the stability of a formulation with insoluble metaphosphate abrasive (König and Mühlemann, 1961).

Marthaler (1965) published the results of a 3-year double-blind clinical trial with children aged 6–14 years; the mean age of the younger group studied was 7 years and that of the older group was 11–12 years. Tooth brushing was unsupervised and no organized effort was made to improve the standard of oral cleanliness of the children participating in the trial. The supplies of toothpaste were not delivered to the participants but were available from the local dental clinics, relying on the cooperation of the children to ask for further supplies. The rest of the family were not automatically supplied with the dentifrice being used by the participant. Initially there were three amine fluoride formulations being tested with differing abrasive systems:

Compound amine fluoride dentifrices	*Abrasive system*
A. 297 + 242 (0·125% F)	IMP
B. 297 + 242 (0·125% F)	BaSO4
Single amine fluoride dentifrice	
C. 297 (0·125% F)	BaSO4
Control dentrifices	
D. —	IMP
E. —	BaSO4

After 18 months, because of their low abrasiveness, pastes B and E containing a barium sulphate abrasive system were replaced by pastes A and D. The amine fluoride pastes were compared for clinical efficacy with a control paste containing a conventional detergent, 1 per cent sodium lauroyl sulphate. In the first 3 months of the trial, test pastes were packed in metal tubes in which they were found to lose approximately 20 per cent of their caries-inhibitory potential due to chemical reactivity between the active ingredients in the paste and the tube. Subsequently they were packed in polythene tubes with no evidence of diminishing cariostatic activity, even after 14 months' storage (König and Mühlemann, 1961).

The supply of paste to the participants was subject to interruption after 18 months of the study. This lapse was due to a number of factors. The result of the first 6-month examination had shown no benefit with use of the test pastes. Many children thought the trial had ended after this interval and did not continue to obtain supplies of paste from the clinics. Owing to diminished cooperation, investigators had ceased supply of the pastes to some of the clinics. At 27 months, when results of the 18-month examination showed promising results, the study revived and supplies of

Table 32. Clinical Trials of Amine Fluoride Dentifrices

Investigators	% Fluoride + Abrasive		Unsupervised (U) or supervised (S) use	Duration of trial	No. of carious surfaces saved per year	Reduction in carious surface increment (%)	Level of statistical significance
Marthaler (1965)	297+242	IMP	U	3 years	(a)* 3–4 (b)* 4	30 24	0·001 0·05
Marthaler (1968)	297	BaSO₄	U	3 years	—	—	—
	297+242	IMP	U	7 years	5–6	26	0·001
	297	BaSO₄	U	7 years	—	—	—
Patz and Naujoks (1970)	297+242 (Elmex)	Not known	U	3 years	0·25	7	—
Franke et al. (1979)	Not known (Elmex)	known	U	7 years	Not known	41†	—
Ringelberg et al. (1979)	(1250 ppm F⁻)	known	U	30 months	0·2	18	NS

* (a), (b) Different age groups.
† Note that this is a combined effect of supervised brushing with fluoride-containing fluid plus unsupervised brushing with toothpaste.

paste were received at regular intervals. The mean number of months calculated for the period when the supply of paste had lapsed was 5–7 months. For some children this period was as long as 12 months.

The statistical planning and design of this study varied from the conventional protocol as suggested by Backer Dirks et al. (1967).

Comparisons with the control group were made only for the test groups using the formulations A and B. After 3 years, reductions in the younger age group for children using the test formulation were of the order of 3–4 surfaces per child compared to the control groups (P < 0·001). Radiographic evidence showed a reduction of 1 surface per child for the test groups. A higher relative reduction was observed for dentinal lesions, indicating an inhibitory effect on caries progression. Detailed analyses of individual surface reductions showed that almost half the percentage reduction in caries increment between test and control group was clinically diagnosed on the approximal surfaces of anterior teeth. The reduction was of the order of 58 per cent or 1–2 surfaces per child for 3 years. A similar finding was made by Jackson and Sutcliffe (1967) who found a reduction of attack on approximal surfaces of incisor teeth to be of the order of 50 per cent with use of a stannous fluoride–calcium pyrophosphate toothpaste. In the older age group a total reduction of 4 surfaces per child in the test group was observed for the trial period, while radiographic examination showed a reduction of 1–2 surfaces per child. The strongest reduction effect in the 11–12-year-olds was noted on the buccolingual surface of teeth. There was no caries-inhibitory effect detectable for the occusal surfaces.

Marthaler (1968) published the results after 7 years for children aged 6–8 years when the study began. The numbers in the group were small. A significant reduction in caries increment for the 7 years was found to be of the order of 5–6 surfaces per child for the test group relative to the control. Radiographic examination revealed a difference in caries increments of the order of 2 surfaces. Approximately 40 per cent of the total increment reduction attributable to the fluoride paste occurred on the approximal surfaces of the buccal segments. The relative reduction effect was greater for dentinal lesions on analysis of radiographic results, indicating a greater inhibitory effect on the progression of early carious lesions to more advanced ones. Interval analysis showed the caries-inhibitory effect of the amine fluoride pastes to be sustained, and even increase, with longer use.

Further studies (*Table* 32) have now been reported. An amine fluoride dentifrice named Elmex is now marketed in a number of European countries, but is not at present on sale in the United Kingdom.

CONCLUSION

In general the results of the studies reviewed in this section show that toothpaste is a useful vehicle whereby fluoride compounds can be applied to teeth. The magnitude of the caries-preventive effect of fluoride in toothpaste has sometimes been overstated by stressing the percentage differences in caries increment between test and control groups. Clinically, the most important fact is the reduction in the actual number of surfaces attacked by caries over a given period of time; this information has been given wherever possible. Furthermore, the results of the follow-up study by Koch (1970) suggest that any caries-inhibitory effect of fluoride toothpaste is reliant on regular and sustained applications. Nevertheless, as the majority of people find that a toothpaste makes tooth cleaning easier and more pleasant, they should be encouraged to use a fluoride toothpaste which has been shown to have some caries-preventive effect. Further research is needed to determine the most suitable means of incorporating fluoride into toothpaste. Consideration should also be given to the best means of convincing people who never use any sort of toothpaste how they would benefit by including a fluoride toothpaste in the oral hygiene régime.

REFERENCES

Andlaw R. J. and Tucker G. J. (1975) A dentifrice containing 0.8 per cent sodium monofluorophosphate in an aluminium oxide trihydrate base. *Br. Dent. J.* **138**, 426–432.
Backer Dirks O., Baume L. J., Davies G. N. and Slack G. L. (1967) Principle requirements for controlled clinical trials. *Int. Dent. J.* **17**, 93–103.
BDA News (1981) 7 April, p. 2.
Beiswanger B. B. and Gish C. W. (1981) A three-year study of the effect of a sodium fluoride–silica abrasive dentifrice on dental caries. *Pharmacol. Ther. Dent.* **6**, 9–16.
Beiswanger B. B., Billings R. J., Sturzenberger O.P. and Bollmer B. W. (1978) The additive anticariogenic effect of an SnF_2–$Ca_2P_2O_7$ dentifrice and APF topical applications. *J. Dent. Child.* **45**, 137.
Bibby B. G. (1945) Test of the effect of fluoride-containing dentifrices on dental caries. *J. Dent. Res.* **24**, 297–303.
Bixler D. and Muhler J. C. (1962) Experimental clinical human caries. *J. Am. Dent. Assoc.* **65**, 482–488.
Bixler D. and Muhler J. C. (1966) Effect on dental caries in children in a non-fluoride area of combined use of three agents containing stannous fluoride: a prophylactic paste, a solution and a dentifrice. II. Results at the end of 24 and 36 months. *J. Am. Dent. Assoc.* **72**, 392–396.
Brudevold F. and Chilton N. W. (1966) Comparative study of a fluoride dentifrice containing soluble phosphate and a calcium-free abrasive. Second year report. *J. Am. Dent. Assoc.* **72**, 889–894.
Brudevold F., McCann H. G., Nilsson R., Richardson B. and Cocklica V. (1967) The chemistry of caries inhibition and challenges in topical treatments. *J. Dent. Res.* **46**, 37–45.
Brudevold F., Savoy A., Gardiner D. E., Spinelli M. and Speirs R. (1963) A study of acidulated fluoride solutions, I. In vitro effects on enamel. *Arch. Oral Biol.* **8**, 167–177.

Capozzi L., Brunetti P., Negri P. L. and Migliorini E. (1967) Enzymatic mechanism of action of some fluorine compounds. *Caries Res.* **1**, 69–77.

Cilley W. A. and Haberman J. P. (1981) Fluoride in enamel and correlation to caries *J. Dent. Res.* IADR Abstr, 1069.

Downer M. C. (1974) *Aspects of the Validity of Diagnosis in the Epidemiology of Dental Caries.* Ph.D. Thesis, University of Manchester.

Downer M. C., Holloway, P. J. and Davies T. G.. H. (1976) Clinical testing of a topical fluoride caries preventive programme. *Br. Dent. J.* **141**, 242–247.

Edlund K. and Koch G. (1977) Effect on caries of daily supervised toothbrushing with sodium monofluorophosphate and sodium fluoride dentifrices after three years. *Scand. J. Dent. Res.* **85**, 41–45.

Ennever J., Peterson J. K., Hester W. R., Segreto V. A. and Radike A. W. (1980) Influence of alkaline pH on the effectiveness of sodium fluoride dentifrices. *J. Dent. Res.* **59** (4), 658–661.

Ericsson Y. (1961) Fluorides in dentifrices. Investigations using radioactive fluorine. *Acta Odontol. Scand.* **19**, 41–77.

Ericsson Y. (1963) The mechanism of monofluorophosphate action on hydroxy-apatite and dental enamel. *Acta Odontol. Scand.* **21**, 341–358.

Fanning E. A., Gotjamanos T. and Vowles N. J. (1968) The use of fluoride dentifrices in the control of dental caries: methodology and results of a clinical trial. *Aust. Dent. J.* **13**, 201–206.

Finn S. B. and Jamison H. C. (1963) A comparative clinical study of three dentifrices. *J. Dent. Child.* **30**, 17–25.

Fogels H. R., Alman J. E., Meade J. J. and O'Donnell J. P. (1979) The relative caries-inhibiting effects of a stannous fluoride dentifrice in a silica gel base. *J. Am. Dent. Assoc.* **99**, 456–459.

Forsman B. (1974) Studies on the effect of dentifrices with low fluoride content. *Community Dent. Oral Epidemiol.* **2**, 166–175.

Franke von W., Künzel W., Treide A. and Blüthner K. (1977) Karieshemmung durch Aminfluorid nach 7 jahren Kollektiv angeleiteter Mundhygiene. *Stomatol. DDR* **27**, 13–16.

Frankl S. N. and Alman J. E. (1968) Report of a three-year clinical trial comparing a toothpaste containing sodium monofluorophosphate with two marketed products. *J. Oral Ther. Pharmacol.* **4**, 443–450.

Gerdin P. O. (1972) Studies in dentifrices, VIII: Clinical testing of an acidulated, non-grinding dentifrice with reduced fluorine content. *Swed. Dent. J.* **67**, 283–297.

Gish C. W. and Muhler J. C. (1965) Combined use of three agents containing stannous fluoride: a prophylactic paste, a solution and a dentifrice. *J. Am. Dent. Assoc.* **70**, 914–920.

Gish C. W. and Muhler J. C. (1971) Effectiveness of a stannous fluoride dentifrice on dental caries. *J. Dent. Child.* **38**, 211–214.

Glass R. L. and Shiere F. R. (1978) A clinical trial of a calcium carbonate base dentifrice containing 0·76% sodium monofluorophosphate. *Caries Res.* **12**, 284–289.

Goaz P. W., McElwaine L. P. and Biswell H. A. (1966) Anticariogenic effect of a sodium monofluorophosphate solution in children after 21 months of use. *J. Dent. Res.* **45**, 286–290.

Goaz P. W., McElwaine L. P., Biswell H. A. and White W. E. (1963) Effect of daily applications of sodium monofluorophosphate solution on caries rate in children. *J. Dent. Res.* **42**, 965–972.

Grøn P. and Brudevold F. (1967) The effectiveness of sodium fluoride dentifrices. *J. Dent. Child.* **34**, 122–127.

Grøn P., Brudevold F. and Aasenden R. (1971) Monofluorophosphate interaction with hydroxyapatite and intact enamel. *Caries Res.* **5**, 202–214.

Halikis S. E. (1966) A pilot study on the effectiveness of a stannous fluoride dentifrice on dental caries in children. *Aust. Dent. J.* Oct., 336–337.

Hargreaves J. A. and Chester C. G. (1973) Clinical trial among Scottish children of an anticaries dentifrice containing 2 per cent sodium monofluorophosphate. *Community Dent. Oral Epidemiol.* **1**, 41–46.

Hargreaves J. A., Chester C. G. and Wagg B. J. (1975) An assessment of children in active and placebo groups, one year after termination of a clinical trial of a 2 per cent sodium monofluorophosphate dentifrice. *Caries Res.* **9**, 291 (abstr.).

Hawes, R. R., Sonnes S. and Brudevold F. (1954) Pilot studies of three topical fluoride application procedures. *J. Dent. Res.* **33**, 661.

Hefferen J. J., Zimmerman M. and Koehler H. M. (1966) Reactions of stannous fluoride with some inorganic compounds. *J. Dent. Res.* **45**, 1395–1402.

Hermann U and Mühlemann H. R. (1958) Inhibition of salivary respiration and glucolysis by an organic fluoride. *Helv. Odontol. Acta* **2**, 28–33.

Hodge H. C., Holloway P. J., Davies T. G. H. and Worthington H. V. (1980) Caries prevention by dentifrices containing a combination of sodium monofluorophosphate and sodium fluoride. *Br. Dent. J.* **149**, 201–204.

Horowitz H. S., Law F. E., Thompson M. B. and Chamberlain S. R. (1966) Evaluation of a stannous fluoride dentifrice for use in dental public health programs—basic findings. *J. Am. Dent. Assoc.* **72**, 408–421.

Howat A. P., Holloway P. J. and Davies T. G. H. (1978) Caries prevention by daily supervised use of a MFP gel dentifrice. *Br. Dent. J.* **145**, 233–235.

Ingram G. S. (1972) The reaction of monofluorophosphate with apatite. *Caries Res.* **6**, 1–15.

Irwin M., Leaver A. G. and Walsh J. P. (1957) Further studies on the influence of surface active agents on decalcification of the enamel surface. *J. Dent. Res.* **36**, 166–172.

Jackson D. and Sutcliffe P. (1967) Clinical testing of a stannous fluoride-calcium pyrophosphate dentifrice in Yorkshire schoolchildren. *Br. Dent. J.* **123**, 40–48.

James M. C. and Anderson R. J. (1967) Clinical testing of a stannous fluoride-calcium pyrophosphate dentifrice in Buckinghamshire schoolchildren. *Br. Dent. J.* **123**, 33–39.

James P. M. C., Anderson R. J., Beal J. F. and Bradnock G. (1977) A 3-year clinical trial of the effect on dental caries of a dentifrice containing 2 per cent sodium monofluorophosphate. *Community Dent. Oral Epidemiol.* **5**, 67–72.

Jordan W. A. and Peterson J. K. (1959) Caries inhibiting value of a dentifrice containing stannous fluoride. Final report of a two-year study. *J. Am. Dent. Assoc.* **58**, 42–44.

Kinkel H. J. and Raich R. (1972) Zur Wirkung einer Na$_2$FPO$_3$—Zahnpasta auf die Karies bei Kindern. *Schweiz. Monatsschr. Zahnheilkd.* **82**, 169–175.

Kinkel H. J. and Stolte G. (1968) Zur Wirkung einer natrium monofluorophosphat—und bromchlorophenhaltigen Zahnpasta im chronischen Tierexperiment und auf die Karies bei Kindern wahrend eines Zwei Jahre langen unüberwachten Gebrauches. *Dtsch. Zahnaerztebl.* **9**, 455.

Koch G. (1967a) Effect of sodium fluoride in dentifrice and mouthwash on the incidence of dental caries in schoolchildren. *Odontol. Revy* **18**, 48–66.

Koch G. (1967b) Effect of sodium fluoride in dentifrice and mouthwash on the incidence of dental caries in schoolchildren. *Odontol. Revy* **18**, 67–71.

Koch G. (1970) Long-term study of the effect of supervised toothbrushing with a sodium fluoride dentifrice. *Caries Res.* **4**, 149–157.

König K. G. and Mühlemann H. R. (1961) Caries inhibiting effect of amine fluoride containing dentifrice tested in an animal experiment and a clinical study. In: Mühlemann H. R. and König K. G. (ed.), *The Present Status of Caries Prevention by Fluorine-containing Dentifrices*. Berne, Huber, pp. 126–130.

Kyes F., Overton N. J. and McKean T. W. (1961) Clinical trials of caries inhibitory dentifrices. *J. Am. Dent. Assoc.* **63**, 189–193.

Lind O. P., Møller I. J., von der Fehr F. R. and Larsen M. J. (1974) Caries-preventive effect of a dentifrice containing 2 per cent sodium monofluorophosphate in a natural fluoride area in Denmark. *Community Dent. Oral Epidemiol.* **2**, 104–113.

Lu K. H., Hanna J. D. and Peterson J. K. (1980) Effect on dental caries of a stannous fluoride-calcium pyrophosphate dentifrice in an adult population: one-year results. *Pharmacol Ther. Dent.* **5**, 11–16.

Mainwaring P. and Naylor M. N. (1978) A three-year clinical study to determine the separate and combined caries inhibiting effects of sodium monofluorophosphate toothpaste and an acidulated phosphate fluoride gel. *Caries Res.* **12**, 202–212.

Marthaler T. M. (1965) The caries-inhibiting effect of amine fluoride dentifrices in children during three years of unsupervised use. *Br. Dent. J.* **119**, 153–163.

Marthaler T. M. (1968) Caries inhibition after seven years of an amine fluoride dentifrice. *Br. Dent. J.* **124**, 510–515.

Mergele M. (1968a) Report I—A supervised brushing study in state institution schools. *Acad. Med. New J. Bull.* **14**, 247–250.

Mergele M. (1968b) Report II—An unsupervised brushing study on subjects residing in a community with fluoride in the water. *Acad. Med. New J. Bull.* **14**, 251–255.

Mobley M. J. and Tepe J. H. (1981) Fluoride uptake from in situ brushing with an SnF_2 and an NaF dentifrice. *J. Dent. Res.* IADR Abstr., 653.

Møller I. J., Holst J. J. and Sørensen E. (1968) Caries reducing effect of a sodium monofluorophosphate dentifrice. *Br. Dent. J.* **124**, 209–213.

Mühlemann H. R. (1967) Die kariesprophylaktische Wirkung der Aminfluoride—10 Jahre Erfahrungen. *Die Quintessenz* 18, Ref. 3192, Issues 5–8.

Mühlemann H. R., Schmid H. and König K. G. (1957) Enamel solubility reduction studies with inorganic and organic fluorides. *Helv. Odontol. Acta* **1**, 23–33.

Muhler J. C. (1960) Combined anticariogenic effect of a single stannous fluoride solution and the unsupervised use of a stannous fluoride-containing dentifrice, II. Results at the end of two years. *J. Dent. Res.* **39**, 955–958.

Muhler J. C. (1961) A practical method for reducing dental caries in children not receiving the established benefits of communal fluoridation. *J. Dent. Child.* **28**, 5–12.

Muhler J. C. (1962) Effect of a stannous fluoride dentifrice on caries reduction in children during a three year study period. *J. Am. Dent. Assoc.* **64**, 216–224.

Muhler J. C. (1970) A clinical comparison of fluoride and antienzyme dentifrices. *J. Dent. Child.* **37**, 501–513.

Muhler J. C. and Radike A. W. (1957) Effect of a dentifrice containing stannous fluoride on dental caries in adults, II. Results at the end of two years of unsupervised use. *J. Am. Dent. Assoc.* **55**, 196–198.

Muhler J. C., Radike A. W., Nebergall W. H. and Day H. G. (1955a) Effect of a stannous fluoride-containing dentifrice on caries reduction in children, II. Caries experience after one year. *J. Am Dent. Assoc.* **50**, 163–166.

Muhler J. C., Radike A. W., Nebergall W. H. and Day H. G. (1955b) A comparison between the anticariogenic effect of dentifrices containing stannous fluoride and sodium fluoride. *J. Am. Dent. Assoc.* **51**, 556–559.

Muhler J. C., Spear L. B., Bixler D. and Stookey G. K. (1967) The arrestment of incipient dental caries in adults after the use of three different forms of SnF_2 therapy: results after 30 months. *J. Am. Dent. Assoc.* **75**, 1402–1406.

Murray J. J. and Shaw L. (1980) A 3-year clinical trial of the effect of fluoride content and toothpaste abrasivity on the caries inhibitory properties of a dentifrice. *Community Dent. Oral Epidemiol.* **8**, 46–51.

Naylor M. N. and Emslie R. D. (1967) Clinical testing of stannous fluoride and sodium monofluorophosphate dentifrices in London schoolchildren. *Br. Dent. J.* **123**, 17–23.

Naylor M. N. and Glass R. L. (1979) A 3-year clinical trial of calcium carbonate dentifrice containing calcium glycerophosphate and sodium monofluorophosphate. *Caries Res.* **13**, 39–46.

Patz von J. and Naujoks R. (1970) Die kariesprophylaktische Wirkung einer amidfluoridhaligen Zahnpaste bei jugendlichen nach dreijährigen unüberwachten Gebrauch. *Dtsch. Zahnaertzl. Zeitschr.* **25**, 617–625.

Peterson J. K. (1979) A supervised brushing trial of sodium monofluorophosphate dentifrices in a fluoridated area. *Caries Res.* **13**, 68–72.

Peterson J., Williamson L. and Casad R. (1975) Caries inhibition with MFP-calcium carbonate dentifrice in fluoridated area. *J. Dent. Res.* **54** (special issue), L85, Abstr. L338.

Reed M. W. (1973) Clinical evaluation of three concentrations of sodium fluoride in dentifrices. *J. Am. Dent. Assoc.* **87**, 1401–1403.

Reed M. W. and King J. D. (1975) A clinical evaluation of a sodium fluoride dentifrice. *Pharmacol. Ther. Dent.* **2**, 77–82.

Ringelberg M. L., Webster D. B., Dixon D. O. and LeZotte D. C. (1979) The caries-preventive effect of amine fluorides and inorganic fluorides in a mouth-rinse or dentifrice after 30 months of use. *J. Am. Dent. Assoc.* **98**, 202–208.

Scola F. P. and Ostrom C. A. (1968) Clinical evaluation of stannous fluoride when used as a constituent of a compatible prophylactic paste, as a topical solution, and in a dentifrice in naval personnel. II. Report of findings after 2 years. *J. Am. Dent. Assoc.* **77**, 594–597.

Shiere F. R. (1976) *The Massachusetts Study. Report of a clinical trial designed to determine the caries inhibition effect of a dentifrice containing 0·76 per cent sodium monofluorophosphate*, 7/15/76. New Jersey, USA, Beecham Products.

Slack G. L. and Martin W. J. (1964) The use of a dentifrice containing stannous fluoride in the control of dental caries. *Br. Dent. J.* **117**, 275–280.

Slack G. L., Berman D. S., Martin W. J. and Hardie J. M. (1967a) Clinical testing of a stannous fluoride-calcium pyrophosphate dentifrice in Essex schoolgirls. *Br. Dent. J.* **123**, 26–33.

Slack G. L., Berman D. S., Martin W. J. and Young J. (1967b) Clinical testing of a stannous fluoride-insoluble metaphosphate dentifrice in Kent schoolgirls. *Br. Dent. J.* **123**, 9–16.

Slack G. L., Bulman J. S. and Osborn J. F. (1971) Clinical testing of fluoride and non-fluoride containing dentifrices in Hounslow school-children. *Br. Dent. J.* **130**, 154–158.

Stookey G. K. and Beiswanger B. B. (1975) Influence of an experimental sodium fluoride dentifrice on dental caries incidence in children. *J. Dent. Res.* **54**(1), 53–58.

Thomas A. E. and Jamison H. C. (1966) Effect of stannous fluoride dentifrices on caries in children: two year clinical study of supervised brushing in children's homes. *J. Am. Dent. Assoc.* **73**, 844–852.

Thomas A. E. and Jamison H. C. (1970) Effect of a combination of two cariostatic agents in children: a three year clinical study of supervised brushing in children's homes. *J. Am. Dent. Assoc.* **81**, 118–124.

Torell P. and Ericsson Y. (1965) Two year clinical tests with different methods of local caries-preventive fluoride application in Swedish schoolchildren. *Acta Odontol. Scand.* **23**, 287–322.

Torell P., Hals E. and Morch T. (1958) Effect of topically applied agents on enamel. *Acta Odontol. Scand.* **16**, 329–341.

Van Huysen G. and Boyd T. M. (1952) Cleaning effectiveness of dentifrices. *J. Dent. Res.* **31**, 575–581.

Weisenstein P. R. and Zacherl W. A. (1972) A multiple examiner clinical evaluation of a sodium fluoride dentifrice. *J. Am. Dent. Assoc.* **84**, 621–623.

Winkler K. C., Backer Dirks O. and Van Amerogen J. (1953) A reproducible method for caries evaluation. Test is a therapeutic experiment with a fluoridated dentifrice. *Br. Dent. J.* **95**, 119–124.

Zacherl W. A. (1972a) Clinical evaluation of neutral sodium fluoride, stannous fluoride, sodium monofluorophosphate and acid fluoride-phosphate dentifrices. *J. Can. Dent. Assoc.* **38**, 35–38.

Zacherl W. A. (1972b) Clinical evaluation of an aged stannous fluoride-calcium pyrophosphate dentifrice. *J. Can. Dent. Assoc.* **38**, 155–157.

Zacherl W. A. (1973) A clinical evaluation of a stannous fluoride and a sarcosinate dentifrice. *J. Dent. Child.* **40**, 451–453.

Zacherl W. A. (1981) A three-year clinical caries evaluation of the effect of a sodium fluoride–silica abrasive dentifrice. *Pharmacol. Ther. Dent.* **6**, 1–7.

Zacherl W. A. and McPhail C. W. B. (1970) Final report on the efficacy of a stannous fluoride–calcium pyrophosphate dentifrice. *J. Can. Dent. Assoc.* **36**, 262–264.

Zipkin I. and McClure F. J. (1951) Complex fluorides: caries reduction and fluoride retention in the bones and teeth of white rats. *Public Health Rep.* **66**, 1523–1532.

CHAPTER 8

FLUORIDE PROPHYLACTIC PASTES
AND DENTAL CARIES

In vitro investigations have shown that small but significant amounts of enamel (approximately $4 \, \mu m$) can be removed when a thorough prophylaxis is carried out with commercially available prophylactic pastes containing the usual abrasive systems (pumice, silica dioxide, zirconium silicate, alumina) (Vrbic et al., 1967; Vrbic and Brudevold, 1970; Stearns, 1973). This loss of surface enamel is undesirable because the surface enamel contains the highest concentrations of fluoride. Fluoride compounds have been incorporated into prophylactic pastes to try to maintain a high fluoride concentration in the surface enamel and to determine whether, in combination with topical fluoride applications, an additional caries-inhibitory effect can be obtained. The following agents have been incorporated into prophylactic pastes: sodium fluoride, stannous fluoride, acidulated phosphate fluoride, stannous hexafluorozirconate.

1. PASTES CONTAINING SODIUM FLUORIDE

Investigations of fluoride prophylactic pastes can be traced to 1946. Bibby et al. (1946) evaluated a paste containing 1 per cent sodium fluoride and pumice in a small group of children and reported a caries increment reduction of 25–43 per cent, depending on the number of treatments given. A second study by the same investigator (Bibby, 1948) with 250 participants in a 1-year study with the above formula did not confirm the findings.

2. PASTES CONTAINING STANNOUS FLUORIDE

With the development of stannous fluoride as a recognized anti-cariogenic agent investigations were carried out to determine its effectiveness when incorporated in a prophylactic paste. Initial in vitro experiments carried out at Indiana University in the USA reported significant reductions in enamel solubility with application of stannous fluoride–pumice prophylactic pastes (Mericle and Muhler, 1963; Whitehurst et al., 1968). The reduction in enamel solubility when a stannous fluoride paste was applied was confirmed by tests investigating an alternative abrasive system of silex–silicone (Segreto et al., 1961; Wolf, 1964). A clinical study to evaluate the effectiveness of this formulation showed that the paste was as effective in preventing dental caries as an 8 per cent topical stannous fluoride solution, but no added benefit resulted from following the prophylaxis by a topical application (Peterson et al., 1963). The investigators suggested that the failure to achieve additional benefits by combined use of the agents might be due to the silicone in the paste forming an anti-wetting film on the tooth surface, thus serving as a barrier to the action of the subsequent topical applications.

Another abrasive, lava pumice, was said to be superior as a cleansing agent and more compatible chemically with stannous fluoride than previously tried abrasive systems (Dudding and Muhler, 1962; Mericle and Muhler, 1963). Using an 8·9 per cent stannous fluoride–lava pumice paste, Bixler and Muhler (1966) reported average reductions of 34 per cent of DMF increments at the end of 1 year for children aged 5–18 years receiving two applications of this prophylactic paste at 6-monthly intervals. Another group in the same study, who were treated with a topical application of an 8 per cent stannous fluoride solution as well as the stannous fluoride prophylactic paste, demonstrated an even greater reduction (approximately 45 per cent DMF surfaces) when the results of the two examiners were averaged. Scola and Ostrom (1968) also investigated semi-annual application of the prophylactic paste followed by a topical application of a 10 per cent stannous fluoride solution and routine use of a 0·4 per cent stannous fluoride dentifrice, in US Navy personnel. They reported a significant reduction in caries increment with combined use of applications. However, in the group treated with only stannous fluoride–lava pumice prophylactic paste a minimal reduction (12 per cent fewer DMF surfaces) was reported which was not statistically significant.

In contrast, Horowitz and Lucye (1966) failed to demonstrate the preventive effect of a stannous fluoride–lava pumice paste or a combination of the paste and topical application of an 8 per cent solution of stannous fluoride in a 2-year study using annual applications for children aged 8–10 years. Independent laboratory investigations by Vrbic et al. (1967) demonstrated minimal uptake of the fluoride ion by enamel from pastes of stannous fluoride–pumice, due to fluoride complexing. These results were confirmed by Melberg and Nicholson (1968) in further in vitro investigations. These workers also observed a rapid loss of available free fluoride ion with time, and an associated increase in pH to approximate neutrality when using this formulation.

A further abrasive system, zirconium silicate, was shown in clinical and laboratory studies to have superior cleaning properties to pumice and subsequent polishing of the tooth surface treated (Muhler et al., 1964; Stookey et al., 1966). Its superior reliability as an abrasive system was reported to be related to its action being self-limiting owing to particle size reduction during the period of application. Mellberg and Nicholson

(1968) found a smaller loss in available free fluoride and increase in pH when zirconium silicate was used in combination with stannous fluoride, as opposed to lava pumice.

In 1970 Muhler et al. published results of an investigation of annual self-application of a 9 per cent stannous fluoride–zirconium silicate prophylactic paste in children aged 6–14 years. The paste was applied with a soft toothbrush under supervision of a dentist. Results after 1 year reported a statistically significant reduction in caries increment for the test group of one surface per child despite large losses of subjects, particularly in the test group. Lang et al. (1970) reported reductions of 2 surfaces per child in 18 months with 6-monthly self-applications of the same formula for children aged 6–10 years living in an area with an optimum level of fluoride in the water. In contrast, Gunz (1971), using the same technique and formulation of prophylactic paste as Muhler et al. (1970), found no difference in caries increment between the test and control groups after one application. The examination was carried out 14 months after the application, but it is unlikely that the slightly greater length of time between application and re-examination explained the negative findings.

Mellberg and Nicholson (1968) considered further the problem of a compatible abrasive system. The results of their in vitro study suggested that an abrasive system of insoluble metaphosphate was not associated with any loss of free fluoride ions from the formula, nor any increase in pH values. Vrbic and Brudevold (1970) found this abrasive system removed significantly less enamel when used in a prophylactic paste. However, while it is less deleterious to the tooth surface than all the other abrasives tested, it is inadequate in practice for the removal of all exogenous tooth stains, and would necessitate the use of two pastes—one with a more abrasive quality for heavy stain removal, and an insoluble metaphosphate paste for routine use.

More recently, 3 studies testing the effectiveness of twice-yearly self-application of 9–10 per cent SnF_2 prophylactic paste have been published (Gish et al., 1975; Woodhouse, 1978 and Beiswanger et al., 1980). Each study lasted three years. While Gish et al. reported statistically significant reductions of 25 per cent (1·3 surfaces) for children living in a fluoridated area and 37 per cent (2·0 surfaces) for children living in a low fluoride area, the reductions in caries increment were lower (16 per cent reduction in DMFS) in the trial of Woodhouse, and no caries reduction was recorded by Beiswanger et al.

In 1969, 250 000 Californian schoolchildren began a school-based preventive programme which involved annual 'brush-ins' with 9 per cent SnF_2 (Zircate) prophylactic paste. The effectiveness of the programme was monitored by Horowitz and Bixler (1976) over a 3-year period. They state that 'the findings of this study are inconclusive and neither fully refute nor support the efficacy of annual self-application of a stannous–fluoride–zirconium silicate paste in preventing dental caries'. Zircate (9 per cent

SnF_2) paste has now been withdrawn from the market (Beiswanger et al., 1980).

3. PASTES CONTAINING ACIDULATED PHOSPHATE FLUORIDE

Following evidence documenting the efficacy of professionally applied acidulated phosphate fluoride in solution and gel forms, Peterson et al. (1969) conducted a 2-year study with children aged 11–13 years in a fluoridated and non-fluoridated community to determine the caries-inhibitory effectiveness of freshy prepared acidulated phosphate fluoride–lava pumice prophylactic paste applied annually. The active agent used was potassium fluoride dihydrate giving a concentration of 2·1 per cent fluoride ions. Two examiners independently examined the entire study population: both consistently found only slightly smaller caries increments in the treated groups than in the control groups in both communities. The differences between test and control groups were not statistically significant except those recorded by one examiner in the non-fluoride area only, who found a reduction of one surface per child in 2 years for the test group relative to the control group ($P < 0.05$). The authors suggested this minimal caries inhibition might be attributed to the neutralization of the acid phosphate fluoride reduction in the paste by the pumice abrasive.

In vitro studies by Mellberg and Nicholson (1968) to determine a stable formulation with good cleaning properties and fluoride deposition in enamel, found a formulation of silicone dioxide paste incorporating (in the liquid phase) 1·2 per cent fluoride ion and having a pH of 3·2 to be adequate. An investigation of this paste was reported by de Paola and Mellberg (1973). The paste was applied semi-annually by dental hygienists for children aged 10–13 years for 2 years. The teeth were given a thorough prophylaxis with a placebo paste prior to application of the fluoride paste which was applied and left for 4 minutes. The active ingredient in the paste was ammonium fluorosilicate giving 1·2 per cent fluoride, and 0·1 M phosphate from monobasic sodium phosphate. At the end of the first year significant reductions of half a surface of a tooth per child were observed in the test group, while at the end of 2 years a reduction of one surface per child was found. For teeth erupting during the study, a reduction in caries increment in the test group of half a surface per child over the 2-year period was reported.

The results of one year's use of the same ammonium silicofluoride (1·2 per cent F) paste (pH 3·0) were reported by Schutze et al. (1974). The subjects of the study were 3–5-year-old children living in fluoridated Baltimore attending a dental clinic for twice-yearly applications of the APF paste. A 9 per cent (0·14 surface) reduction was reported after 1 year.

Table 33. Clinical Trials of Prophylactic Pastes containing Fluoride

Investigators	Active ingredient	Abrasive system	pH	Duration (yrs)	Age	Application	Statistically significant reductions		
							Tooth surfaces	%	P
Bibby (1946)	1% NaF + H$_2$O$_2$	Pumice	4·0	1	(a) 6–15 (b) 6–14	(a) Semi-annual (b) 3 times/year	* *	25 42	* *
Bibby (1948)	,,			1	6–15	3 times/year	—	—	—
Gish and Muhler (1965)	8·9% SnF$_2$	Lava pumice	*	1	6–14	Annual	1–2	39–41	<0·0001
Bixler and Muhler (1966)	,,		*	3	5–18	Semi-annual	3–4	29–38	0·001
Horowitz and Lucye (1966)	,,		*	2	8–10	Annual	—	—	—
Peterson et al. (1963)	17·5% SnF$_2$	Silex		2		(a) Semi-annual (b) Annual	* *	42 34	* *
Scola and Ostrom (1968)	,,	Lava pumice	*	2	19–20	Semi-annual	—	—	—
Muhler et al. (1970)	9% SnF$_2$	Zirconium Silicate	*	1	6–14	Annual	1	64	<0·001
Lang et al. (1970) Gunz (1971)	,,			$1\frac{1}{2}$ $1\frac{1}{6}$	6–10	Semi-annual Annual	2 —	38–42 —	—
Peterson et al. (1969)	Potassium fluoride dihydrate (2·1% F) + 4·6% orthophosphoric acid	Lava pumice	*	2	11–13	Annual (a) Fluoride area (b) Non-fluoride area	(a) — (b) 1	— 21	— 0·05
De Paola and Mellberg (1973)	Ammonium fluorosilicate (1·2% F) + 0·1 M phosphate solution	Silica	3·2	2	10–13	Semi-annual	1	21	<0·01

* Data not given.

131

4. PASTES CONTAINING HEXAFLUOROZIRCONATE

Researchers at Indiana University developed a new compound, stannous hexafluorozirconate, which was reported to be effective in reducing the acid solubility of enamel and reducing dental caries. The original data from preliminary in vitro and laboratory experiments have not been published. Independent in vitro investigations of this compound by Shannon (1969) confirmed that hexafluorozirconate did reduce enamel solubility. Results of two preliminary investigations with children who received semi-annual topical applications of stannous hexafluorozirconate showed decided reduction in dental caries (Muhler et al., 1968). Concentrations of 16 and 24 per cent stannous hexafluorozirconate in solution with semi-annual applications showed a 16 per cent lower incidence of DMF surfaces for the latter concentration after 12 months. However, the number and magnitude of negative incremental caries scores that appear in the data are disconcerting. Results have not been substantiated by independent investigators.

Horowitz and Heifetz (1970) have reported toxic reactions after use of stannous hexafluorozirconate in a zirconium silicate prophylactic paste. Irritation and subsequent inflammation of the gingiva occurred, and in extreme cases frank necrosis of the soft tissue was produced (Peterson et al., 1967). Muhler et al. (1968) reported no toxic reactions in study participants with application of the same formula providing there was careful preparation of the solution, allowing complete dissolution of the compound to permit part of the tin to be chemically stabilized by forming complexes with zirconium. Muhler maintained that lack of care in preparation of stannous hexafluorozirconate gave a high concentration of tin in the paste, which was responsible for the adverse soft-tissue reactions.

Recently pilot studies of self-administration of stannous fluoride–zirconium silicate pastes in the USA as a public health measure have reported that 48 per cent of the children who treated themselves with the paste experienced disturbing systematic reactions, such as nausea, vomiting and headaches (Horowitz and Heifetz, 1970).

Controlled professional applications of prophylactic pastes have reported few toxic reactions. As with all topical applications of stannous fluoride, a prophylactic paste containing this compound was found to give transitory blanching and minor irritation of the gingivae in some studies, as well as a degree of staining of the teeth. As one of the major functions of a prophylactic paste is cleansing and stain removal, this latter side-effect detracted from the acceptability of this active ingredient, unless staining effects were modified. The results of the clinical trials with fluoride prophylactic pastes published to date (summarized in *Table* 33) have not established beyond doubt that 6-monthly or yearly prophylaxes with these agents result in caries inhibition.

REFERENCES

Beiswanger B. B., Mercer V. H., Billings R. J. and Stookey G. K. (1980) A clinical caries evaluation of a stannous fluoride prophylactic paste and solution. *J. Dent. Res.* **59**, 1386–1391.

Bibby B. G. (1948) Fluoride mouthwashes, fluoride dentifrices and other uses of fluorides in control of caries. *J. Dent. Res.* **27**, 367–373.

Bibby B. G., Zander H., Mckelleget M. and Labunsky B. (1946) Preliminary reports on the effects on dental caries of the use of sodium fluoride in a prophylactic cleaning mixture and in a mouthwash. *J. Dent. Res.* **25**, 207–211.

Bixler D. and Muhler J. C. (1966) Effect on dental caries in children in a nonfluoride area of combined use of three agents containing stannous fluoride: a prophylactic paste, a solution, and a dentifrice. II. Results after 24 and 36 months. *J. Am. Dent. Assoc.* **72**, 392–396.

De Paola P. F. and Mellberg J. R. (1973) Caries experience and fluoride uptake in children receiving semi-annual prophylaxis with an acidulated prophylaxis fluoride paste. *J. Am. Dent. Assoc.* **87**, 155–159.

Dudding N. J. and Muhler J. C. (1962) Technique of application of stannous fluoride in a compatible prophylactic paste and as a topical agent. *J. Dent. Child.* **24**, 219–224.

Gish C. W., Mercer V. H., Stookey G. K. and Dahl L. O. (1975) Self-application of fluoride as a community preventive measure: rationale, procedures and 3-year results. *J. Am. Dent. Assoc.* **90**, 388–397.

Gish C. W. and Muhler J. C. (1965) Effect on dental caries in children in a natural area of combined use of three agents containing stannous fluoride, a prophylactic paste, a solution and dentifrice. *J. Am. Dent. Assoc.* **70**, 914–920.

Gunz G. M. (1971) The effect of self-applied fluoride paste. *J. Public Health Dent.* **31**, 177–181.

Horowitz H. S. and Bixler D. (1976) The effect of SnF_2-$ZrSiO_4$ prophylactic paste on dental caries: Santa Clara County, Calif. *J. Am. Dent. Assoc.* **92**, 369–373.

Horowitz H. S. and Heifetz S. B. (1970) The current status of topical fluorides in preventive dentistry. *J. Am. Dent. Assoc.* **81**, 166–177.

Horowitz H. S. and Lucye H. S. (1966) A clinical study of stannous fluoride in a prophylaxis paste and as a solution. *J. Oral Ther.* **3**, 17–25.

Lang L. A., Thomas H. G., Taylor J. A. and Rothar R. E. (1970) Clinical efficacy of a self-applied stannous fluoride prophylactic paste. *J. Dent. Child.* **37**, 211–216.

Mellberg J. R. and Nicholson C. R. (1968) In vitro evaluation of an acidulated phosphate fluoride prophylaxis paste. *Arch. Oral Biol.* **13**, 1223–1234.

Mericle M. R. and Muhler J. C. (1963) Studies concerning the antisolubility effectiveness of different stannous fluoride prophylaxis paste mixtures. *J. Dent. Res.* **42**, 21–27.

Muhler J. C., Bixler D. and Stookey G. K. (1968) The clinical effectiveness of stannous hexafluorozirconate as an anticariogenic agent. *J. Am. Dent. Assoc.* **76**, 558–563.

Muhler J. C., Dudding N. J. and Stookey G. K. (1964) The clinical effectiveness of a particular size distribution of zirconium silicate for use as a cleaning and polishing agent for oral hard tissues. *J. Periodontol.* **35**, 481–485.

Muhler J. C., Kelley G. E., Stookey G. K., Linds F. I. and Harris N. O. (1970) The clinical evaluation of a patient-administered stannous fluoride hexafluorozirconate prophylactic paste on children. I. Results after one year in the Virgin Islands. *J. Am. Dent. Assoc.* **81**, 142–145.

Peterson J. K., Jordan W. A. and Snyder J. R. (1963) Effectiveness of stannous fluoride-silex-silicone prophylaxis paste: two year report. *Northwest Dent.* **42**, 276–278.

Peterson J. K., Horowitz H. S., Jordan W. A. and Pugnier V. (1967) Effectiveness of acidulated phosphate fluoride and stannous zirconium hexafluoride in prophylactic pastes. Abstracted International Association of Dental Research Programs and Abstracts of Papers, No. 277 (March).

Peterson J. K., Horowitz H. S., Jordan W. A. and Pugnier V. (1969) Effectiveness of an acidulated phosphate fluoride-pumice prophylactic paste: a two year report. *J. Dent. Res.* **48**, 346–350.

Schutz H. J., Forrester D. J. and Balis S. B. (1974) Evaluation of a fluoride prophylaxis paste in a fluoridated community. *J. Can. Dent. Assoc.* **40**, 675–683.

Scola F. P. and Ostrom C. A. (1968) Clinical evaluation of stannous fluoride when used as a constituent of a compatible prophylactic paste, as a topical solution and in a dentifrice in naval personnel, II. Report of findings after two years. *J. Am. Dent. Assoc.* **77**, 594–597.

Segreto V. A., Harris N. O. and Hester W. R. (1961) A stannous fluoride, silex, silicone dental prophylaxis paste with anticariogenic potentialities. *J. Dent. Res.* **40**, 90–96.

Shannon I. L. (1969) Stannous hexafluorozirconate and enamel solubility. *J. Dent. Child.* **36**, 175–180.

Stearns R. I. (1973) Incorporation of fluoride by human enamel, III. In vivo effects of non-fluoride and fluoride prophylactic pastes and APF gels. *J. Dent. Res.* **52**, 30–35.

Stookey G. K., Hudson J. R. and Muhler J. C. (1966) Studies concerning the polishing properties of zirconium silicate in enamel. *J. Periodontol.* **37**, 200–207.

Vrbic V. and Brudevold F. (1970) Fluoride uptake from treatment with different fluoride prophylaxis pastes and from the use of pastes containing soluble aluminium salt followed by a topical application. *Caries Res.* **4**, 158–167.

Vrbic V., Brudevold F. and McCann H. G. (1967) Acquisition of fluoride by enamel from fluoride pumice pastes. *Helv. Odontol. Acta* **11**, 21–26.

Whitehurst V. E., Stookey G. K. and Muhler J. C. (1968) Studies concerning the cleaning, polishing and therapeutic properties of commercial prophylactic pastes. *J. Oral Ther.* **4**, 181–191.

Wolf R. G. (1964) Effect of stannous fluoride prophylaxis paste on enamel solubility. *J. Dent. Res.* **43**, 168–174.

Woodhouse A. D. (1978) A longitudinal study of the effectiveness of self applied 10% stannous fluoride paste for secondary schoolchildren. *Austral. Dent. J.* **23**, 422–428.

CHAPTER 9

TOPICAL FLUORIDES AND DENTAL CARIES

Topical fluorides have been used as caries-preventive agents in dental practice for over 30 years. During this period four main types of preparations have been advocated: neutral sodium fluoride solutions, stannous fluoride solutions, acidulated phosphate fluoride agents, and varnishes containing fluoride. The aim of this chapter is to review the results of clinical trials concerning the effectiveness of the various fluoride agents in reducing the incidence of dental caries.

NEUTRAL SODIUM FLUORIDE SOLUTION

In 1940 Volker et al. showed that in vitro the solubility of enamel could be appreciably reduced by treating it with a fluoride solution. The first clinical study was started by Bibby in 1941 using a 0·1 per cent aqueous NaF solution. After prophylaxis and drying of teeth, applications for 7–8 minutes were made three times a year at 3–4-monthly intervals. One year later the caries increment in the experimental quadrant was 45 per cent lower than that found in the opposing control quadrant (Bibby, 1943).

In 1942 Knutson began a series of clinical trials using a different technique which required four visits within a short period. After prophylaxis and drying a 2 per cent aqueous NaF solution was applied for 3 minutes. Knutson concluded that maximum reduction in caries was achieved from four treatments at weekly intervals and suggested that the series of applications should be carried out at the ages of 3, 7, 10 and 13 years to coincide with the eruption of teeth (Knutson, 1948). A 2 per cent aqueous NaF solution has generally been used, although Galagan and Knutson (1948) showed that a 1 per cent NaF solution was equally effective. Many of the subsequent studies have followed Knutson's technique; nearly all reported a reduction in caries varying from 4·9 per cent (Jordan et al., 1959) to 58 per cent (Davies, 1950). A few reports (Arnold et al., 1944; Kutler and Ireland, 1953) produced negative findings but these studies were carried out on adults.

An important question to ask of the Knutson technique is whether the reduction in caries is only a short-term reduction of a year or so or whether it has a long-term preventive effect. In 1942 Knutson and Armstrong began a study involving children aged 7–15 years. The results after 3 years were published in 1946 and are summarized in *Table* 34. The percentage reduction in DF surfaces between study and control teeth was

Table 34. Results of a 3-year Study of 242 Children aged 7–15 Years treated with Sodium Fluoride
(Knutson and Armstrong, 1946)

Quadrant	No. of caries-free teeth (1942)	New DF teeth (1945)	DF surfaces in new DF teeth	DF surfaces in previous DF teeth	Total new DF surfaces	% difference* in DF surfaces
Treated	1870	214	287	216	503	32·8
Untreated	1888	338	464	284	748	

* The percentage difference between total new DF surfaces in treated and untreated quadrants has been calculated without reference to the total number of teeth treated.

Table 35. Results of a 3-year Study of 242 Children aged 7–15 Years treated with Sodium Fluoride
(Knutson and Armstrong, 1946)

Quadrant	Total no. of teeth	New DF teeth	Percentage new DF teeth*
Treated	2086	430	20·6
Untreated	2172	622	28·6

* The new DF teeth are expressed as percentages of the total number of teeth in treated and untreated quadrants.

33 per cent. However, the procedure of working out the percentage reduction between study and control quadrants does not take into account the total number of teeth involved. If the number of new carious teeth is given as a percentage of the total number of teeth present in treated and untreated quadrants (*Table* 35), the difference in caries incidence between treated and untreated teeth amounts to 8 per cent.

Sundvall-Hagland et al. (1959) studied the effectiveness of Knutson's technique on caries incidence in the deciduous dentition. Their findings after 3 years are given in *Table* 36, from which it will be seen that there was a marked fall-off in inhibition of caries. After 3 years the reduction in mean DMF surfaces increment between the control and experimental sides was 7·5 per cent. In contrast, Bergman (1953), in a study of 11–12-year-old children, concluded that caries inhibition on the treated side after 3 years was 43 per cent.

Table 36. Results of a 3-year Study of 102 Children aged $2\frac{1}{2}$ years treated with Sodium Fluoride (*Sundvall-Hagland et al., 1959*)

Period (yrs)	No. of children	Mean DMF surfaces increment on treated side	Mean DMF surfaces increment on control side	Percentage in DMF surfaces
1	107	4·6	5·7	19
2	104	7·5	8·7	14
3	102	9·9	10·7	7·5

STANNOUS FLUORIDE SOLUTION

In Vitro Studies

Buonocore and Bibby (1945) conducted a series of experiments to determine which fluoride salt was the most effective in reducing enamel solubility; they concluded that lead fluoride was appreciably more effective in reducing enamel solubility than was sodium fluoride. However, Muhler and van Huysen (1947) carried out in vitro studies of a similar nature using many different reagent solutions and concluded that tin fluoride was the most effective and that lead fluoride and sodium fluoride had about the same absorption qualities for enamel. Much of the work on stannous fluoride has been carried out by Muhler and his colleagues at the University of Indiana, following the finding that stannous fluoride in a concentration of 10 ppm in drinking water given to rats fed on a cariogenic diet was superior to 10 ppm of sodium fluoride in reducing caries (Muhler and Day, 1950). It was also claimed that stannous fluoride was three times more effective than sodium fluoride in preventing dissolution of calcium and phosphorus from enamel by dilute acids

(Muhler et al., 1950). Since that time, however, later work using the electron microscope has shown that stannous ions form a coating on the enamel surface (Scott, 1960); this coating has no protective action against the carious process and it has been suggested that stannous ions may actually reduce fluoride uptake (Brudevold et al., 1967).

Clinical Studies

The recommended procedure for application of stannous fluoride solution begins with a thorough prophylaxis and drying of the teeth. A freshly prepared 8 per cent solution of stannous fluoride is applied continuously to the teeth with cotton-wool so that the teeth are kept moist for 4 minutes. Gish et al. (1957) studied 554 7-year-olds in Montgomery County, Indiana. After 8 months children who had received one application of SnF_2 had an average DMF teeth increment of 0·60 compared with an average DMF teeth increment of 0·76 in children who had received four applications of 2 per cent NaF. This gave a 21 per cent difference, although in absolute terms a difference of 0·16 DMF teeth is clinically insignificant. However, Gish et al. (1957) considered that the results indicated a considerable advantage in using 8 per cent SnF_2 as only one treatment was required and this could be fitted in more conveniently with the patient's recall appointments. Over a 5-year period (1957–1962) Muhler, working with Gish and Howell, compared single, annual applications of 8 per cent SnF_2 with a series of four applications of 2 per cent NaF every 3 years. Over the 5-year period the caries increment in the SnF_2 group was approximately 35 per cent less than the increment in the NaF group. No control group was examined, although Gish et al. (1962) suggested that the caries increment in the SnF_2 group was 56 per cent lower than the 'national average' increment for the United States.

Other investigators have found stannous fluoride to be effective, although the percentage reductions reported have generally been less than that obtained by Muhler and his co-workers. On the other hand, some studies in America and Sweden have reported negative results. These studies are tabulated in *Table 37*.

The study by Houwink et al. (1974) involved 22 pairs of monozygotic twins. The teeth of one child were treated twice yearly with SnF_2 solution (yielding 1 per cent F) over a period of 9 years. When the children were 16 years old the result was that treated children had 37 per cent fewer lesions than the controls. Five years after the last application 18 pairs were examined once more. In 3 pairs the controls had received full dentures. The caries experience of the remaining 15 pairs is summarized in *Table 38*. Although during the period without treatment the study group had a very slightly higher mean annual increment than the control group, the effect of the 9 years' treatment was still apparent 5 years after treatment had stopped. The increment over the 14-year period was still 23·8 per cent

Table 37. Comparison of the Results of Stannous Fluoride Studies

Author	Study period (yrs)	Reduction in DMF surfaces (%)
Compton et al. (1959)	1	28
Jordan et al. (1959)	2	38
Law et al. (1961)	1	24
Mercer and Muhler (1961)	1	51
Burgess et al. (1962)	2	29
Harris (1963)	1	23
Torell (1965)	1	None
Wellock et al. (1965)	1	None
Horowitz and Lucye (1966)	2	None
Houwink et al. (1974)	9	37

lower in the study group than in the control. Thus, there is a divergence of opinion as to the effectiveness of stannous fluoride as a caries-preventive agent. A disadvantage of stannous fluoride is that it causes brown pigmentation of teeth, particularly in hypocalcified areas and around margins of restorations. It can also cause gingival irritation. Because stannous fluoride is unstable in aqueous solution it has to be freshly prepared for each treatment.

ACIDULATED PHOSPHATE AGENTS

In Vitro Studies

As far back as 1947 Bibby reported that as the pH of the solution was lowered fluoride was absorbed into enamel more effectively. Brudevold et al. (1963) studied the effect of prolonged exposure of enamel to sodium fluoride in acid sodium phosphate solutions. They concluded that the fluoride concentration in enamel increased with decrease in the pH of the solution. Mellberg (1966) reported that after a 10-minute exposure of a cut tooth section to an acid phosphate fluoride solution there was a high fluoride concentration in the inner layers of enamel.

Clinical Studies

Acidulated phosphate solutions, containing 1·23 per cent available fluoride in 0·1 M phosphoric acid at pH 2·8, are applied in a similar manner to stannous fluoride solution. The first clinical trial was started in 1961 by Wellock and Brudevold (1963). After 2 years children in the study group had approximately 66 per cent fewer carious surfaces than children in the control group. Bitewing radiographs were used to aid diagnoses.

Table 38. DFS Increment in 15 Pairs of Monozygotic Children during SnF$_2$ Treatment (1957–1966) and during 5 years without Treatment (1966–1971) (Houwink et al., 1974)

	Period with treatment		Period without treatment		Total DFS 1957–1971	
	Mean DFS	Mean DFS/year	Mean DFS	Mean DFS/year	Total	Mean DFS/year
Study	14·8	1·6	12·7	2·5	27·5	2·0
Control	24·6	2·7	11·5	2·3	36·1	2·6

Table 39. Results of Two 1-year Studies of APF Gels

Authors	Age of children (yrs)		No. of children	DMF teeth increment	Percentage reduction in DMF teeth
Szwejda et al. (1967)	7	Test	182	0·67	—
		Control	188	0·65	
Bryan and Williams (1968)	8–11	Test	121	0·93	45·0
		Control	122	1·69	

140

Parmeijer et al. (1963), in a study of 77 children aged 4–10 years, compared the effectiveness of a solution of neutral sodium fluoride with an acidulated phosphate fluoride (APF) solution used on opposite sides of the mouth. On the right side (APF) 45 new DMF surfaces were recorded, whereas on the left side (NaF) 92 new surfaces were found; it was therefore concluded that APF was 50 per cent more effective than neutral NaF as a caries-preventive agent. Further studies (Wellock et al., 1965; Cartwright et al., 1968) have reported reductions of 44–49 per cent in new DMF teeth in children given annual or bi-annual applications of APF solution compared with control groups receiving treatment with tap water only.

One of the problems of carrying out the topical fluoride applications so far described is that the teeth must be kept moist for 4 minutes, which means that the solution must be applied with cotton-wool to each tooth approximately every 30 seconds. To overcome this problem workers experimented with wax or plastic trays in which blotting paper soaked in the solution could be applied to the teeth which would then be continuously surrounded by the fluoride agent. Other workers introduced a gelling agent (usually methyl cellulose or hydroxyethyl cellulose) which removed the need for the blotting-paper inserts. The disadvantage of using trays is that one can never be absolutely sure that all the surfaces of the teeth, particularly the approximal areas, have been completely covered by the fluoride agent. Gentle pressure should be maintained on the tray to force the gel approximally. The gels are thixotropic, that is they convert to a sol and flow more easily under pressure.

Szwejda et al. (1967) carried out the first published clinical trial of APF gels on 7-year-old children. They observed no reduction in caries increment after one year. In contrast, Bryan and Williams (1968) reported a 45 per cent reduction in DMF teeth after a single application of APF gel in foam rubber trays. The results of these two studies are summarized in *Table* 39. Ingraham and Williams (1970) carried out a 2-year study to compare the effectiveness of APF solutions and gels in reducing caries experience. Their results are shown in *Table* 40. It was concluded that the greatest reduction in caries experience occurred using the APF gels (over 50 per cent); the APF solutions were approximately only half as effective as the gels. However, one of the aspects of this study which makes it rather difficult to interpret is the difference between the groups in baseline DMF teeth values. Although the authors state that there was no statistical difference between the groups at the start of the study, *Table* 40 indicates that there was a 0·44 difference between groups 2 and 4A in the baseline DMF teeth values.

The largest APF study so far carried out is that by Horowitz and Doyle (1971). After 3 years a total of 681 Hawaiian children aged 10–12 years had taken part continuously in the study. A summary of the results is given in *Table* 41. The greatest reduction in caries increment was obtained with the APF solutions rather than the APF gels, in contrast to the

Table 40. Results of 2-year Study of 238 Children aged 6–11 Years treated with APF Agents (*Ingraham and Williams, 1970*)

Description of group	No. of children	Baseline DMF teeth	Percentage difference in baseline DMF teeth (from 4A)	DMF teeth increment	Percentage reduction in DMF teeth
1. Prophylaxis only	63	1·49	31	1·76	—
2. APF solution on cotton-wool	57	1·58	39	1·44	18·2
3. APF solutions in trays with paper inserts	62	1·27	11	1·34	23·9
4A. APF gel in bees-wax trays	28	1·14	—	0·86	51·1
4B. APF gel in foam rubber trays	28	1·43	25	0·82	53·4
4. A + B	56	1·29	13	0·84	52·3

Table 41. Results of 3-year Study of 681 Children aged 10–12 Years treated with APF Agents (*Horowitz and Doyle, 1971*)

Description of group	No. in group	Baseline DMF teeth	DMF teeth increment	Percentage reduction in DMF teeth after 3 years
1. Control: annual prophylaxis only	170	5·15	3·62	—
2. Annual prophylaxis plus APF gel	182	4·96	3·06	15·6
3. Annual prophylaxis plus APF solution	167	5·05	2·68	26·8
4. Bi-annual prophylaxis plus APF solution	162	4·93	2·24	40·3

findings of Ingraham and Williams (1970). The caries increment in the gel group was 15 per cent lower than that in the control group which was not statistically significant. In absolute terms this meant a difference in DMF teeth increment of 0·6 teeth over a 3-year period, or a caries prevention of 0·2 teeth per person per year. The results for the APF solutions were more favourable; a bi-annual prophylaxis and APF solution application achieved a 40 per cent reduction compared with that in the children in the control group who received an annual prophylaxis only. However, Horowitz (1969), in a discussion of the findings after 2 years, suggested that the extra work involved in carrying out 6-monthly applications may not be justified in terms of the extra caries reduction achieved. He reported that it would be necessary to treat approximately 6 children with the solution twice a year rather than once a year to prevent one more decayed tooth or surface. As each prophylaxis and application took approximately 30 minutes this means that one dentist or dental hygienist would have to work 3 extra hours a year to prevent one more decayed tooth or surface among 6 children.

The study by Horowitz and Doyle (1971) involved a large number of children from Hawaii, was meticulously reported, and lasted for a longer period of time than any previous topical fluoride study so far published. However, one aspect of the procedure which may have influenced the results was that after the prophylaxis and prior to the fluoride application the teeth were not thoroughly dried with cotton-wool or air; instead the gel was applied to the teeth in wax trays after the children had removed as much saliva as they could from their mouths by rapid inspiration of air through clenched teeth. Initially this investigation involved approximately 1100 children aged 10–12 at the start of the study. By the third year the number of children who had been seen at each yearly examination had fallen to 681. Although the fluoride applications ceased at the end of the third year a further series of examinations was carried out in 397 children $2\frac{1}{2}$–3 years after the last fluoride treatment had been given in order to measure the long-term caries-preventive effect of APF agents. It was concluded that there was only a slight fall-off in caries protection throughout the post-treatment period (Horowitz et al., 1971). This is the only study so far reported which has attempted to measure the long-term effect of APF agents applied topically either annually or semi-annually.

On the other hand, two studies have reported that application of aqueous NaF, acidulated APF or stannous fluoride produced insignificant reductions in caries increments compared with control groups. Averill et al. (1967), in a 2-year study in Rochester, New York, compared the caries-preventive effect of a 2 per cent aqueous sodium fluoride solution, a 4 per cent stannous fluoride solution and a 2 per cent acidulated phosphate-buffered sodium fluoride solution (pH 4·4) used for topical application in 483 children initially aged 7–11 years old. Each agent was applied twice yearly. Children in the control group received topical applications of distilled water flavoured with wintergreen. The DMFS increment over the 2-year period was 4·4 in the control group, 3·9 in the aqueous NaF group, 4·1 in the SnF_2 group and 4·5 in the APF group.

Similar findings were reported by Cons et al. (1970), who carried out a 3-year study on 1948 7–8-year-old children from Albany, New York. The children were divided into five groups. Children in the control group had distilled water applied for 30 seconds; those in the stannous fluoride group had 8 per cent SnF_2 applied for 4 minutes. Two APF agents were used, a solution and a gel; both contained 1·23 per cent NaF at pH 3 in 0·1 M phosphoric acid and were applied for 4 minutes. All these children first received a prophylaxis with pumice, the teeth were then dried with compressed air and isolated cotton-wool holders and salivary ejectors. The agent was applied annually and after treatment the children were asked to avoid eating, drinking or rinsing for 30 minutes. Children in the fifth group received a prophylaxis and then one series of four applications of 2 per cent aqueous sodium fluoride after the method described by Knutson. At the end of the third year 1412 children remained in the study. The results (*Table* 42) showed that, for DMF teeth only the differences between gel and control groups were statistically significant (P < 0·05), but the magnitude of the difference was less than 0·5 teeth per child, over the 3-year period. None of the treated groups differed significantly from the control when DMFS increments for first permanent molars were compared (*Fig.* 18). The authors concluded that, considering their own results, together with a large number of other reports on topical fluoride, it was obvious that the mechanism by which topical fluoride retards cavitation is not yet fully understood. They suggested that additional laboratory and

Table 42. Number of Children, Mean Net Increment and Difference from Control by Group for Permanent Teeth and First Molar Surfaces, over a 3-year Period (*Cons et al., 1970*)

Group	No.	Increment	Difference	P
Teeth				
Control	311	1·99	—	—
NaF	270	1·66	0·33	*
SnF_2	273	1·83	0·16	*
APF sol.	280	1·66	0·33	*
APF gel	278	1·50	0·49	<0·05
First Permanent Molar Surfaces				
Control	311	3·82	—	—
NaF	270	3·41	0·41	*
SnF_2	273	3·52	0·30	*
APF sol.	280	3·88	−0·06	*
APF gel	278	3·14	0·68	*

*P > 0·05.

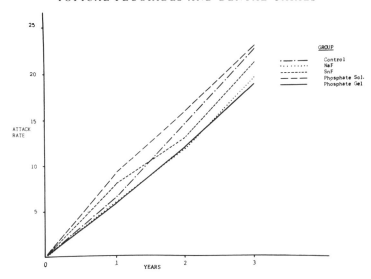

Fig. 18. Per cent number of first permanent molar surfaces affected by caries over a 3-year period. (From Cons et al., 1970.) (*Copyright by the American Dental Association. Reprinted by permission.*)

clinical research would be necessary to establish the superiority of any given fluoride preparation and the scheduling of topical applications. This conclusion is in accord with that reached by Horowitz and Heifetz (1970), who remarked that the results of the various studies using acidulated phosphate fluoride agents show that it can reduce the incidence of dental caries. However, further long-term studies are needed to determine the exact degree of caries reduction conferred by these agents and the best method and frequency of applying them. APF agents are stable in plastic containers and cause no tooth discoloration or gingival irritation.

FLUORIDE VARNISHES

In recent years varnishes incorporating fluoride have been produced in an attempt to maintain the fluoride ion in intimate contact with the enamel surface for a longer period of time than is achieved by APF agents. Finally, three materials have been used in clinical trials: Duraphat, Elmex Protector and Epoxylite 9070.

Fluoride lacquer, or Duraphat, was first used by Heuser and Schmidt (1968). This fluoride varnish yields 2·26 per cent F^- from a suspension of sodium fluoride in an alcoholic solution of natural varnish substances. The manufacturers claim that it is remarkably water tolerant, so that it covers even moist teeth with a well-adhering film of varnish. Riethe and Weinmann (1970), using 75 Osborne–Mendel rats, reported that both Duraphat and an amine fluoride gel showed similar short-term caries-inhibitory properties in rats. Amine fluoride 297, similar to that used in Reithe and Weinmann's study, had a self-polymerizing polyurethane varnish added to it and was marketed under the name of Elmex Protector. Although amine fluoride has been shown to have caries-inhibitory properties when incorporated in a toothpaste (Marthaler, 1968), no large-scale clinical studies have been carried out to determine whether Elmex Protector has a caries-preventive effect. Rock (1974), in a 2-year study involving 100 children aged 11–13 years, concluded that this material was ineffective as a caries-preventive agent; after 2 years 19·3 per cent of test teeth and 20·5 per cent of control teeth became carious.

Epoxylite 9070 has been described as a long-lasting topical fluoride coating. The type of fluoride used in this preparation is disodium monofluorophosphate, which is incorporated into a soft, flexible, polyurethane-based adhesive coating. Before the Epoxylite 9070 coating is applied, a normal prophylaxis is carried out and then the tooth surfaces should be cleaned with an acid-based cleanser, Epoxylite Cavity Cleanser 9070-C. Although it has been claimed that Epoxylite 9070 has shown a reduction in caries of laboratory rats of up to 60 per cent (Lee et al., 1972), Rock (1972), in a 1-year study of 11–13-year-old children, reported that Epoxylite 9070 produced no significant reduction in the incidence of occlusal caries between test and control group.

Following the early work on Duraphat by Heuser and Schmidt (1968), the clinical potential of this material has been tested in two main ways. The fluoride content of surface enamel after topical application of Duraphat has been measured in vitro and in vivo, and the inhibition of caries in children taking part in clinical trials where Duraphat has been applied annually or semi-annually has been assessed.

In an in vitro study, Koch and Peterson (1972) measured the uptake of fluoride by enamel treated with Duraphat for 1–12 hours, using 20 non-carious premolars extracted for orthodontic reasons. The highest concentrations of fluoride were found in the outermost layer. In the experimental group the mean concentration in this layer ranged between 3800 and 2250 ppm F compared with about 1150 ppm F for the control group. After exposure of the enamel to the varnish for 6–12 hours, the concentrations in all the layers down to a depth of 80 μm were significantly higher than the corresponding values in the control parts.

In a further in vitro study, fluoride concentrations in deciduous enamel were determined after a single application of Duraphat (Edenholm. et al., 1977). Eight deciduous teeth were tested: each one was sectioned vertically to give a test and control part. The test parts were exposed for 24 hours to the fluoride varnish. Three teeth were then analysed for fluoride content immediately and 5 were stored for 1 week in synthetic saliva to study the fluoride leakage. After 24 hours' exposure to Duraphat, an increase in enamel F concentration of about 5000 ppm F had taken place in the outermost 3–4-micron enamel layer, although the increase in the inner-most enamel layer studied (a depth of about 20 microns) showed an increase of only about 1500 ppm F. After storing for 1 week in synthetic saliva, a high fluoride leakage was reported, about half the fluoride uptake had been washed away from the outermost layer, and at a depth of about 15 microns no difference between study and control groups was reported.

Bang and Kim (1973) reported their findings for 19 adults who required the extraction of non-carious teeth. The varnish was applied to the tooth surface in vivo and the teeth were extracted 1 week later. A tooth which had been extracted from the same subject prior to topical treatment served as a control. Using an electron microprobe they showed that the fluoride content of surface enamel was significantly higher in the treated teeth compared with the control teeth. Furthermore, using X-ray and electron diffraction techniques, calcium fluoride could not be detected in surface enamel of treated teeth, suggesting that most of the fluoride in the enamel surfaces was probably in the form of fluorapatite, although absorption and mechanical bonding, particularly in roughened enamel surfaces, could also account for some of the fluoride detected by the electron probe.

Petersson (1975) used an acid-etch technique and assessed the fluoride content in enamel of 58 pairs of homologous teeth extracted after being treated in vivo by a variety of topical fluorides. The highest F uptake (< 1250 ppm) occurred after Duraphat varnish had been applied 3 times at weekly intervals. A substantial penetration of fluorine to about 100 μm was observed. Using an ion probe technique, Petersson (1975) showed that fluorine taken up from varnish appeared to be gradually lost from the outermost enamel, but was more permanently retained at depths in excess of about 0·3 μm.

Stamm (1974) went one stage further and measured fluoride uptake by an in vivo enamel biopsy method and a half-mouth technique. The teeth were cleaned and Duraphat was applied to right or left maxillary teeth in 35 subjects. The untreated teeth served as a control. After 5 weeks, the outer 8–12-μm layer of enamel was removed by an in vivo enamel biopsy of both the treatment and the control teeth. The results indicated that the outer enamel of teeth treated with the fluoride varnish contained a mean fluoride level of 1203 ppm compared with the mean fluoride level in the control teeth of 612 ppm.

Heuser and Schmidt (1968) treated 224 children aged 13–14 years and reported a 30 per cent reduction in the incidence of caries 15 months after a single administration of Duraphat, compared with the caries increment in 163 untreated controls. A contrary result was reported by Maiwald and Geiger (1973) who tested the same material in 179 children aged 11 years; 174 children of similar age acted as a control. After 23 months they reported that the varnish had no effect on caries incidence if applied once a year, but obtained a reduction of 45 per cent when used every 4 months.

Hetzer and Irmisch (1973) determined the effect of five applications of Duraphat over a 3-year period on 72 children aged $9\frac{1}{2}$ years (group 1) and 67 children aged $10\frac{1}{2}$ years (group 2), with 137 children of comparable ages acting as controls. The children in the test group were given oral hygiene instruction and parental involvement was encouraged. Children brushed their own teeth before being treated at the local clinic; in this way 35 children were treated in 60–70 minutes. It is not known whether bitewing radiographs were taken. In group 1 there was an 18 per cent reduction in DMFS scores over untreated controls (5·0 DMFS as against 6·1 DMFS) and in group 2 a 43 per cent reduction in DMFS scores was reported (4·3 as against 7·6).

Koch and Petersson (1975) studied the effect of semi-annual applications of Duraphat to the teeth of 60 15-year-old children over a period of 1 year. Sixty-two children of similar age acted as a control group. All these children were exposed to the local dental health programme of mouth rinsing with 0·2 per cent NaF solution every 2 weeks. Before the varnish was applied all teeth were cleaned with pumice and rubber cup and the approximal surfaces were also cleaned with dental floss and toothpicks. A clinical and radiographic examination of all children was performed immediately prior to the first application of varnish and repeated 1 year later. In the test group, the mean DMFS score was 31·0 at baseline and this increased to 31·9 at the first-year examination. The baseline score for the control group (27·4) was lower than for the test group, but increased to 31·3 by the end of the first year. The mean percentage reduction in caries increment was approximately 75 per cent. The percentage reduction on occlusal surfaces was similar to that recorded on approximal and free smooth surfaces. The authors suggested that the excellent effects on the occlusal surfaces might be the result of the adhesiveness of the varnish and concluded that the short time needed for application, and the low application frequency, make the varnish practical as a preventive measure.

The speed and ease with which Duraphat can be applied suggests that it may have a place in the prevention of caries in primary and first permanent molar teeth, although the clinical trials so far reported have concerned children aged 9–15 years.

A recent study (Murray et al., 1977) measured the caries-inhibitory effect of applying Duraphat every 6 months for 2 years to the teeth of 5-year-old children attending 9 schools. A half-mouth technique was used involving two varnishes supplied by the manufacturers. In 5 schools varnish A was applied to the left molars and varnish B to the right molars. In the remaining 4 schools varnish B was applied to the left side and varnish A applied to the right side. After the clinical examinations had been completed the code was broken: varnish A was Duraphat (23 000 ppm F) and varnish B was the placebo (less than 12 ppm F).

Over the 2-year trial period 694 new dmf surfaces were recorded on deciduous molars treated with the placebo compared with 643 new dmf surfaces on teeth treated with Duraphat, a reduction of 7·4 per cent. In addition 124 surfaces were affected on first permanent molars treated with the placebo compared with 80 carious surfaces on teeth coated with Duraphat—a reduction of 37 per cent.

COMBINATIONS OF TOPICAL FLUORIDE THERAPY

Combinations of fluoride toothpaste with mouthrinses (Ashley et al., 1977; Triol et al., 1980) and topical gel applications (Lind et al., 1976; Luoma et al., 1978; Mainwaring and Naylor, 1978) have been investigated. The effect on 2-year dental caries increment of an 0·02 per cent APF rinse (100 ppm F$^-$) (Ashley et al., 1977) and a sodium monofluorophosphate toothpaste (0·76 per cent MFP, yielding 1000 ppm F$^-$) was assessed, both alone and in combination, in a double-blind controlled clinical trial in a low-fluoride community. Although the greatest reduction in caries (27 per cent, 1·5 DFS/child) occurred in the group receiving both fluoride toothpaste and fluoride rinse, there was no statistical difference among the three experimental groups (fluoride toothpaste alone showed a saving of 1·2 DFS/child and fluoride mouthrinses alone gave a saving of 0·8 DFS/child over the 2-year period).

A 2½-year trial involving the use of an MFP toothpaste in combination with a range of mouthrinses containing 0, 0·025, 0·05 or 0·1 per cent sodium fluoride concluded that there was an additive effect (Triol et al., 1980). The greatest reduction occurred with the most concentrated fluoride rinse, but the difference among the three fluoride mouthrinsing groups was not statistically significant.

Two 3-year studies concluded that the unsupervised use of Na MFP toothpaste was as effective in reducing caries as twice annual, professionally applied, treatments of APF gel. Further, the reductions in caries obtained by the combined use of fluoride toothpaste and gel applications were not significantly greater than the use of fluoride toothpaste or gel applications alone (Lind et al., 1976; Mainwaring and Naylor, 1978). In contrast a 2-year study, involving the use of stannous fluoride alone, annual APF application alone and both treatments in combination (but no placebo group), concluded that there was no difference between the single therapy groups, but that the combined therapy produced significantly less caries and therefore had an additive effect (Luoma et al., 1978). All these studies were carried out in low-fluoride areas.

Horowitz (1980) gave information on studies conducted by the National Institute of Dental Research into combinations of fluoride procedures. One study concerned a combination of APF gel self-application and NaF fluoride rinsing in a fluoride area. The children in the test group applied APF gel (1·23 per cent F) in custom-fitted trays on 5 consecutive days, three times during the first year of the study—a total of 15 gel-tray treatments. In addition they rinsed for 1 minute once a week in school for 3 school years with a 0·2 per cent NaF solution. Children in the control group engaged only in mouthrinsing with a placebo solution (Heifetz et al., 1979). After 30 months 131 children in the test group had developed 30 per cent fewer DMF surfaces, in teeth present in the mouth at the time of the baseline examination, than 135 children in the control group. It was concluded that although the gel-tray procedure used was expensive and may lack economic practicality, the findings of the study corroborate the effectiveness of self-administered topical fluoride procedures in an optimally fluoridated community.

Horowitz (1980) concluded that 'there is increasing evidence that various combinations of fluoride agents produce additive anticariogenic effects. In order to achieve maximal caries protection additional studies should be done to determine other effective combinations of fluoride and to verify the effects of those that have already been tested. It is also important to learn the contribution of the various components of the combinations to the total cariogenic effect.' It must be borne in mind that as sales of fluoride toothpastes presently comprise 80 per cent of total toothpaste sales in the United States and over 95 per cent in the United Kingdom, all current studies of various fluoride combinations inherently represent evaluations of combined fluoride therapies, assuming that the participants continue to use a dentifrice of their choice.

REFERENCES

Arnold F. A. jun., Dean H. T. and Singleton D. W. jun. (1944) Effect on caries incidence of a single topical application of a fluoride solution to the teeth of young adult males of a military population. *J. Dent. Res.* **23**, 155.

Ashley F. P., Mainwaring P. J., Emslie R. D. and Naylor M. N. (1977) Clinical testing of a mouthrinse and a dentifrice containing fluoride. *Br. Dent. J.* **143**, 333–338.

Averill H. M., Averill J. E. and Ritz A. G. (1967) A two year comparison of three topical fluoride agents. *J. Am. Dent. Assoc.* **74**, 996–1001.

Bang S. and Kim Y. J. (1973) Electron microprobe analysis of human tooth enamel coated in vivo with fluoride-varnish. *Helv. Odontol. Acta* **17**, 84–88.

Bergman G. (1953) The caries inhibiting action of sodium fluoride. Experimental studies *Acta Odontol. Scand.* **11**, Suppl. 12.

Bibby B. G. (1943) The effect of sodium fluoride applications on dental caries. *J. Dent. Res.* **22**, 207.

Bibby B. G. (1947) A consideration of the effectiveness of various fluoride mixtures. *J. Am. Dent. Assoc.* **34**, 26.

Brudevold F., McCann H. G., Nilsson R., Richardson B. and Coklica V. (1967) The chemistry of caries inhibition problems and challenges in topical treatments. *J. Dent. Res.* **46**, 37.

Brudevold F., Savory A., Gardner D. E., Spinelli M. and Speirs R. (1963) A study of acidulated fluoride solutions I. In vitro effects on enamel. *Arch. Oral Biol.* **8**, 167.

Bryan E. T. and Williams J. E. (1968) The cariostatic effectiveness of a phosphate-fluoride gel administered annually to schoolchildren. *J. Public Health Dent.* **28**, 182.

Buonocore M. G. and Bibby B. G. (1945) Effects of various ions on enamel solubility. *J. Dent. Res.* **24**, 103.

Burgess R. C., Mondrow T. G., Nikiforuk G. and Compton F. H. (1962) Topical stannous fluoride as a caries preventative for pre-school children. *J. Can. Dent. Assoc.* **28**, 312.

Cartwright H. V., Lindahl R. L. and Bawden J. W. (1968) Clinical findings on the effectiveness of stannous fluoride and acid phosphate fluoride as caries reducing agents in children. *J. Dent. Child.* **35**, 36.

Compton F. H., Burgess R. C., Mondrow T. G., Grainger R. M. and Nikiforuk G. (1959) The Riverdale pre-school dental project. *J. Can. Dent. Assoc.* **25**, 478.

Cons N. C., Janerich D. T. and Senning R. S. (1970) Albany topical fluoride study. *J. Am. Dent. Assoc.* **80**, 777–781.

Davies G. N. (1950) Dental caries control and the general practitioner. *N.Z. Dent. J.* **46**, 25.

Galagan D. J. and Knutson H. W. (1948) Effect of topically applied fluoride on dental caries experience, VI. Experiments with sodium fluoride and calcium chloride; widely spaced applications; use of different solution concentrations. *Public Health Rep.* **63**, 1215.

Gish C. W., Howell C. L. and Muhler J. C. (1957) A new approach to the topical application of fluorides for the reduction of dental caries in children. *J. Dent. Res.* **36**, 784.

Gish C. W., Muhler J. C. and Howell C. L. (1962) A new approach to the topical application of fluorides for the reduction of dental caries in children. Results at the end of five years. *J. Dent. Child.* **29**, 65.

Harris R. (1963) Observations on the effect of eight per cent stannous fluoride on dental caries in children. *Aust. Dent. J.* **8**, 335.

Heifetz S. B., Franchi G. J. Mosley G. W. et al. (1979) Combined anticariogenic effect of fluoride gel-trays and fluoride mouthrinsing in an optimally fluoridated community. *Clin. Prev. Dent.* **1**, 21–3, 28.

Hetzer G. and Irmisch B. (1973) Kariesprotektion durch Fluorlack (Duraphat)—Klinische ergebnisse und erfahrungen. *Dtsch. Stomatol.* **23**, 917–922.

Heuser H. and Schmidt H. F. M. (1968) Deep impregnation of dental enamel with a fluorine lacquer for prophylaxis of dental caries. *Stoma* **2**, 91.

Horowitz H. S. (1969) Effect on dental caries of topically applied acidulated phosphate-fluoride: results after two years. *J. Am. Dent. Assoc.* **78**, 568.

Horowitz H. S. (1980) Established methods of prevention. *Br. Dent. J.* **149**, 311–318.

Horowitz H. S. and Doyle J. (1971) The effect on dental caries of topically applied acidulated phosphate-fluoride: results after 3 years. *J. Am. Dent. Assoc.* **81**, 166.

Horowitz H. S. and Heifetz S. B. (1970) The current status of topical fluorides in preventive dentistry. *J. Am. Dent. Assoc.* **81**, 166.

Horowitz H. S. and Lucye H. S. (1966) A clinical study of stannous fluoride in a prophylaxis paste and as a solution. *J. Oral Ther. Pharmacol.* **3**, 17.

Horowitz H. S., Doyle J. and Kan M. C. W. (1971) Retained anti-caries protection from topically applied acidulated phosphate fluoride: 30 and 36 month post treatment effects. IADR Abstr. **213**, No. 642.

Houwink B., Backer Dirks O. and Kwant G. W. (1974) A nine year study of topical applications with stannous fluoride in identical twins and the caries experience five years after ending the applications. *Caries Res.* **8**, 27.

Ingraham R. Q. and Williams J. E. (1970) An evaluation of the utility of application and cariostatic effectiveness of phosphate-fluorides in solution and gel states. *J. Tenn. Dent. Assoc.* **50**, 5.

Jordan W. A., Snyder J. R. and Wilson V. (1959) A study of a single application of eight per cent stannous fluoride. *J. Dent. Child.* **26**, 355.

Jordan W. A., Wood O. B., Allison J. A. and Irwin V. D. (1946) Effects of various numbers of topical applications of sodium fluoride. *J. Am. Dent. Assoc.* **33**, 1385.

Knutson J. W. (1948) Sodium fluoride solutions: technic for application to the teeth. *J. Am. Dent. Assoc.* **36**, 37.

Knutson J. W. and Armstrong W. D. (1946) The effect of topically applied sodium fluoride on dental caries experience. III. Report of findings for the third study year. *Public Health Rep.* **61**, 1683.

Koch G. and Petersson L. G. (1972) Fluoride content of enamel surface treated with a varnish containing sodium fluoride. *Odont. Revy* **23**, 437.

Koch G. and Petersson L. G. (1975) Caries preventive effect of a fluoride-containing varnish (Duraphat) after 1 year's study. *Community Dent. Oral Epidemiol.* **3**, 262–266.

Kutler B. and Ireland R. L. (1953) Effect of sodium fluoride application on the dental caries experience in adults. *J. Dent. Res.* **32**, 458.

Law F. E., Jeffreys M. H. and Sheary H. C. (1961) Topical applications of fluoride solutions in dental caries control. *Public Health Rep.* **76**, 287.

Lee H., Ocumpaugh D. E. and Swartz M. L. (1972) Sealing of developmental pits and fissures, II. Fluoride release from flexible fissure sealers. *J. Dent. Res.* **51**, 183.

Lind O. P., Möller I. J., Fehr F. R. von der and Larsen M. J. (1974) Caries preventive effect of a dentifrice containing 2 per cent sodium monofluorophosphate in a natural fluoride area in Denmark. *Community Dent. Oral Epidemiol.* **2**, 104–113.

Luoma H., Murtomaa H., Nuuja T. et al. (1978) A simultaneous reduction of caries and gingivitis in a group of schoolchildren receiving chlorhexidine-fluoride applications: results after 2 years. *Caries Res.* **12**, 290–298.

Mainwaring P. J. and Naylor M. N. (1978) A three year study to determine the separate and combined caries-inhibiting effects of sodium monofluorophosphate toothpaste and an acidulated phosphate-fluoride gel. *Caries Res.* **12**, 202–212.

Maiwald J. H. and Geiger L. (1973) Topical application of a fluoride protective varnish for caries prophylaxis. *Dtsch. Stomatol.* **23**, 56.

Marthaler T. M. (1968) Caries inhibition after seven years of unsupervised use of an amine fluoride dentifrice. *Br. Dent. J.* **124**, 510.

Mellberg J. R. (1966) Fluoride uptake by intact human tooth enamel from acidulated fluoride phosphate preparations. *J. Dent. Res.* **45**, 303.

Mercer V. H. and Muhler J. C. (1961) Comparison of a single application of stannous fluoride with a single application of sodium fluoride or two applications of stannous fluoride. *J. Dent. Child.* **28**, 84.

Muhler J. C. and Day H. C. (1950) Effects of SnF_2, NaF on incidence of dental lesions in rats fed caries producing diets. *J. Am. Dent. Assoc.* **41**, 528.

Muhler J. C. and van Huysen G. (1947) Solubility of enamel protected by sodium fluoride and other compounds. *J. Dent. Res.* **26**, 119.

Muhler J. C., Boyd T. M. and van Huysen G. (1950) Effect of fluorides and other compounds on the solubility of enamel, dentine and tri-calcium phosphate. *J. Dent. Res.* **29**, 182.

Murray J. J., Winter G. B. and Hurst C. P. (1977) Duraphat fluoride varnish: a 2-year clinical trial in 5-year-old children. *Br. Dent. J.* **143**, 11–17.

Parmeijer J. H. N., Brudevold F. and Hunt E. E. (1963) A study of acidulated fluoride solutions, III. The cariostatic effect of repeated topical sodium fluoride applications with and without phosphate. A pilot study. *Arch. Oral Biol.* **8**, 183.

Petersson L. G. (1975) On topical application of fluorides and its inhibiting effect on caries. *Odontol. Revy* **26**, Suppl. 34.

Riethe P. and Weinmann K. (1970) Caries inhibition with fluoride gel and fluoride varnish in rats. *Caries Res.* **4**, 63.

Rock W. P. (1972) Fissure sealants: results obtained with two different sealants after only one year. *Br. Dent. J.* **133**, 146.

Rock W. P. (1974) Fissure sealants: further results of clinical trials. *Br. Dent. J.* **136**, 317.

Scott D. B. (1960) Electron-microscope evidence of fluoride-enamel reaction. *J. Dent. Res.* **39**, 1117.

Stamm J. W. (1974) Fluoride uptake from topical sodium fluoride varnish measured by an in vivo enamel biopsy. *J. Can. Dent. Assoc.* **40**, 501–505.

Sundvall-Hagland I., Brudevold F., Armstrong W. D., Gardner D. E. and Smith F. A. (1959) Comparison of the increment of fluoride in enamel and the reduction in dental caries resulting from topical fluoride applications. *Arch. Oral Biol.* **1**, 74.

Szwejda L. F., Tossy C. V. and Below D. M. (1967) Fluorides in community programmes: results from a fluoride gel applied topically. *J. Public Health Dent.* **27**, 192.

Torell P. (1965) Two year clinical tests with different methods of local caries-preventive fluorine application in Swedish schoolchildren. *Acta Odontol. Scand.* **23**, 287.

Triol C. W., Kranz S. M., Volpe A. R., Frankl S. N., Alman J. E. and Allard R. L. (1980) Anticaries effect of a sodium fluoride rinse and an MFP dentifrice in a non-fluoridated area: a thirty-month study. *Clin. Prev. Dent.* **2**, 13–15.

Volker J. F., Hodge H. C., Wilson H. J. and van Voorkis S. N. (1940) The absorption of fluorides by enamel, dentine, bone and hydroxyapatite as shown by the use of the radioactive isotope. *J. Biol. Chem.* **135**, 543.

Wellock W. D. and Brudevold F. (1963) A study of acidulated fluoride solutions, II. The caries inhibiting effect of single annual applications of an acidic fluoride and phosphate solution. A two year experience. *Arch. Oral Biol.* **8**, 179.

Wellock W. D., Maitland A. and Brudevold F. (1965) Caries increments, tooth discoloration, and state of oral hygiene in children given single annual applications of acid phosphate fluoride and stannous fluoride. *Arch. Oral Biol.* **10**, 453.

CHAPTER 10

REPEATED SELF-APPLICATIONS OF FLUORIDE AGENTS AND THE EFFECT OF TOPICAL FLUORIDES ON SURFACE ENAMEL

The traditional approach to the administration of topical fluorides requires that each child be treated individually by a dentist or dental hygienist; this is expensive in terms of dental manpower requirements. Englander et al. (1967) considered that, by using custom-fitted polyvinyl mouthpieces, multiple topical fluoride applications could be carried out much more cheaply, supervised by trained personnel in the classroom. The purpose of this chapter is to examine the evidence concerning the effect of multiple applications of topical fluorides on, firstly, the incidence of caries, and secondly the concentration of fluoride in surface enamel.

CLINICAL STUDY USING MOUTHPIECES IN LOW-FLUORIDE AREA

The first study by Englander et al. (1967) involved 574 children aged 11–14 years, from Cheektowaga, N.Y. They were divided into three groups: the first group applied an acidulated 1·1 per cent NaF gel (pH 4·5) in custom-fitted maxillary and mandibular applicators for 6 minutes each school day for 2 academic years; the second group used the same technique as the first group, but substituted a neutral 1·1 per cent NaF gel (pH 7·0). The third group was the control group: applicators were not made for this group and no NaF or placebo gels were applied. Maxillary and mandibular applicators were constructed for every child in the NaF gel groups by vacuum drawing heat-softened sheets of thermoplastic polyvinyl over models poured from alginate impressions of the jaws. The children placed about 5–10 drops of NaF gel into each mouthpiece from an individual plastic container. The applicators were checked by dental hygienists to ensure that they were properly coated with gel and then both applicators were inserted by each child for 6 minutes. After the applicators were removed, the children rinsed their mouths, washed their applicators and stored them in cardboard boxes. The teeth were not dried at the beginning of an application and no attempt was made to brush the teeth immediately before or after application. All children were provided with fluoride-free toothpaste for home use throughout the study.

Initial clinical examinations were carried out in September 1964 and final examinations were concluded in June 1966. All clinical examinations were carried out by the same examiner who was unaware to which group each child belonged. Of the 369 children in the NaF gel groups initially, 305 (83 per cent) continued to participate regularly throughout the 21-month study. The average child received a total of 246 6-minute applications (range 200–277 applications). Almost a quarter of these children had to have their arch applicators re-made during the study. The three groups were balanced with respect to age, sex and initial DMF, PI and OHI scores. DMFT and DMFS increments over the 21 months of the study for continuous participants are recorded in *Table* 43.

The per cent difference in caries increments for the acidulated NaF phosphate group compared with the control group was 64 per cent in terms of DMFT and 75 per cent in terms of DMFS. The comparable figures for the plain NaF gel compared with the control were 67 per cent and 80 per cent. There was no difference in caries increment between the NaF gel groups. There were no changes observed in the PI scores and OHI scores among the three groups over the study period.

The NaF topical applications ceased in June 1966. A further study was carried out in May 1968 to assess the residual anti-caries effect 23 months later: 379 children were available for re-examination. Caries increments in these children for the 44-month period are given in *Table* 44. It was concluded from this study that children who had received at least 200 daily topical fluoride treatments, with either an acidulated or plain NaF gel, over a period of 21 months continued to have significantly lower caries increments, 23 months after treatment had been discontinued, than were found in an untreated control group.

Certain aspects of these results require further consideration. Firstly, as pointed out by Englander et al. (1969), caries increments for 1964–1966 given in *Table* 44 differ from those originally reported (*Table* 43). Thus, the 379 children who participated in the study over the entire study period of 44 months cannot be regarded as representative of the 500 children who completed the first 21 months of the project. For example, the DMF increments for the NaF groups after 21 months in *Table* 43 are 1·00 and 0·90: the DMF increments for the same groups over a 44-month period in *Table* 44 are 1·02 and 1·10.

Secondly, the DMF increment in the control group over the first period (2·39) was almost three times greater than in the second period (0·83). In fact this latter increment was very similar in magnitude to those obtained in the NaF gel groups during the first 21 months of the study (0·77 and 0·83).

FLUORIDE CONTENT OF EXFOLIATED DECIDUOUS TEETH

A further aspect of this study concerned the amount of fluoride incorporated into the outer layer of enamel as a result of repeated topical

Table 43. Mean Caries Increments in Children, aged 11–14 Years at the Start of the Study, continuously participating in the Study for 21 Months (Englander et al., 1967)

| | Controls | | | Acidulated NaF phosphate gel | | | Plain NaF gel | |
No.	DMFT increment	DMFS increment	No.	DMFT increment	DMFS increment	No.	DMFT increment	DMFS increment
195	2·75	4·39	154	1·00	1·1	151	0·90	0·89

Table 44. Mean Caries Increments in Children, aged 11–14 Years at the Start of the Study, continuously participating in the Study for 44 Months* (Englander et al., 1969)

| Year | No. | Controls | | No. | Acidulated NaF phosphate gel | | No. | Plain NaF gel | |
		DMFT	DMFS		DMFT	DMFS		DMFT	DMFS
1964–1966 (21 months)	137	2·39	3·69	127	0·77	0·71	115	0·83	0·78
1966–1968 (23 months)		0·83	2·80		0·24	1·04		0·27	1·25
1964–1968* (44 months)		3·23	6·58		1·02	1·83		1·10	1·99

* These figures are taken from the original paper, Tables 2, 3 and 4 (Englander et al., 1969). Adding the increments for the first and second parts of the study does not give the same result as taking the total increment over the 44-month period.

fluoride applications. Exfoliated deciduous teeth were collected from the Cheektowaga children. A total of 131 deciduous teeth were collected (Mellberg et al., 1967a, b). The teeth treated with acidulated phosphate fluoride gel during the second year had an average of 172 6-minute treatments over the two school years. The average F concentration in their outer 80 µm of enamel was strikingly greater than that of the teeth collected during the first year (these had received only 44 treatments) and of the untreated teeth (*Fig.* 19).

The teeth treated with the neutral NaF collected during the second year of the study had received an average of 168 treatments before exfoliation. They also contained higher F concentrations in their outer enamel when compared with teeth collected in the first year and with untreated teeth (*Fig.* 20). However, the fluoride increase using neutral NaF was not as pronounced as it was from the acidulated phosphate NaF.

Furthermore, the teeth in each gel group were placed in six subgroups according to the number of applications received before exfoliation. The

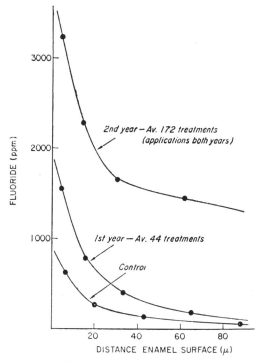

Fig. 19. Average fluoride concentrations in deciduous enamel treated with acid-phosphate-fluoride gel. (From Mellberg et al., 1967b.) (*Reproduced from 'Archives of Oral Biology', by kind permission of the Editor and Pergamon Press.*)

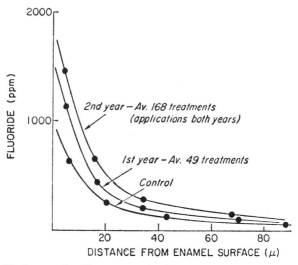

Fig. 20. Average fluoride concentration in deciduous enamel treated with neutral fluoride gel. (From Mellberg et al., 1967b.) (*Reproduced from 'Archives of Oral Biology', by kind permission of the Editor and Pergamon Press.*)

teeth in both NaF gel groups showed a progressive increase in enamel F concentration that varied with the number of treatments received before exfoliation. The increase for the acidulated phosphate fluoride group was more marked than for the neutral group, particularly in the deeper enamel layers. It was suggested that this finding might have an important clinical implication because greater subsurface F concentrations should favour a more lasting anti-caries effect and possibly retard the progression of carious lesions. However, the results of the clinical study (*Tables* 43 and 44) showed that there was no difference between the neutral NaF group and the acidulated phosphate NaF group in terms of DMF increment after 21 months or 44 months.

CLINICAL STUDY USING MOUTHPIECES IN OPTIMUM FLUORIDE AREA

Englander and co-workers (1971) reported the results of a second trial involving repeated topical application of sodium fluoride in mouthpieces, this time in children continuously resident in Charlotte State, an area with 1 ppm F in the drinking water. The study began in 1966 when 896 children aged 11–15 years volunteered to participate in the study. They were divided into two groups. The first group applied acidulated 1·1 per cent NaF gel drops (pH 4·5) in custom-fitted maxillary and mandibular applicators for 3 minutes on Mondays, Wednesdays and Fridays for 3 academic years (a maximum of 258 applications). The teeth were not dried before the applications and they were not brushed immediately before or afterwards. The second group were not provided with mouthpieces and no placebo gel was used. All children were supplied with a fluoride-free toothpaste for home use throughout the study.

Initially it was intended that all children should be examined by one examiner, but in the event two examiners were used. The baseline examinations were carried out during the period October 1966 to February 1967 and the final dental examination took place in May 1969. Each examiner restricted his examinations to the children he had examined initially and the results were presented separately: 557 children (62 per cent of the original sample) were seen on both occasions. Children in the treated group received on average 255 applications (range 222–258). The baseline DMFS score was slightly higher in the NaF group than the control group (3·98 as against 3·35); apart from this the two groups were balanced initially with respect to age, sex and mean number of intact tooth surfaces. Considering only those 557 children who completed the trial, the initial DMFS scores were 3·99 for the study group and 3·37 for the control. The mean caries increments over the 30 months of the study are summarized in *Table* 45. Combined data from the two examiners showed that the increment in the study group was 0·63 less than in the control group over the 30-month period, but results differed between the two examiners. Examiner A saw mostly 12-year-old children and the DMFS increment in the study group was 1·05 lower than in the control. Forty-two per cent of the total increment reported by examiner A resulted from surfaces that changed from caries-free to filled. In contrast, examiner B reported a difference in increment between the two groups of only 0·28 DMFS, which was not statistically significant. Furthermore, over 90 per cent of the total DMF increment reported by examiner B was attributed to newly filled surfaces, suggesting that these children had a much higher level of dental care than those seen by examiner A. In such circumstances, there is a possibility that some of these fillings were placed for prophylactic reasons in pits and fissures that would have been considered non-carious by the standards of diagnosis used by the examiners in the study, and if this had in fact occurred to any great extent the likelihood of detecting an effect of the test agent would have been reduced.

The results from both examiners show that children living in a fluoridated area have a low caries experience (the mean DMFS scores for children aged 13–17 years who had completed the study was 5·56 in the NaF group and 5·57 in the control group). The data obtained from examiner A suggested that the 255 NaF application over the 30 months of the study had further reduced the caries incidence of children who had ingested fluoridated drinking water from birth. The overall results are equivocal, however, because the data from examiner B did not show

Table 45. Mean DMFS Increments for Children, aged 11–15 Years initially, continuously participating in the Study for approximately 30 Months (*Englander et al., 1971*)

| | Control | | Acidulated NaF phosphate | |
	No.	DMFS	No.	DMFS
Combined examiners	220	2·20	337	1·57
Examiner A	91	3·07	123	2·02
Examiner B	129	1·59	214	1·31

Table 46. Caries Increments in Children from New Orleans completing 2 Years of the Study (*Heifetz et al., 1970a*)

| Group | No. of children | Teeth | | Surfaces | |
		Mean DMF· increment	Per cent difference from control	Mean DMF increment	Per cent difference from control
A Non-fluoride prophylaxis and placebo solution	148	2·45	−7·8	4·26	−10·6
B Non-fluoride prophylaxis and APF solution	123	2·26	+6·9	3·81	−3·1
C No prophylaxis APF solution	136	2·62		4·13	
D No prophylaxis APF gel	161	2·19	−10·6	3·94	−7·5

160

a clinically or statistically significant difference in the mean caries increments of treated and control groups.

FLUORIDE CONTENT OF DECIDUOUS AND PERMANENT TEETH

As in the study in Cheektowaga, exfoliated deciduous teeth from Charlotte children participating in the study were collected and analysed for fluoride content. In addition 89 premolars that had been extracted for orthodontic reasons were studied (Mellberg et al., 1970). In all 106 untreated exfoliated deciduous teeth and 212 deciduous teeth from children who had received 20–237 topical NaF treatments were analysed (*Fig.* 21). The topically treated teeth had a higher mean fluoride content than the untreated teeth. At a depth of 5 μm untreated teeth showed approximately 900 ppm F, whereas teeth receiving 221 treatments of acidulated NaF gel contained approximately 2400 ppm F. At a depth of 60 μm the difference between the groups had diminished considerably, but

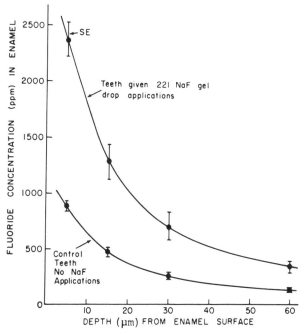

Fig. 21. Average fluoride concentration in deciduous enamel from an optimum fluoride area, treated with acid-phosphate-fluoride gel. (From Mellberg et al., 1970.) (*Copyright by the American Dental Association. Reprinted by permission.*)

the treated enamel had about 200 ppm F more than the untreated enamel. Comparisons with data obtained from the previous study in a non-fluoride area (*Figs.* 19 and 20) showed that at 5 μm the fluoride content in deciduous enamel which had not received any topical fluoride treatment was about 900 ppm in a fluoride area and about 650 ppm in a non-fluoride area. Thus the continuous consumption of fluoridated water from birth appeared to add an extra 200–300 ppm F to the outer layer of deciduous enamel.

Seventy-seven permanent teeth that had received 35–258 topical fluoride treatments were also analysed for fluoride content and compared with that found in 12 untreated permanent teeth. The pattern of increased fluoride uptake in the permanent teeth as the number of topical treatments increased was similar to that found in the deciduous teeth. The permanent

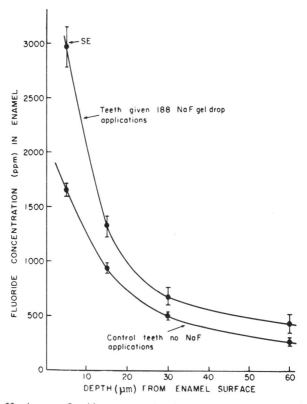

Fig. 22. Average fluoride concentration in permanent enamel from an optimum fluoride area, treated with acid-phosphate-fluoride gel. (From Mellberg et al., 1970.) (*Copyright by the American Dental Association. Reprinted by permission.*)

teeth which had received no topical fluoride treatment had, however, a higher initial fluoride concentration than the deciduous teeth (*Fig.* 22). At 5 μm the control permanent teeth from the fluoridated area contained 1650 ppm F in the enamel, almost twice that found in deciduous enamel at the same depth (900 ppm F). It was concluded from these studies that although the enamel of permanent teeth given a comparable number of topical fluoride treatments reached a higher final fluoride concentration than deciduous enamel, this was because the permanent enamel before the treatment contained very much more fluoride than deciduous enamel before treatment. In fact, permanent enamel seemed to acquire less fluoride from topical treatment than did deciduous enamel. This conclusion was in accord with in vitro experiments that show the amount of fluoride acquired by deciduous and permanent teeth from topical treatment to be dependent on the initial fluoride concentration (Nicholson and Mellberg, 1969).

It must be stressed that the studies by Englander and co-workers involved a very large number of APF gel applications—approximately 250 over a period of 21–30 months. Inevitably this demands a very high degree of motivation on the part of the children, the teaching staff and the supervisory personnel. Horowitz and Heifetz (1970) concluded that 'although the results of the study in Cheektowaga have added much to our knowledge of ultimate decay-preventive benefits that can be achieved through self-administered topical fluoride procedures—it is doubtful if a daily application procedure can realistically be considered as a feasible public health measure'. In addition, the amount of fluoride ingested must be considered when repeated topical applications of fluoride agents are advocated. In the study by Horowitz et al. (1974) the various procedures were pre-tested before the trial started, and it was reported that 8 ml of 1·23 per cent solution contain 98·4 mg F. This was almost twice the amount of fluoride (50 mg) that the investigators estimated would be safe for children to use under non-professional supervision. Therefore, as a precautionary measure, the concentration of fluoride in the APF solution was reduced to 0·6 per cent. However, only 4 ml of APF gel were needed to wet all the teeth, so the fluoride concentration in the gel was left at 1·23 per cent. Although it is inevitable that a small proportion of the fluoride agent will be ingested, it is important, when using topical fluorides, to ensure that as much of the agent as possible is removed from the mouth once the teeth have been treated (*see* pp. 242–5).

CLINICAL STUDIES INVOLVING REPEATED APPLICATIONS BY TOOTHBRUSHING

Other studies in this field have been concerned with the effect of self-application of topical fluoride agents by toothbrushing, usually 4–10 times a year. Bullen et al. (1965, 1966) reported a study of 464 children who had brushed with a 1·23 per cent APF fluoride or placebo solution at school under supervision at least seven times over a 2-year period. Results after the first year showed that caries in deciduous teeth was unaffected by the fluoride application, but that caries in the first permanent molars was 38 per cent lower in the study group than in the control (2·6 DMFS against 1·6 DMFS). However, the results after 2 years were not so encouraging: the DMFS increment was 6·0 in the control group compared with 5·1 in the study group—a difference of 15 per cent.

Heifetz et al. (1970a) reported the results of an intended 3-year study to test the effect of self-application of various topical fluoride treatments in 1043 children aged 13–14 years in New Orleans, a low-fluoride area. Four groups were defined: Group A, the control group, brushed their teeth with a non-fluoride prophylaxis paste and then brushed with a placebo solution; Group B brushed with the same prophylaxis paste and then brushed with a flavoured APF solution containing 0·6 per cent F with a pH of 3·0; Group C brushed with the 0·6 per cent APF solution without using the prophylaxis paste first; Group D brushed with the prophylaxis paste and then with an APF gel containing 1·25 per cent F at a pH of 3·0. The brushings were carried out five times a year at school at approximately 2-monthly intervals and were supervised by trained housewives. Each supervisor was able to instruct up to 10 children simultaneously. Children were taught to use a systematic toothbrushing method: a total of 30 seconds was given to each quadrant of the mouth when using the prophylaxis paste and two separate brushings of 21 seconds to every quadrant when brushing with the solution or gel.

After 2 years only 568 of the original 1043 school participants remained in the trial. The same dentist who examined the children at the baseline examination also carried out the follow-up examination. All four groups were balanced with respect to caries experience at the start of the trial. The caries increments after 2 years are given in *Table* 46 and fail to show a caries-preventing effect of brushing with a 0·6 per cent APF solution or a 1·23 per cent APF gel. Because none of the procedures demonstrated any caries-preventive benefits and because of the large attrition of subjects, the study was discontinued after the second year.

However, a second study by Horowitz and co-workers (1974) in São Paulo, Brazil, produced a significant result. Of the 1279 children aged 11–14 years who participated in the study, 566 children completed the 3-year trial. The study design was broadly similar to the New Orleans investigation, but in São Paulo five groups were used. Group A (controls) brushed with a non-fluoride prophylactic paste and then with a placebo solution; Group B brushed with the same paste and then with an APF solution (0·6 per cent F, pH 3); Group C brushed with the solution without first brushing with the prophylactic paste; Group D brushed with the paste and then with an APF gel (1·23 per cent F, pH 3); Group E brushed with the APF gel without first brushing with the paste. Fifteen brushings spaced evenly throughout the 3 years were carried out in school, controlled by supervisory personnel. The results for the children continuously participating in the trial are summarized in *Table* 47.

The differences in DMFS increments from the controls in treatment groups B, C and D were statistically significant at $P < 0.01$. The differences between group E and the controls were not statistically significant at the 0·05 level, but closely approached significance. Although none of the differences between the treatment groups was statistically significant, children who brushed with prophylaxis paste and then with APF gel (group D) showed the greatest caries inhibition (3·8 surfaces less than the control). Children in group E who used the same gel, but did not use prophylaxis paste first, developed on average 1·65 more DMF surfaces over the 3-year period, suggesting that the prophylaxis paste was important. However, the findings with the APF solution in groups B and C do not support the value of prior tooth cleaning. Possibly, molecular diffusion of the solution to the tooth surface, unlike the gel, was not impaired by the presence of debris or plaque.

In comparing the contrary findings of the São Paulo and New Orleans studies, Horowitz et al. (1974) mentioned three important non-controllable variables which could perhaps explain how a limited but real treatment effect observed at one study site can be obscured at another. Firstly, they reported that São Paulo children were more enthusiastic and cooperated more fully in toothbrushing than did the New Orleans children and thus may have given themselves better treatments. Secondly, professionally applied topical fluorides and fluoride toothpastes were much more available in New Orleans than they were in Brazil. Thirdly, much more restorative treatment had been carried out in New Orleans than in São Paulo. The investigators therefore had to accept the diagnoses of caries in terms of fillings placed by local dentists at a disproportionate rate in the two studies. This problem of 'preventive fillings' was observed by Englander et al. in their Charlotte study.

Marthaler et al. (1970) also obtained a positive reduction in caries increment when children brushed 48 times over 2 years with an amine fluoride gel containing 1·25 per cent F. At the end of the experimental period those brushing with this gel had 1·8 fewer DF surfaces than did children brushing with the control gel.

Mellberg et al. (1974) tested the effectiveness of semi-annual applications of an acidulated phosphate fluoride prophylaxis paste to the teeth of 12–13-year-old children living in a non-fluoride area. The results for 313 children (157 study, 156 control) who had completed the 3-year study showed that the total DFS increment was 21 per cent lower in the study group (4·7) than in the control group (6·0). The greatest inhibition occurred on buccolingual surfaces—these were also the surfaces expected to receive the greatest exposure to fluoride paste. Lowest reductions were

Table 47. Caries Experience in Children, initially aged 11–14 Years, participating in an APF Toothbrushing Study in Brazil for 3 Years
(Horowitz et al., 1974)

Group	No. in group	Initial DMFS	Final DMFS	Mean DMFS increment over 3 years	Mean fewer DMFS/child	Per cent inhibition in increment
A Non-fluoride prophylaxis and placebo solution	117	11·44	22·92	11·48		
B Non-fluoride prophylaxis and APF solution	117	12·09	20·59	8·50	2·98	26·0
C No prophylaxis APF solution	108	12·10	20·58	8·48	3·00	26·1
D Non-fluoride prophylaxis APF gel	116	11·37	19·05	7·68	3·80	33·1
E No prophylaxis APF gel	108	11·34	20·67	9·33	2·15	18·7

Table 48. Mean Fluoride Concentrations in Deciduous Enamel in Children who brushed 1–9 Times with APF Prophylaxis Paste, compared with Control Teeth (Mellberg et al., 1974)

Group	No. of teeth	ppm F at four depths (μm)			
		5	15	30	60
Untreated	52	702	339	163	85
Paste-treated	710	752	362	174	86

observed on occlusal and proximal surfaces of posterior teeth. The authors suggested that future studies should emphasize the brushing of posterior teeth in particular in order to deposit sufficient fluoride on these teeth. They also measured the fluoride concentration of deciduous teeth exfoliated during the study and the results in ppm F at four depths in enamel are given in *Table* 48. Fluoride was significantly greater in treated teeth only at the 5 μm depth (752 ppm F as against 702 ppm F).

The maximum mean fluoride concentration was obtained after only two brushings: further applications did not build up higher fluoride levels. Almost all of the increased fluoride was lost within 6 months from anterior teeth and within 2–3 months from posterior teeth. Although it is stated that deciduous teeth were collected from all children in the study, no explanation is given for the fact that 14 times more teeth were collected from the study group than the control, even though there were similar numbers of children in both groups.

FLUORIDE UPTAKE IN PERMANENT TEETH OF ADULTS

No studies have been reported on the effect of repeated topical fluoride applications in adults. However, in vivo fluoride uptake by enamel in adults following a single fluoride application was studied by Heifetz and co-workers (1970b). Forty white male inmates of a US Federal Penitentiary aged 18–39 years, who had at least three pairs of homologous teeth scheduled for extraction, were selected for the study.

Group I subjects received on the control half of the mouth a prophylaxis using a non-fluoride pumice paste. One week later, teeth on the control side were extracted. After a period of 2 weeks, to allow time for healing, the test half of the mouth was given a prophylaxis using the same abrasive paste followed immediately by a topical application of an acidulated phosphate fluoride (APF) solution containing 1·23 per cent fluoride. One week later, teeth on the test side were extracted. Following the same sequence of half-mouth treatments and extractions, subjects in Group II were given a topical application of a 10 per cent stannous fluoride (SnF_2) solution containing 2·42 per cent fluoride; subjects in Group III were given a prophylaxis with an acidulated phosphate fluoride–silicon dioxide paste, pH 3·2, containing 1·2 per cent fluoride in its liquid phase; and subjects in Group IV were given a prophylaxis with a stannous fluoride–zirconium silicate paste, pH approximately 2·3, containing 4·8 per cent fluoride in its liquid phase. Information on the general compositions of both fluoride prophylaxis pastes has been reported (Mellberg and Nicholson, 1968; Smith, 1970). For Groups III and IV, teeth on the control side were given the test treatment using the respective prophylaxis paste minus all active agents; the pH of the placebo pastes was neutral. A summary of the study design is given in *Fig.* 23.

In-vivo FLUORIDE UPTAKE BY ENAMEL OF TEETH OF HUMAN ADULTS

SCHEMA OF TREATMENTS IN THE STUDY

Study Group	Treatments	
	Control side	Test side
I	Prophy. with non–F paste	Prophy. with same paste + APF sol. (1.23% F)
II	Prophy. with non–F paste	Prophy. with same paste + 10% SnF_2 sol. (2.42% F)
III	Prophy. with silicon dioxide paste	Prophy. with APF–silicon dioxide paste (1.2% F)*
IV	Prophy. with zirconium silicate paste	Prophy. with SnF_2–zirconium silicate paste (4.8% F)*

* % in liquid phase on w/w basis

SEQUENCE FOR TREATMENTS (Rx)

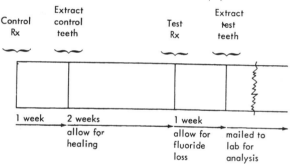

Control Rx	Extract control teeth		Test Rx	Extract test teeth
1 week	2 weeks allow for healing		1 week allow for fluoride loss	mailed to lab for analysis

Fig. 23. Outline of treatment by Heifetz et al. (1970b). (*Reproduced from 'Archives of Oral Biology', by kind permission of the Editor and Pergamon Press.*)

A total of 204 teeth were sent for laboratory analysis. One block of sound enamel was cut from each tooth and mounted with paraffin on the end of a plastic rod, exposing only the intact enamel surface. Four thin layers of enamel were then removed using $0.5\ HClO_4$ solution and the fluoride content determined by the method described by Nicholson (1966) and used in the study of Cheektowaga children referred to in the first part of this chapter. The results of this investigation are shown in *Fig.* 24. It is apparent that all the curves of fluoride acquisition at depths deeper than $15\,\mu m$ are essentially flat. In clinical terms the graphs show that: (1) fluoride uptake occurred at the enamel surface in Group I (APF solution) and Group III (APF–silicon dioxide paste); (2) the gains quickly diminished as the depth of subsurface enamel increased; (3) no clear-cut increase in fluoride content was found in Groups II (SnF_2 solution) and IV

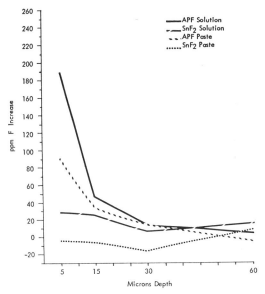

Fig. 24. Fluoride intake in homologous teeth for individuals according to study group and micron depth. (Heifetz et al., 1970b.) (*Reproduced from 'Archives of Oral Biology', by kind permission of the Editor and Pergamon Press.*)

(SnF$_2$–zirconium–silicate paste) at any depth of enamel. It was concluded that, after one application, the enamel of teeth of adults does not acquire a substantial amount of fluoride from any of the applications tested.

FLUORIDE GRADIENTS IN ENAMEL AFTER VARIOUS FORMS OF TOPICAL FLUORIDE APPLICATION

Following the work by Heifetz et al. (1970b), the effect of various forms of topical applications on the surface enamel of premolars—in children aged 11–14 years—was reported by Petersson (1976). After topical application, *in vivo*, the teeth were extracted and a macroscopic stepwise acid etching technique was used to determine the F-concentration in enamel to depths of 40–200 μm. Daily mouth-rinsing for 21–100 days with 0·025 per cent F or 0·05 per cent F solutions resulted in an insignificant increase of fluoride in the outer layer. Topical application of 2 per cent sodium fluoride, 8 per cent stannous fluoride, 2 per cent APF gel showed a moderate F uptake of 100–450 ppm, but limited to the first 10 μm of enamel. The highest F uptake (550–2000 ppm F) was observed when Duraphat F varnish was applied three times at weekly intervals. (Other studies involving Duraphat and surface enamel are referred to on pp. 146–147.)

Very high concentrations of fluoride in enamel were reported by Baijot-Stroobants and Vreven (1980) following topical application of fluoride agents. Using a 'non-destructive physical technique based on prompt activation by proton bombardment' they reported that 30 minutes after an application of an amine fluoride solution the enamel fluoride concentration reached 4460 ppm F. Acidulated phosphate fluoride gels gave a mean increase in enamel F of 1774–3277 ppm F, whereas application of amine fluoride and monofluorophosphate gels showed very little gain. The increase in fluoride was not permanent: follow-up studies showed that the F concentration returned to normal 2–6 weeks after treatment. In this study the teeth were treated for 4 minutes; after application the patient did not rinse, and abstained from eating and drinking for 30 minutes. The fluoride concentration was measured after 30 minutes and then every hour for 6 hours. It does seem possible that remnants of soft high fluoride deposits might have remained on the tooth surface and possibly affected the results of the study.

Intermediate treatment with dicalcium phosphate dihydrate (DCPD) before topical fluoride therapy was said by Chow et al. (1981) to produce significant amounts of permanently bound fluoride *in vivo*. A microbiopsy technique was used to measure the enamel fluoride content before, one month after and 3 months after an application of an APF solution alone or in combination with a DCPD pretreatment on the maxillary incisors of 50 4th grade children aged 10–11 years. One month after treatment there was no significant difference between APF and control groups, but the DCPD/APF treatment produced a mean fluoride uptake of approximately 1000 ppm F.

Brudevold et al. (1967) hypothesized that the cariostatic effectiveness of a topical fluoride agent is proportional to its ability to deposit F as fluorapatite in enamel. However, as Heifetz et al. (1970b) have remarked, clinical evidence in support of this hypothesis is limited; furthermore, some of the published findings are difficult to reconcile with this hypothesis. There is no doubt that the fluoride concentration varies in different parts of the tooth (Weatherell et al., 1977), and that there is a steep gradient from the enamel surface to the innermost part of enamel. These natural variations explain some of the differences in results reported by different workers. Further studies are required to determine how important a factor is the concentration of fluoride in the outermost layer of enamel in rendering a tooth resistant to caries.

REFERENCES

Baijot-Stroobants J. and Vreven J. (1980). In-vivo uptake of topically applied fluoride by human dental enamel. *Archs Oral Biol.* **25**, 617–621.

Brudevold F., McCann H. G., Nilsson R., Richardson B. and Cocklica Vera (1967) The chemistry of caries inhibition. Problems and challenges in topical treatments. *J. Dent. Res.* **46**, 37–45.

Bullen D. C. T., McCombie N. F. and Hole L. W. (1965) One year effect of supervised toothbrushing with an acidulated fluoride-phosphate solution. *J. Can. Dent. Assoc.* **31**, 231–235.

Bullen D. C. T., McCombie C. F. and Hole L. W. (1966) Two year effect of supervised toothbrushing with an acidulated fluoride-phosphate solution. *J. Can. Dent. Assoc.* **35**, 89–93.

Chow L. C., Guo M. K., Hsieh C. C. and Hong Y. C. (1981) Apatitic fluoride increase in enamel from a topical treatment involving intermediate $CaHPO_4.2H_2O$ formation: an in-vivo study. *Caries Res.* **15**, 369–376.

Englander H. R., Carlos J. P., Senning R. S. and Mellberg J. R. (1969) Residual anticaries effect of repeated topical sodium fluoride applications by mouthpieces. *J. Am. Dent. Assoc.* **78**, 783–787.

Englander H. R., Keyes P. H., Gestwicki M. and Sultz H. A. (1967) Clinical anticaries effect of repeated topical sodium fluoride applications by mouthpieces. *J. Am. Dent. Assoc.* **75**, 638–644.

Englander H. R., Sherrill L. T., Miller B. G., Carlos J. P., Mellberg J. R. and Senning R. S. (1971) Incremental rates of dental caries after repeated topical sodium fluoride applications in children with lifelong consumption of fluoridated water. *J. Am. Dent. Assoc.* **82**, 354–358.

Heifetz S. B., Horowitz H. S. and Driscoll W. S. (1970a) Two-year evaluation of a self-administered procedure for the topical application of acidulated phosphate-fluoride; final report. *J. Public Health Dent.* **30**, 7–12.

Heifetz S. B., Mellberg J. R., Winter S. J. and Doyle J. (1970b) In vivo fluoride uptake by enamel of teeth of human adults from various topical fluoride procedures. *Arch. Oral Biol.* **15**, 1171–1181.

Horowitz H. S. and Heifetz S. B. (1970) The current status of topical fluorides in preventive dentistry. *J. Am. Dent. Assoc.* **81**, 166–177.

Horowitz H. S., Heifetz S. B., McClendon B. J., Viegar A. R., Guimares L. O. C. and Lopes E. S. (1974) Evaluation of self-administered prophylaxis and supervised toothbrushing with acidulated phosphate-fluoride. *Caries Res.* **8**, 39–51.

Marthaler T. M., Konig K. G. and Muhlemann H. R. (1970) The effect of a fluoride gel used for supervised toothbrushing 15 or 30 times per year. *Helv. Odontol. Acta* **14**, 67–77.

Mellberg J. R. and Nicholson C. R. (1968) In vitro evaluation of an acidulated phosphate fluoride prophylaxis paste. *Arch. Oral Biol.* **13**, 1223–1234.

Mellberg J. R., Englander H. R. and Nicholson C. R. (1967a) Acquisition of fluoride in vivo by deciduous enamel from daily topical fluoride applications. A preliminary report. *J. Oral Ther. Pharmacol.* **3**, 330–334.

Mellberg J. R., Englander H. R. and Nicholson C. R. (1967b) Acquisition of fluoride in vivo by deciduous enamel from daily topical sodium fluoride applications over 21 months. *Arch. Oral Biol.* **12**, 1139–1148.

Mellberg J. R., Petersson J. K. and Nicholson C. R. (1974) Fluoride uptake and caries inhibition from self-application of an acidulated phosphate fluoride prophylaxis paste. *Caries Res.* **8**, 52–60.

171

Mellberg J. R., Nicholson C. R., Miller B. G. and Englander H. R. (1970) Acquisition of fluoride in vivo by enamel from repeated topical sodium fluoride applications in a fluoridated area: Final Report. *J. Dent. Res.* **49**, 1473–1477.

Nicholson C. R. (1966) Multicell diffusion trays for determining inorganic fluoride in physiological materials. *Anal. Chem.* **38**, 1966–1967.

Nicholson C. R. and Mellberg J. R. (1969) Effect of natural fluoride concentration of human tooth enamel on fluoride uptake in vitro. *J. Dent. Res.* **48**, 302–306.

Petersson L. C. (1976) Fluorine gradients in outermost surface enamel after various forms of topical application of fluorides in vivo. *Odont. Revy* **27**, 22–50.

Smith C. E. (1970) Brush-in: self applied topical fluorides. *Ohio Dent. J.* **44**, 188–190.

Weatherell J. A., Deutsch D., Robinson C. and Hallsworth A. S. (1977) Assimilation of fluoride by enamel throughout the life of the tooth. *Caries Res.* **11** (Suppl. I) 85–115.

CHAPTER 11

FLUORIDE MOUTHRINSING AND DENTAL CARIES

In the early 1940's it was appreciated that tooth enamel could take up fluoride ions from water solutions and that this rendered the enamel more resistant to acid solution. Over the next 40 years this topical method has proved very successful at preventing dental caries, and many permutations and combinations of the concentration of fluoride in the solution, the type of fluoride compound used, and the frequency and mode of application have been studied. Concentrated fluoride solutions have to be applied by trained personnel, usually in a surgery (*see* Chapter 9), but weak solutions may be applied by the individuals themselves as a dentifrice (Chapter 7) or as a mouthrinse. This chapter will discuss fluoride mouthrinses.

As with most of the early investigations into fluoride and caries, the first trials of fluoride mouthrinses were carried out in the USA. Since then results of clinical trials in at least 13 different countries have been reported, and the results of the main studies are given in *Tables* 49 and 50. These trials have been sufficiently favourable for dental public health officials to adopt fluoride mouthrinsing as the main alternative to water fluoridation in community prevention in many areas of the world, e.g.. Sweden, Norway, Denmark, Cuba and Eire. Heifetz (1978) ranked fluoride mouthrinsing as the most cost-effective community procedure out of 6 alternatives for topical fluoride therapy (Chapter 16).

CLINICAL TRIALS OF FLUORIDE MOUTHRINSING

Tables 49 and 50 give the results of 24 studies into the effectiveness of fluoride mouthrinsing where the results were expressed as reduction in DMFS increments in permanent teeth. The way in which these trials were organized varied. In the best organized, the children were randomly distributed to control and test groups within each school and class, and the active and control rinses had similar appearance and taste. In some trials the unit for allocation to groups was the school or class, which allows the possibility of interschool or interclass factors influencing the results. Most studies lasted 2–3 years, and those lasting less than 1 year have been omitted.

The effectiveness of fluoride mouthrinsing on the primary dentition has not been properly investigated because it is difficult to conduct such studies on pre-school children. Ripa and Leske (1979) found that caries increment in primary teeth (dfs) was reduced by 20 per cent in children

Table 49. Results of Clinical Trials of Mouthrinsing with Fluoride Solutions Containing Sodium Fluoride (NaF)

Study	F concentration (ppm)	Rinsing frequency	Age at baseline	No. completing trial	Length of trial (mths)	DFMS Caries increment Control	Test	Per cent caries reduction
Bibby et al. (1946)	1000*	3/wk	18–21	31	12	5·6	6·1	9 (increase)
Roberts et al. (1948)	45*	2/wk	12	187	12	2·4	3·0	25 (increase)
Torell and Ericsson (1965)	225	1/day	10	160	24	10·0	5·1	49
Torell and Ericsson (1965)	900	1/2 wk S	10	172	24	10·0	7·9	22
Koch (1967)	2225	1/2 wk S	10	85	36	21·1	16·1	23
Koch (1967)	2225	3–7/yr S	7	117	36	6·2	4·6	25
Koch (1967)	225	2–9/yr S	8–10	114	24	4·9	4·8	2
Horowitz et al. (1971)	900	1/wk S	6	129	20	1·3	1·1	16
Horowitz et al. (1971)	900	1/wk S	11	117	20	2·9	1·7	44
Brandt et al. (1972)	900	2/wk S	11–12	94	21	7·0	4·0	43
Moreira and Tumang (1972)	450	3/wk S	7	50	24	7·5	4·0	47
Moreira and Tumang (1972)	450	1/wk S	7	50	24	7·5	5·7	25
Moreira and Tumang (1972)	450	1/2 wk S	7	50	24	7·5	5·8	23
Aasenden et al. (1972)	200†	1/day S	8–11	114	36	12·3	9·0	27
Heifetz et al. (1973)	3000	1/wk S	10–12	126	24	7·5	4·7	38
Rugg-Gunn et al. (1973)	225	1/day S	11–12	222	34	10·2	6·6	36
Gallagher et al. (1974)	1800	1/wk S	10–11	306	24	4·4	2·9	34
Maiwald and Padron (1977)	900	1/2 wk S	6	100	88	11·6	5·1	56
De Paola et al. (1977)	1000**	1/day S	10–12	158	24	7·6	4·4	41
Luoma et al. (1978)	200‡	1/day S	11–15	32	24	6·3	4·2	32
Ripa et al. (1978)	900	1/wk S	7–12	750	24	3·2	2·6	20
Ringelberg et al. (1979)	250	1/day S	11	179	30	6·3	4·8	23

S. School only.
* pH 4·0.
† Rinse swallowed (1 mg F).
** pH 4·4.
‡ With buffer (pH 5·9).

Table 50. Results of Clinical Trials of Mouthrinsing with Fluoride Solutions Containing Acidulated Phosphate Fluoride (APF), Stannous Fluoride (SnF_2), Ammonium Fluoride and Amine Fluoride (Amine F)

Study	F compound	F concentration (ppm)	Rinsing frequency	Age at baseline	No. completing trial	Length of trial (mths)	DMFS Caries increment Control	Test	Per cent caries reduction
Frankl et al. (1972)	APF	200*	1/day S	14	246	24	8.7	6.8	22
Aasenden et al. (1972)	APF	200*	1/day S	8–11	109	36	12.3	8.7	30
Heifetz et al. (1973)	APF	3000	1/wk S	10–12	133	24	7.5	5.5	27
Kani et al. (1973)	APF	500	1/day S	10	95	36	7.5	5.9	21
Packer et al. (1975)	APF	200	1/day S	8	80	28	2.7	1.9	27
Packer et al. (1975)	APF	1000	1/wk S	8	108	28	2.7	1.6	41
Laswell et al. (1975)	APF†	200	1/day S	8	106	28	1.6	1.3	23
Laswell et al. (1975)	APF†	1000	1/wk S	8	120	28	1.6	0.9	46
Finn et al. (1975)	APF	100	2/day	8–13	150	26	6.9	5.6	18
Finn et al. (1975)	APF	200	2/day	8–13	142	26	6.9	4.9	29
Ashley et al. (1977)	APF	100	1/day S	12	245	24	5.6	4.8	14
Radike et al. (1973)	SnF_2†	250	1/day S	8–13	348	20	2.9	1.8	38
McConchie et al. (1977)	SnF_2	100	1/day S	10	248	24	5.8	4.6	20
McConchie et al. (1977)	SnF_2	200	1/day S	10	248	24	5.8	4.8	17
De Paola et al. (1977)	NH_4F	1000**	1/day S	10–12	159	24	7.6	4.4	42
Ringelberg et al. (1979)	Amine F	250‡	1/day S	11	162	30	6.3	4.9	22

S, In school only.
* Rinse swallowed (1 mg F).
† In F area.
** pH 5.0.
‡ pH 4.4.

aged 6–9 years at the start of a 2-year trial which tested weekly supervised rinsing with 0·2 per cent sodium fluoride solution.

EFFICACY RELATED TO TYPE OF FLUORIDE COMPOUND USED

Sodium fluoride has been the most frequently tested fluoride compound (*Table* 49): such solutions would tend to have a neutral pH. Two early studies (Bibby et al., 1946; Roberts et al., 1948) suggested that acidified sodium fluoride solutions were ineffective in preventing caries. It was not until Brudevold et al. (1963) had shown that acidulated phosphate fluoride (APF) solutions were likely to prevent caries that these solutions, with low pH, were tested as mouthrinses (*Table* 50). Only two trials have provided direct comparisons of NaF and APF mouthrinses (Aasenden et al., 1972; Heifetz et al., 1973). While in the first trial the effectiveness of the NaF and APF rinses was very similar, the trial of Heifetz et al. (1973) indicated that NaF was slightly more effective but the difference between NaF and APF was not statistically significant. From these studies, and a comparison of *Tables* 49 and 50, it can be concluded that APF mouthrinses have not been shown to be superior to those containing NaF.

Stannous fluoride-containing mouthrinses have been tested in two trials but no direct comparison with other compounds has been made. They do not appear to be superior to NaF-containing rinses. De Paola et al. (1977) compared directly a daily rinse containing ammonium fluoride (NH_4F, pH 5·0) with a NaF rinse acidulated to pH 4·4. Caries reductions were high and virtually the same (42 per cent and 41 per cent respectively). Likewise, caries reductions after using a daily mouthrinse containing amine fluoride appeared to be as effective as a rinse containing NaF at neutral pH—22 per cent and 23 per cent respectively (Ringelberg et al., 1979). No reports of rinses containing sodium monofluorophosphate (the most common fluoride compound in toothpaste sold in the UK) appear to have been published.

The possibility of enhancing the effectiveness of NaF mouthrinses by the addition of ions such as Al, Mn, Fe, Mg, Zr and K has been studied by Swedish research workers for over 20 years (Fjaestad-Seger et al., 1961; Nyström et al., 1961; Torell and Siberg, 1962; Gerdin and Torell, 1969; Torell and Gerdin, 1977). Although some results suggest effectiveness may be increased by the presence of various combinations of the above ions, their superiority to simple NaF mouthrinses has not been established.

In summary, alternative compounds to NaF have a less pleasant taste, necessitate careful formulation of flavouring agents, are more expensive and have not been shown to be more effective than neutral NaF solution. Sodium fluoride, therefore, is the compound of choice at present.

EFFICACY RELATED TO FLUORIDE CONCENTRATION

The concentration of fluoride in the mouthrinses tested in the trials listed in *Tables* 49 and 50 varied between 45 ppm F (Roberts et al., 1948) to 3000 ppm F (Heifetz et al., 1973): 3000 ppm F is 0·3 per cent F. Although, in general, the fluoride concentration in mouthrinses tends to vary inversely with rinsing frequency because of the hazard in frequent swallowing of concentrated solutions, four trials have tested different F concentrations but with the same frequency of rinsing. Koch (1967) found, with very infrequent rinsing (3 times per year), a 25 per cent caries reduction with high F concentration (2225 ppm F) and no reduction with low F concentration (225 ppm F). On the other hand, Forsman (1974) found that there was no difference in effectiveness between a 900 ppm F and a 110 ppm F rinse when the rinsing frequency was once a week in school. She suggested that since the efficacy was the same, rinses with lower F concentration might be particularly suitable for pre-school children.

The trial of Finn et al. (1975) suggested that doubling the F concentration from 100 to 200 ppm F, in an APF rinse which was used twice a day all year, resulted in greater caries reduction (29 per cent compared with 18 per cent). However, McConchie et al. (1977) reported that this direct relationship between concentration and efficacy did not apply to SnF_2 rinses since caries reductions were similar in the two groups rinsing each day in school with either a 100 ppm F or a 200 ppm F rinse.

EFFICACY RELATED TO FLUORIDE CONCENTRATION AND FREQUENCY OF RINSING

In *Table* 51, per cent caries reductions obtained in the trials listed in *Tables* 49 and 50 have been categorized according to fluoride concentration and rinsing frequency. The negative results of the pioneering trials of Bibby et al. (1946) and Roberts et al. (1948) have been excluded. Although throughout this review, and in Table 51 in particular, effectiveness in caries prevention has often been expressed as per cent caries reduction (PCR), this is largely because PCR is a convenient single statistic. For a fuller assessment of the effectiveness of a preventive measure the absolute values for test and control increments and the difference between them in the number of tooth surfaces prevented should be examined. This is important because factors such as age of subjects, level of caries experience in that community, the proportion of caries occurring in anterior teeth and the diagnostic standards of the examiner can all influence the percentage reductions obtained. However, despite its limitations, the PCR remains a useful and often quoted statistic for comparing results of clinical trials.

Table 51. Per cent Caries Reductions (DMFS) obtained in Clinical Trials of Fluoride Mouthrinsing according to (A) Fluoride Concentration of the Rinse and (B) Rinsing Frequency

	DMFS Caries reductions (%)			
	Fluoride concentrations (ppm F)			
Frequency	100	200–250	450–1000	1800–3000
Daily, all year	18*	49		
		29*		
Daily, at school	14*	27	21*	
	20†	30*	41*	
		22*	42**	
		36*		
		38†		
		32		
		23		
		27*		
		23*		
		17†		
		22‡		
3/wk			47	
2/wk			43	
1/wk			44	27*
			16	38*
			25	34*
			20	
			41*	
			46*	
1/2 wks			22	23
			23	
			56	
3–4/yr		2		25

* APF.
† SnF$_2$.
** NH$_4$F.
‡ Amine F.

As far as fluoride concentration in the rinse is concerned, the equivocal findings presented in the previous section appear to be supported by the data presented in *Table* 51. Most trials have tested concentrations in the range 200–1000 ppm F and there is little indication that increasing the F concentration in a mouthrinse increases its effectiveness.

The frequencies of rinsing tested have varied widely—from twice per day (Finn et al., 1975) to 3 times per year (Koch, 1967). Only two trials have tested more than one frequency with other factors (e.g. F concentration) remaining constant. Koch (1967) found that a 2225 ppm F mouthrinse was equally effective if taken once every 2 weeks in school (17 times per year) as when taken 3–4 times per year. On the other hand, Moreira and Tumang (1972) found a 47 per cent caries reduction in children rinsing 3 times per week compared with reductions of 25 per cent and 23 per cent in children rinsing once a week or once every 2 weeks, respectively. With the exception of the very long study of Maiwald and Padron (1977) in Cuba, data presented in *Table* 51 suggest that a rinsing frequency of once a week (or more frequently) would lead to a greater caries-preventive effect than rinsing every 2 weeks (or less frequently).

The results of the three trials in which both F concentration and rinsing frequency have been varied have been contradictory. Torell and Ericsson (1965) found that a 225 ppm F NaF rinse used daily at home resulted in a 49 per cent reduction, over twice the reduction found after rinsing with a stronger solution every 2 weeks in school. However, Packer et al. (1975) and Laswell et al. (1975) found the reverse trend with an APF rinse.

In conclusion, rinsing frequency would appear to be a more important variable than the concentration of fluoride, which does not appear to be of great importance. Rinsing once a week or more is likely to be more effective than less frequent rinsing.

DURATION OF RINSING, QUANTITY OF RINSE AND SWALLOWING

In most trials, the duration of rinsing was either 1 or 2 minutes; sometimes this period was subdivided into 2 or 3 rinses of shorter duration. Ten ml was the most commonly used quantity of rinse which was then expectorated into a cup, although in the trials of Aasenden et al. (1972) and Frankl et al. (1972) 5 ml was dispensed and swallowed after rinsing for 1 minute.

Ten ml of a 1000 ppm F solution contain 10 mg fluoride; even so, if this quantity was swallowed every day, the fluoride ingested from this source would be less than occurs in some high-fluoride areas, e.g. Bartlett in Texas (*see* Chapter 13). Mouthrinses are, in the main, for topical fluoride therapy and should not be swallowed. The most susceptible age group is 6 years and under, since the aesthetically important incisor teeth may be at risk of developing fluorosis up to this age. Because of this risk, several workers have investigated the amount of rinse swallowed by children of different ages. Ericsson and Forsman (1969) concluded that below 3 years of age swallowing reflexes were inadequate and rinsing was not recommended. Between ages 4 and 7 years F retention was 22–24 per cent (*Table* 52), although the under 5-year-olds could rinse for only 30 seconds. Very similar findings were published by Forsman (1974), reinforcing the recommendation of Ericsson and Forsman (1969) that rinsing with a

Table 52. Retention of Fluoride from NaF Mouthrinses by Children in Two Studies

Age (yrs)	No. of children	Rinsing time (sec)	F retention (mg)	F retention (%)
	Ericsson and Forsman (1969): 7 ml of 245 ppm F rinse			
4–5	10	30	0·42	24
5–7	20	60	0·35	22
	Forsman (1974): 7 ml of 110 ppm F rinse			
4	5	30	0·17	22
4	5	60	0·23	29
6	10	60	0·16	20

110 ppm F (0·025 per cent NaF) rinse every week should be completely free from risk in children above 4 years of age.

Birkeland (1973) found that 10–11-year-old children retained significantly less fluoride after rinsing with 7 ml than after rinsing with 10 ml, and concluded from these, and F activity studies, that 7 ml was the most suitable quantity. The F retention in his study was 14 per cent, the same figure as that obtained from analysis of 406 returned rinses during a 3-year clinical trial of daily rinsing with 7·5 ml of solution in 12–15-year-old children (Rugg-Gunn et al., 1973). Hellström (1960) found that 19 per cent of fluoride in 10 ml of rinse was retained in 7–15-year-olds, while Parkins (1972) recorded a 7 per cent retention after adults had rinsed with 5 ml of solution.

A rinsing time of 1–2 minutes would appear suitable for all ages above 5 years. Five ml may be a sufficient amount of rinse for young children, 7 ml for 10–15-year-olds, while older children and adults may require 10 ml. Rinsing is not suitable for children under 4 years, and caution is needed when recommending rinsing for 4–6-year-old children.

CARIES PREVENTION IN DIFFERENT TEETH AND TYPES OF TOOTH SURFACE

It is well established that the per cent reduction in caries following water fluoridation is greater in free smooth surfaces (buccal and lingual) and least in fissure surfaces (see p. 17). This pattern has also been observed in fluoride mouthrinsing trials. The caries increment recorded in the different types of tooth surface in adolescent schoolchildren who have rinsed daily in school for 3 years with a 225 ppm F rinse is shown in Fig. 25. The per cent caries reductions were highest for free smooth surfaces and anterior approximal surfaces (55 and 56 per cent respectively). However, because the incidence of caries in these surfaces is so much lower, the number prevented from becoming carious is small in comparison with fissure or

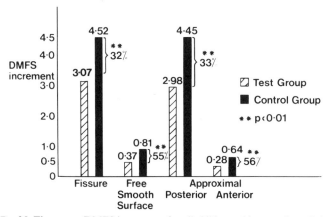

Fig. 25. Three-year DMFS increments for all children taking part in a clinical trial of daily rinsing with 0·05 per cent NaF, given for each surface type separately (From Rugg-Gunn et al., 1973.) (*Reproduced by kind permission of the Editor, 'British Dental Journal'*.)

posterior approximal surfaces. The per cent reduction for fissure caries is surprisingly high at 32 per cent.

In the same trial, the effect of fluoride mouthrinsing was assessed in the quarter of the children with the highest DMFS scores at baseline. The caries reduction in free smooth and anterior approximal surfaces was very high (72 and 67 per cent), but the reduction on fissure surfaces was low (18 per cent) and non-significant (*Fig.* 26). This may be due in part to the high caries prevalence in fissure surfaces, tending towards caries saturation in these surfaces. The majority of caries prevention occurred on posterior approximal surfaces (nearly 1 DMFS per subject per year).

Horowitz et al. (1971) also found substantial caries reductions in all types of tooth surface after weekly rinsing with a 900 ppm F rinse, while in children with very high caries increment Koch (1967) observed no reduction in fissure surfaces but substantial reductions in other surfaces. Ashley et al. (1977) also found only 5 per cent caries reduction in fissure surfaces compared with 54 per cent reduction in other surfaces.

Koch (1967) observed that anterior teeth benefit most from fluoride mouthrinsing, but his observation that caries reduction was greater in lower teeth (28 per cent) than in upper teeth (19 per cent), possibly due to pooling of rinse in the floor of the mouth, was not substantiated by Rugg-Gunn et al. (1973), who found equal reductions in both jaws. They were aware of Koch's results and urged the children to rinse thoroughly.

In addition to a 30 per cent reduction in carious cavities, Rugg-Gunn et al. (1973) also found an 18 per cent reduction in the increment of pre-cavitation carious lesions. Fluoride's action will be discussed further in

181

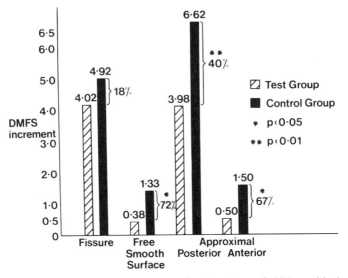

Fig. 26. Three-year DMFS increments for the quarter of children with the highest initial DMFS at the beginning of a clinical trial of daily rinsing with 0·05 per cent NaF, given for each surface type separately. (From Rugg-Gunn et al., 1973.) (*Reproduced by kind permission of the Editor, 'British Dental Journal'.*)

Chapter 14, but suffice it to say that it is uncertain whether this reduction in pre-cavitation carious lesions resulted from an increased rate of healing of these lesions in the fluoride group or a decreased rate in their formation, or both. Nevertheless, Hirschfield (1978) concluded that regular use of fluoride mouthrinses appeared to be effective at reducing decalcification of teeth undergoing orthodontic treatment.

There has been some discussion whether the presence of plaque on the tooth surfaces enhances the caries-preventive action of fluoride (Luoma et al., 1978). It would appear likely that the beneficial effect of plaque as a 'biological fluoride applicator', resulting in higher enamel fluoride levels in plaque-covered areas, is likely to be at least equalled by the detrimental effect of plaque as an essential ingredient in the aetiology of caries and gingivitis. This view is, to some extent, supported by Aasenden et al. (1972) who found that although caries increment was correlated with debris score in both control and test groups, the per cent caries reductions following the use of a fluoride mouthrinse were approximately the same in subjects with low, medium or high debris scores. In other words, the presence of plaque appeared to neither enhance nor diminish the effectiveness of fluoride mouthrinses.

POSSIBLE LACK OF CONTINUING EFFECT AFTER RINSING CEASES

Only Koch (1969) and McConchie et al. (1977) have re-examined subjects who took part in fluoride mouthrinse trials a year or two after the trials had ceased. Koch (1967, 1969) observed a 22 per cent reduction in caries (4·4 tooth surfaces) during the 3 years of the trial, but during the next 2 years, during which the children did not rinse, the test group developed slightly more caries than the control group children (*Table* 53). This finding has been frequently quoted as indicating that protection conferred by fluoride mouthrinsing is transitory and lost as soon as the rinsing ceases. However, four factors should be mentioned. First, that the children in Koch's trial were 10 years old at the beginning of the study and premolars, second molars and upper canine teeth are likely to have erupted towards the end of the 3-year rinsing period. Most British trials are timed to begin 2 years later, with children aged 12 years, to coincide with the eruption of these teeth. Secondly, caries increments were very high in this trial (nearly 7 new carious surfaces per year per child): the caries challenge would therefore seem to be overpowering, a view supported by the fact that no protection was conferred on fissure surfaces during the 3-year trial in contrast to the findings from other trials. Thirdly, since the test group children developed less caries than those in the control group during the 3-year trial, they had more sound surfaces at risk of attack during the next 2 years. Fourthly, at the end of the 5-year period, children in the test group still had lower caries experience than those in the control group.

McConchie et al. (1977) examined children one year after they had completed a 2-year trial testing daily rinsing with stannous fluoride. The level of caries inhibition (16–22 per cent) observed during the 2 years was maintained at the end of the third year. However, the one-year post-trial period is short for adequate evaluation of the permanency or otherwise of the caries-preventive effect of fluoride mouthrinses, and further information is required from other trials on this important point.

Table 53. Number of New Carious Tooth Surfaces in 69 Test and 71 Control Group Children during a 3-year Clinical Trial of Fortnightly Mouthrinsing with a 0·5 per cent NaF (2225 ppm F) Solution, and during the Subsequent 2 Years (*Koch, 1969*)

	Test	Control	Difference	Difference (%)
During 3 yrs of trial	15·7	20·0	4·4	22
During 2 subsequent yrs	13·7	13·1		
During all 5 years	29·3	33·1	3·8	11

ADVERSE EFFECTS FROM FLUORIDE MOUTHRINSING

Koch and Lindhe (1967) reported that fortnightly mouthrinsing with a 2225 ppm F solution by children in the test group of a clinical trial (Koch, 1967) resulted in a higher level of gingival inflammation compared with the control children who rinsed with distilled water. However, these comparisons should be interpreted with caution since no baseline gingival data were available.

Subsequently at least 6 reports have found no increase in gingival inflammation resulting from fluoride mouthrinse therapy, although none of these tested fluoride levels as high as 2225 ppm F. Frandsen et al. (1972) and Birkeland et al. (1973) found no detrimental effect after children had rinsed weekly with a 900 ppm F solution. Rugg-Gunn et al. (1973) and Ashley et al. (1977) also found no difference in gingival inflammation between children taking part in their fluoride mouthrinsing clinical trials. The possibility that amine fluoride rinses might reduce plaque quantity and therefore gingival inflammation has been investigated by Ringelberg et al. (1977) and Stoller et al. (1977). In both studies subjects rinsed with 250 ppm F solutions. While Stoller et al. (1977) found significantly less inflammation in subjects who rinsed twice a day, no difference was found by Ringelberg et al. (1977) when the subjects rinsed once a day. No case of allergy to fluoride in mouthrinses has been substantiated (Torell and Ericsson, 1974).

It is recognized that stannous fluoride solution may occasionally stain teeth. Radike et al. (1973) reported that some yellow stain was observed on the teeth of children with poor oral hygiene and that this was somewhat more noticeable in test group children. McConchie et al (1977) also reported staining of teeth in a very small proportion of children taking part in a trial of daily rinsing with SnF_2 mouthrinses (100 and 200 ppm F), but did not mention whether the children were in either of the two active groups or the placebo group.

COMPARISON OF EFFECTIVENESS WITH OTHER METHODS OF FLUORIDE THERAPY

The classical 2-year study of Torell and Ericsson (1965) in Sweden indicated that fluoride mouthrinsing is likely to be among the most effective methods of topical fluoride therapy (*Fig.* 27). Caries reductions were greater in the children who rinsed than in children who received clinical topical application of fluoride or who used a fluoride toothpaste. Ringelberg et al. (1979) also found that mouthrinses were more effective than toothpastes. Holm et al. (1975) found that daily chewing of a fluoride

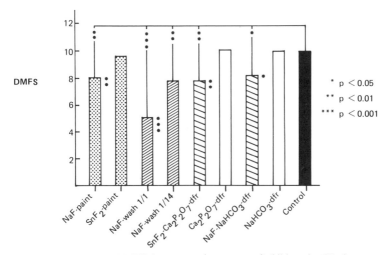

Fig. 27. Two-year DMFS increments in groups of children in Göteborg, Sweden, who received a variety of fluoride preventive measures both in school and at home.

NaF-paint, Topical application of 2 per cent NaF by Knutson's method; SnF_2-paint, Single topical application of 10 per cent SnF_2; NaF-wash 1/1, Daily mouthrinse with 0·05 per cent NaF; NaF-wash 1/14, Fortnightly mouthrinse with 0·2 per cent NaF; SnF_2-$Ca_2P_2O_7$-dfr, Home use of dentifrice containing SnF_2 and calcium pyrophosphate; $Ca_2P_2O_7$-dfr, Control for above SnF_2 dentifrice; NaF–$NaHCO_3$-dfr, Home use of dentifrice containing NaF and sodium bicarbonate; $NaHCO_3$-dfr, Control for above NaF dentifrice; Control, Main control group.

(From Torell and Ericsson, 1965.) (*Reproduced by kind permission of the Editor, 'Acta Odont. Scand'.*)

tablet was no more effective than weekly fluoride rinsing. However, the trend which they observed in favour of the rinsing programme was supported by Poulsen et al. (1981), who found that fortnightly rinsing in school with 0·2 per cent NaF was more effective than daily use of a 0·5 mg F tablet at school. Ollinen (1966) and Rosenkrantz (1967) recorded that rinsing or brushing with the same concentration of fluoride solution performed in school with the same frequency was of equal effectiveness. Ashley et al. (1977) observed that the effectiveness of daily supervised brushing with a dentifrice in school or rinsing in school was apparently equal, although Koch (1967) found that supervised daily brushing with fluoride toothpaste in school was twice as effective as fortnightly mouth-rinsing in school.

In summary, it would appear that mouthrinsing is at least as effective as alternative methods of topical fluoride therapy. Its effectiveness may be greater than other methods if rinsing is performed frequently (e.g. daily).

EFFECTIVENESS OF FLUORIDE MOUTHRINSES IN COMBINATION WITH OTHER METHODS OF CARIES PREVENTION

The percentage caries inhibition does not appear to be reduced when mouthrinsing is performed in fluoridated areas (Radike et al., 1973; Laswell et al., 1975), although the absolute number of tooth surfaces saved by the rinsing alone is likely to be less. Both Ashley et al. (1977) and Ringelberg et al. (1979) observed a small additional effect in children who used both a fluoride dentifrice and a fluoride mouthrinse. Ringelberg et al. (1976) also found a slight additive effect with a fluoride mouthrinse and twice-yearly brushing with an APF prophylactic paste.

It would appear, therefore, that combinations of types of fluoride therapy increase the preventive effect but the benefit is less than the sum of effects of the individual methods.

SUMMARY

A wide range of types of fluoride compound, concentration of fluoride and frequency of rinsing has been tested in many areas of the world. From the results it can be concluded that fluoride mouthrinses are amongst the most effective methods of topical fluoride therapy. As with other topical methods, effectiveness may diminish after rinsing ceases. Neutral sodium fluoride has been the most commonly tested compound, and because of its effectiveness, ease of formulation, low cost, ease of storage, and lack of taste or possible staining, it is the agent of choice. Effectiveness increases with frequency of rinsing, but substantial reductions are observed with weekly rinses. Fluoride concentrations between 200 and 100 ppm F would seem effective and safe, although rinsing with concentrations around 110 ppm F might be preferable for children under 6 years. Gingival inflammation is unaffected by rinses at concentrations less than 2225 ppm F. Because the organization of mouthrinsing programmes in schools is relatively easy (Little, 1969; Horowitz, 1973; Leske and Ripa 1977), they have become the method of choice in many community preventive programmes (see Chapter 16). However, in some communities even this level of cooperation may not be forthcoming.

REFERENCES

Aasenden R, De Paola P. F. and Brudevold F. (1972) Effects of daily rinsing and ingestion of fluoride solutions upon dental caries and enamel fluoride. *Arch. Oral Biol.* **17**, 1705–1714.

Ashley F. P., Mainwaring P. J., Emslie R. D. and Naylor M. N. (1977) Clinical testing of a mouthrinse and a dentifrice containing fluoride. *Br. Dent. J.* **143**, 333–338.

Bibby B. G., Zander H. A., McKelleget M. and Labunsky B. (1946) Preliminary reports on the effect on dental caries of the use of sodium fluoride in a prophylactic cleaning mixture and in a mouthwash. *J. Dent. Res.* **25**, 207–211.

Birkeland J. M. (1973) Intra- and interindividual observations on fluoride ion activity and retained fluoride with sodium fluoride mouthrinses. *Caries Res.* **7**, 39–55.

Birkeland J. M., Jorkjend L. and von der Fehr F. R. (1973) The influence of fluoride mouth rinsing on the incidence of gingivitis in Norwegian children. *Community Dent. Oral Epidemiol.* **1**, 17–21.

Brandt R. S., Slack G. L. and Waller D. F. (1972) The use of sodium fluoride mouthwash in reducing the dental caries increment in eleven year old English school children. *Proc. Br. Paedodont. Soc.* **2**, 23–25.

Brudevold F., Savory A., Gardner D. E., Spinnelli M. and Spiers R. (1963) A study of acidulated fluoride solutions—I. 'In vitro' effects on enamel. *Arch. Oral Biol.* **8**, 167–177.

De Paola P. F., Soparkar P., Foley S., Bookstein F. and Bakkhos Y. (1977) Effect of high concentration ammonium and sodium fluoride rinses on dental caries in schoolchildren. *Community Dent. Oral Epidemiol.* **5**, 7–14.

Ericsson Y. and Forsman B. (1969) Fluoride retained from mouthrinses and dentifrices in preschool children. *Caries Res.* **3**, 290–299.

Finn S. B., Moller P., Jamison H., Regattier L. and Manson-Ling L. (1975) The clinical cariostatic effectiveness of two concentrations of acidulated phosphate fluoride mouthwash. *J. Am. Dent. Assoc.* **90**, 398–402.

Fjaestad-Seger M., Norstedt-Larsson K., and Torell P. (1961) Försök med enkla metoder för klinisk fluorapplikation. *Sver. Tandläk-Förb. Tidn.* **53**, 169–180.

Forsman B. (1974) The caries preventing effect of mouthrinsing with 0.025% sodium fluoride solution in Swedish children. *Community Dent. Oral Epidemiol.* **2**, 58–65.

Frandsen A. M., McClendon B. J., Chang J. J. and Creighton W. E. (1972) The effect of oral rinsing with sodium fluoride on the gingiva of children. *Scand. J. Dent. Res.* **80**, 445–448.

Frankl S. N., Fleisch S. and Diodati R. R. (1972) The topical anticariogenic effect of daily rinsing with an acidulated phosphate fluoride solution. *J. Am. Dent. Assoc.* **85**, 882–886.

Gallagher S. J., Glassgow I. and Caldwell R. (1974) Self-application of fluoride by rinsing. *J. Public Health Dent.* **34**, 13–21.

Gerdin P. -O. and Torell P. (1969) Mouthrinses with potassium fluoride solutions containing manganese. *Caries Res.* **3**, 99–107.

Heifetz S. B. (1978) Cost-effectiveness of topically applied fluorides. In: Burt B. A. (ed.), *The Relative Efficiency of Methods of Caries Prevention in Dental Public Health.* Ann Arbor, University of Michigan, pp. 69–104.

Heifetz S. B., Driscoll W. C. and Creighton W. E. (1973) The effect on dental caries of weekly rinsing with a neutral sodium fluoride mouthwash. *J. Am. Dent. Assoc.* **87**, 364–368.

Hellström I. (1960) Fluorine retention following sodium fluoride mouthwashing. *Acta Odontol. Scand.* **18**, 263–278.

Hirschfield R. E. (1978) Control of decalcification by the use of fluoride mouthrinses. *J. Dent. Child.* **45**, 458–460.

Holm G. -B., Holst K., Koch G. and Widenheim J. (1975) Fluoridtuggtablett nytt hjalpmedel i kariesprofylaktiken. *Tandläkartidningen* **67**, 354–361.

Horowitz H. S. (1973) The prevention of dental caries by mouthrinsing with solutions of neutral sodium fluoride. *Int. Dent. J.* **23**, 585–590.

Horowitz H. S., Creighton W. E. and McClendon B. J. (1971) The effect on human dental caries of weekly oral rinsing with a sodium fluoride mouthwash. *Arch. Oral Biol.* **16**, 609–616.

Kani M., Fujioka M., Nagamine Y., Fuji K., Kani T. and Matsumura T. (1973) The effect of mouthwash on human dental caries during three years of regular usage with acidulated sodium fluoride solution. *J. Dent. Health (Jap.)* **23**, 244–250.

Koch G. (1967) Effect of sodium fluoride in dentifrice and mouthwash on incidence of dental caries in schoolchildren. *Odontol. Revy* **18**, suppl. 2.

Koch G. (1969) Caries increment in schoolchildren during and two years after end of supervised rinsing of the mouth with sodium fluoride solution. *Odontol. Revy* **20**, 323–330.

Koch G. and Lindhe J. (1967) The effect of supervised oral hygiene on the gingiva of children. The effect of sodium fluoride. *J. Periodont. Res.* **2**, 64–69.

Laswell H. R., Packer M. W. and Wiggs J. S. (1975) Cariostatic effects of fluoride mouthrinses in a fluoridated community. *J. Tenn. St. Dent. Assoc.* **55**, 198–200.

Leske G. S. and Ripa L. W. (1977) Guidelines for establishing a fluoride mouthrinsing caries preventive program for school children. *Public Health Rep.* **92**, 240–244.

Little E. J. (1969) A system of fluoride mouthrinsing in schools. *J. Irish. Dent. Assoc.* **15**, 103–105.

Luoma H., Murtomaa H., Nuuja T., Nyman A., Nummikoski P., Ainamo J. and Luoma A.-R. (1978) A simultaneous reduction of caries and gingivitis in a group of schoolchildren receiving chlorhexidine-fluoride applications; results after 2 years. *Caries Res.* **12**, 290–298.

Maiwald H.-J and Padron F. S. (1977) The results of collective caries prevention by mouth-rinsing with a 0.2% sodium fluoride solution after 88 months. *Stomatol. DDR* **27**, 835–840.

McConchie J. M., Richardson A. S., Hole L. W., McCombie F. and Kolthammer J. (1977) Caries-preventive effect of two concentrations of stannous fluoride mouthrinse. *Community Dent. Oral Epidemiol.* **5**, 278–283.

Moreira B.-H. W. and Tumang A. J. (1972) Prevencao da carie dentaria atraces de bochechos com solucoes de fluoreto de sodio a 0.1%. *Rev. Bras. Odontol.* **29**, 37–42.

Nyström S., Bramstang S. and Torell P. (1961) Munsköljning med zirkoniumfluorid- eller jarnfluoridlösingar. *Sven. Tandläk. Tidskr.* **54**, 217–220.

Ollinen P. (1966) Munsköljning eller borstning med olika fluoridlösingar. *Sver. Tandläk-Förb. Tidn.* **58**, 913–918.

Packer M. W., Laswell H. R., Doyle J., Naff H. H. and Brown F. (1975) Cariostatic effects of fluoride mouthrinses in a non-fluoridated community. *J. Tenn. State Dent. Assoc.* **55**, 22–26.

Parkins F. M. (1972) Retention of fluoride with chewable tablets and a mouthrinse. *J. Dent. Res.* **51**, 1346–1349.

Poulsen S., Gadegaard E. and Mortensen B. (1981) Cariostatic effect of daily use of fluoride-containing lozenge compared to fortnightly rinses with 0.2% sodium fluoride. *Caries Res.* **15**, 236–242.

Radike A. W., Gish C. W., Peterson J. K., King J. D. and Segreto V. A. (1973) Clinical evaluation of stannous fluoride as an anticaries mouthrinse. *J. Am. Dent. Assoc.* **86**, 404–408.

Ringelberg, M. L. and Webster D. B. (1977) Effects of an amine fluoride mouthrinse and dentifrice on the gingival health and the extent of plaque of schoolchildren. *J. Periodontol.* **48**, 350–353.

Ringelberg M. L., Conti A. J. and Webster D. B. (1976) An evaluation of single and combined self-applied fluoride programs in schools. *J. Public Health Dent.* **36**, 220–236.

Ringelberg M. L., Webster D. B., Dixon D. O. and LeZotte D. C. (1979) The caries-preventive effect of amine fluorides and inorganic fluorides in a mouthrinse or dentifrice after 30 months of use. *J. Am. Dent. Assoc.* **98**, 202–208.

Ripa L. W. and Leske G. S. (1979) Two years' effect on the primary dentition of mouthrinsing with a 0.2% neutral NaF solution. *Community Dent. Oral Epidemiol.* **7**, 151–153.

Ripa L. W., Leske G. S. and Levinson A. (1978) Supervised weekly rinsing with a 0.2% neutral NaF solution: results from a demonstration program after two school years. *J. Am. Dent. Assoc.* **97**, 793–798.

Roberts J. F., Bibby B. G. and Wellock W. D. (1948) The effect of an acidulated fluoride mouthwash on dental caries. *J. Dent. Res.* **27**, 497–500.

Rosenkrantz F. (1967) Kariesprophylaktischer Vergleich zwischen Mundspülen und Zähneputzen mit Natrium fluoridlösung. *Odontol. Tidskr.* **75**, 528–534.

Rugg-Gunn A. J., Holloway P. J. and Davies T. G. H. (1973) Caries prevention by daily fluoride mouthrinsing. *Br. Dent. J.* **135**, 353–360.

Stoller N. H., Cohen D. W. and Yankell S. L. (1977) Clinical evaluations of an amine fluoride mouthrinse on gingival inflammation and plaque accumulation. *J. Periodontol.* **48**, 650–653.

Torell P. and Ericsson Y. (1965) Two-year clinical tests with different methods of local caries-preventive fluorine application in Swedish school-children. *Acta Odontol. Scand.* **23**, 287–322.

Torell P. and Ericsson Y. (1974) The potential benefits derived from fluoride mouth rinses. In Forester D. J. and Schultz E. M. (eds), *International Workshop on Fluoride and Dental Caries Reductions*, Baltimore, Md, University of Maryland, pp. 113–166.

Torell P. and Gerdin P.-O. (1977) Fortnightly fluoride rinsing combined with topical painting of fluoride solutions containing Al-, Fe-, and Mn-ions. *Scand. J. Dent. Res.* **85**, 38–40.

Torell P. and Siberg A. (1962) Mouthwash with sodium fluoride and potassium fluoride. *Odontol. Revy* **13**, 62–71.

CHAPTER 12

THE PHYSIOLOGY OF FLUORIDE

AVAILABILITY OF FLUORIDE

Fluorine is the most electronegative of all chemical elements. It has an atomic weight of 19·0 and an atomic number of 9. Combined chemically in the form of fluorides, chiefly as fluorspar (CaF_2), fluorapatite ($Ca_{10}[PO_4]_6F_2$) or cryolite (Na_3AlF_6), it is seventeenth in the order of abundance of elements in the earth's crust (Fleischer, 1953). Barth (1947) estimated that the earth's crust contained 880 ppm. Most studies have shown that the level of fluoride in soil decreases from below upwards, the mean fluoride content varying between 200 and 290 ppm (Vinogradov, 1954). Fluoride also occurs in sea water, in concentrations ranging from 0·8 to 1·4 ppm (Thompson and Taylor, 1933; Wattenberg, 1943; Kappana et al., 1962). It is present in nearly all fresh ground waters, though the concentration in some water supplies is very small. The range of fluoride levels in drinking water varies in different parts of the world. In Africa areas have been reported with as much as 95 ppm in the drinking water (Tanganyika Government Chemist, 1955); the range in the USA is given as 0–16 ppm (WHO, 1970), whilst in England the range is 0–5·8 ppm (Heasman and Martin, 1962).

Additional fluorides are widely distributed in the atmosphere originating from the dusts of fluoride-containing soils (Williamson, 1953), from gaseous industrial wastes (MacIntire et al., 1952), from the burning of coal fires in populated areas (Cholak, 1959), and from gases emitted in areas of volcanic activity (Noguchi et al., 1963). Thus fluoride, in varying concentrations, is freely available in nature. It is difficult to understand how any form of life, in land, sea or air, evolved and survived unless it was fully able to cope with continuous uptake from its environment. The fluoride content of plants remains remarkably constant whether they are grown in soil with much or little fluoride (McClure, 1949a). There is no consistent difference in the fluoride content of the soft tissues of fresh-water and salt-water fish: very little fluoride appears in cow's milk and the amount is increased only slightly, if at all, by the addition of large amounts of fluoride to the drinking water or grain ration (McClure, 1949a). Negligible amounts of fluoride are stored in human soft tissues and these concentrations do not rise with increased levels of fluoride in the individual's drinking water (Smith et al., 1960). It is clear that no serious imbalance can or does exist between the life processes and ordinary amounts of fluoride acquired from the environment.

190

INTAKE OF FLUORIDE

Assuming a water fluoride content of 1 ppm, the average intake from all sources in the United Kingdom would be about 3·2 and 2·2 mg per day for men and women respectively (Longwell, 1957). In children aged 5–14 years the intake is 1·2 mg (Ministry of Health, 1962). McClure (1949a) determined the fluoride content in different types of food. Certain types of fish, for example dried mackerel and dried salmon, contain large amounts of fluoride (84·5 ppm and 19·3 ppm respectively). Tea leaves contain on average 97·0 ppm F. Whole potatoes contain 6·4 ppm F. McClure (1949a) considered that about 0·3–0·5 mg F were provided by the ordinary mixed solid foods of the American adult. In a further study of daily intake of fluoride from food and drinking water containing 1 ppm F, McClure (1949a) estimated that the total daily intake of a 10–12-year-old child would be 0·016–0·069 mg per kg of body weight. Thus for a 50-kg person the total daily intake would be 0·8–3·5 mg. More recently, Singer et al. (1980) have estimated the mean fluoride intake for young American males to be 0·91 mg F/day in unfluoridated Kansas City and 1·72 mg F/day in fluoridated Atlanta, USA.

ABSORPTION OF FLUORIDE

Fluoride is readily absorbed into the body. Absorption occurs mainly from the stomach, is passive in nature, and no active transport mechanism is involved. Carlson et al. (1960a) demonstrated that 1 mg of fluoride labelled with ^{18}F and ingested by two adult humans was rapidly absorbed. The maximum plasma radiofluoride concentration was reached within 60 minutes.

Absorption can also occur from the lungs by inhalation of fluoride dusts and gases. A third and very rare route of absorption is through the skin. Fluoride absorption may occur when hydrogen fluoride is applied to the skin: however, the resulting burn to the skin is more serious than is the fluoride that is absorbed (Goodman and Gilman, 1965). It is rapidly excreted via the kidney. Human studies have shown that between 20 and 30 per cent of an ingested fluoride dose was found in the urine within 3–4 hours (Carlson et al., 1960b; Ericsson, 1958; Hodge and Smith, 1965). Animal experiments have shown that fluoride is removed from the gastro-intestinal tract by simple diffusion (Zipkin and Likins, 1957; Stookey et al., 1964)

Soluble fluorides in drinking water will be absorbed nearly completely, regardless of the level of fluoride in the water supply (McClure et al., 1945; Largent, 1960). The question has been raised whether fluoride in milk is as readily available as it is in water. Ericsson (1958), using ^{18}F, found that at concentrations of 1 and 4 ppm F the absorption of fluoride from milk was slower than that from water, but that the ultimate percentage absorbed was nearly the same whether fluoride was supplied in milk or in water. Tea is a rich natural source of fluoride. The average fluoride concentration in tea leaves is approximately 100 ppm. Approximately 90 per cent of the fluoride from this source is extracted after infusion, so that the fluoride concentration of the infusion is around 1 ppm F (Ham and Smith, 1950). The absorption of fluoride from food depends on the solubility of the inorganic fluorides in the diet and on the calcium content of the diet. If calcium (as calcium phosphates or calcium carbonate) or aluminium compounds are added, the fluoride absorption is markedly reduced—to about 50 per cent. In such cases the fluoride is bound in a less soluble form and faecal excretion increases (Hodge and Smith, 1965).

EXCRETION OF FLUORIDE

Fluoride is excreted in the urine, lost through sweat and excreted in the faeces. It occurs in traces in milk, saliva, hair and tears. The principal route of fluoride excretion is via the urine and the urinary fluoride level is widely regarded as one of the best indices of fluoride intake. Human urinary fluoride concentrations depend on the drinking water concentrations. This was first shown by McClure and Kinser (1944), who measured the urinary fluoride concentration from 1900 young males from areas where the fluoride concentration in the drinking water varied from 0·5 to 5·1 ppm and has been repeatedly confirmed (*Fig.* 28).

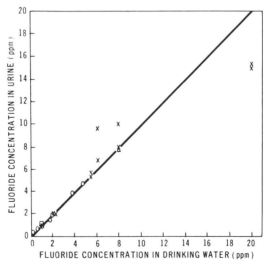

Fig. 28. Relation between fluoride concentration in the urine of humans and that in the water supplies used. (*Reproduced from 'Fluorides and Human Health' (WHO Monograph Series No. 59), by courtesy of the World Health Organisation.*)

192

The mechanisms by which fluoride is excreted by the kidney remain unknown. The clearance of fluoride is less than that of inulin (Chen et al., 1956; Carlson et al., 1960a). Thus presumably, less fluoride is excreted in the urine than is filtered at the glomerulus, and the implication is that fluoride is reabsorbed from the tubules. Whether tubular secretion of fluoride occurs is not known (Goodman and Gilman, 1965).

Fluoride is rapidly excreted from the body. Even small amounts, for example 1·5 mg (Hodge and Smith, 1965) or 5 mg (Zipkin and Leone., 1957) taken in a glass of water are absorbed and excreted so rapidly that 20 per cent of the fluoride can be found in the urine after 3 hours (*Fig.* 29). Using ^{18}F Carlson et al. (1960b) and Ericsson (1958) found that up to 30 per cent of a 1-mg dose was detectable in the urine in 4 hours. The very rapid rate of excretion is one of the most protective factors in severe fluoride poisoning: usually either death occurs within 4 hours or the individual recovers. The critical period is short because F is rapidly removed from the blood stream and extracellular fluid via the kidney and because skeletal deposition is extremely rapid.

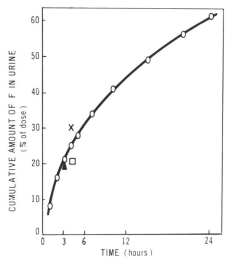

Fig. 29. Cumulative secretion of fluoride in the urine of man following the oral administration of sodium fluoride. (*Reproduced from 'Fluorides and Human Health' (WHO Monograph Series No. 59), by courtesy of the World Health Organisation.*)

In the relatively unexposed individual about half a single dose of fluoride is excreted in the urine in the following 24 hours and about half is deposited in the skeleton. Largent (1960) collected samples of everything he ate and drank and of everything he excreted, over a period of several

193

months, so that he was able to make definitive measurements of the retention of fluoride when daily doses of 1–18 mg of fluoride were ingested. This fluoride balance study showed that fluoride retention followed closely a simple straight line indicating storage of 50 per cent of the absorbed fluoride (*Fig*. 30).

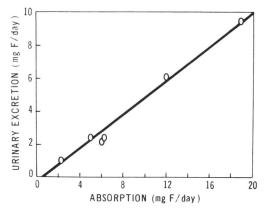

Fig. 30. Relation between absorption and urinary excretion of fluoride. (After Machle and Largent, 1943.) (*Reproduced from 'Fluorides and Human Health' (WHO Monograph Series No. 59), by courtesy of the World Health Organisation.*)

Younger individuals, who have a greater proportion of their skeleton available to the circulation and who are actively laying down bone mineral, excrete a lower percentage of a given dose of fluoride than do adults. Infants excrete 40 per cent of the F ingested daily (Ham and Smith, 1954). Longwell (1957) reported that children in the London area aged 5–6 years excreted half as much F in the urine as did those aged 10–12 years (0·16 mg per 24 hours compared with 0·35 mg per 24 hours).

STORAGE OF FLUORIDE

Fluoride is stored in the hard tissues of the body. It has been detected in every specimen of bone or tooth analysed. The extent of fluoride uptake in different parts of the skeleton and dentition depends upon the amounts ingested and absorbed, the duration of fluoride exposure and the type, region and metabolic activity of the tissue concerned. Therefore there is a great disparity in fluoride levels, both between individuals and between different types of mineralized structures. Even within tissues which appear structurally homogeneous, concentrations may vary markedly over distances of only a few microns.

UPTAKE OF FLUORIDE IN HARD TISSUE

The incorporation of fluoride slightly alters the chemical composition of bone and tooth mineral; the carbonate and citrate contents are lowered and the magnesium level increased; the Ca/P ratio, however, remains unchanged (Weidmann and Weatherell, 1970). Fluoride enters the mineralized tissues by replacing certain ions and groups normally associated with hydroxyapatite crystallites. Neuman and Neuman (1958) proposed a three-stage mechanism to describe the entry of ions into the apatite crystal lattice, which is considered to be surrounded by a hydration shell. The first stage is that fluoride ions exchange with one of the ions or polarized molecules present in this loosely integrated hydration shell. The second stage involved the exchange of fluoride in the hydration shell with an ion group at the surface of the apatite crystal. The ionic exchange would occur between fluoride ions and hydroxyl and bicarbonate groups and also with fluoride ions already present in the crystal. Finally, ions present in the crystal surface might migrate slowly into vacant space in the crystal interior during recrystallization.

FLUORIDE CONTENT OF BONE

Because fluoride ions are able to enter the hydroxyapatite lattice, fluoride concentration in living human bone builds up slowly with age. Smith et al (1953) studied post-mortem specimens of rib cortex which seemed to indicate a linear increase in fluoride concentration with age. Jackson and Weidmann (1958) studied post-mortem specimens of rib cancellum and found that fluoride tended to accumulate less readily in older specimens and stated that a plateau level of fluoride concentration was reached at about the age of 55 years. The value of the plateau level depended on the fluoride intake: in West Hartlepool where fluoride content in drinking water is 1·5–2·0 ppm, the plateau level was 4000 ppm, whereas in Leeds (F in drinking water is 0·1 ppm) the plateau level was 2000 ppm (*Fig.* 31). Results of studies by Blayney et al. (1962) also showed that the fluoride content of bone was related to the fluoride intake. Work by Weatherell (1966), using compact bone from the femora of persons living in an area containing 0·1 ppm F, suggested that a plateau level was not reached, but that the fluoride content increased with age (*Fig.* 32).

The distribution of fluoride within bone is not uniform. It is highest in those areas of most active growth; for example, endosteal and periosteal surfaces usually have a higher fluoride content than the central parts of compact bone (Weidmann and Weatherell, 1959). The two main facts arising from the literature are, firstly, fluoride content of bone increases with age and, secondly, fluoride content of bone increases with increasing fluoride concentration in the drinking water.

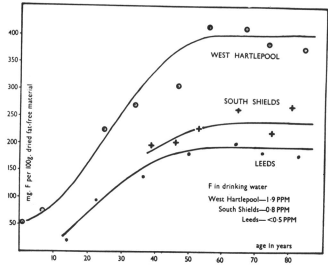

Fig. 31. Fluoride content in post-mortem samples of human rib bone in areas with different fluoride levels in the water supply. *Note*: Data on vertical axis are given as mg F/100 g dried, fat-free material. Multiply by 10 to get ppm F. (From Jackson and Weidmann, 1958.) (*Reproduced by courtesy of the Editor, 'Journal of Pathology and Bacteriology'.*)

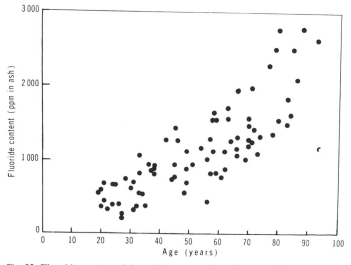

Fig. 32. Fluoride content of femoral compacta from humans of different ages living in low-fluoride areas. (From Weatherell, 1969.) (*Reproduced from 'Mineral Metabolism in Paediatrics', edited by Barltrop D. and Burland W. L., by kind permission of Blackwell Scientific Publications, 1969.*)

FLUORIDE CONTENT OF ENAMEL
AND DENTINE

Fluoride uptake in dental tissues also increases with age and with increasing fluoride concentration in the water supplies, but the fluoride content of dentine and enamel is considerably lower than that found in bone from the same individual. Jackson and Weidmann (1959) showed that in human premolar enamel from West Hartlepool (F = 1·5–2·0 ppm) fluoride concentration increased from 170 ppm F at 10 years and reached a plateau level of 350 ppm at 30 years of age. In contrast, human premolar enamel from Leeds (F = 0·1 ppm) contained 50 ppm F at 10 years and reached a plateau level of 100 ppm F at 30 years of age (*Fig.* 33).

Dentine was found to contain four times more fluoride than enamel. The concentration of fluoride in premolar dentine from West Hartlepool increased from 400 ppm at 10 years to 1200 ppm at 55 years, whereas premolar dentine from Leeds contained 100 ppm F at 10 years and increased to 400 ppm at 55 years (*Fig.* 34). These results were obtained by averaging samples of whole enamel and dentine and the general pattern of the results has been confirmed by Jenkins and Speirs (1954), Jenkins (1963) and Armstrong and Singer (1963).

However, results of studies using whole enamel and dentine obscure the fact that the fluoride content of these tissues is not uniform. After the tooth is fully formed, fluoride is chiefly incorporated at tissue surfaces. The highest concentration of fluoride in dentine is found adjacent to the odontoblastic layer (Yoon et al., 1960). The concentration of fluoride in the outer level of enamel is about four to five times higher than deeper layers. Moreover this differential was present in unerupted teeth and, at least in low fluoride areas, was independent of age. Isaac et al. (1958) concluded that when the fluoride content of the water supply is increased from 0·1 ppm to 5·1 ppm there is a considerable increase in the amount of fluoride deposited in the enamel during tooth formation. Fluoride concentration in the outer layer of enamel in areas with 0·1 ppm F in the water supply increased from 500 ppm F in the under 20-year age group to 1000 ppm F in the over 50-year age group. In areas with 1 ppm F in the water supply fluoride concentration in the outermost layer of enamel increased from 900 ppm F in the under 20-year age group to 1600 ppm F in the over 50-year age groups. In areas with 5 ppm F in the water supply the outer level of enamel contained 3200 ppm F and this value did not increase significantly with age, suggesting that this figure represents fluoride saturation of enamel. Studies by Weatherell and Hargreaves (1965) and by Hallsworth and Weatherell (1969) have shown the distribution of fluoride in enamel and how the concentration of fluorides decreases from the surface inwards to the enamel dentine junction (*Figs.* 35 and 36).

Little et al. (1967) examined enamel from people aged 20–50 years living in areas with less than 0·5 ppm F in the water supply. They concluded that

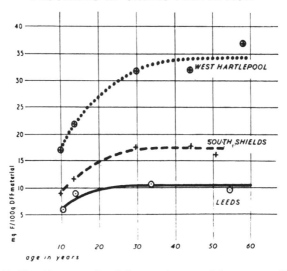

Fig. 33. Fluoride content in whole premolar enamel from persons living in areas with different fluoride levels in the water supply. *Note*: Data on vertical axis are given as mg F/100 g dried, fat-free material. Multiply by 10 to get ppm F. (*Reproduced by courtesy of the Editor, 'British Dental Journal'.*)

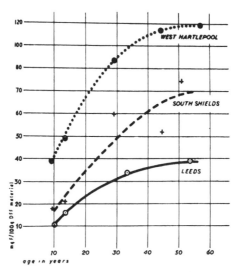

Fig. 34. Fluoride content in whole premolar dentine from persons living in areas with different fluoride levels in the water supply. *Note*: Data on vertical axis are given as mg F/100 g dried, fat-free material. Multiply by 10 to get ppm F. (From Jackson and Weidmann, 1959.) (*Reproduced by courtesy of the Editor, 'British Dental Journal'.*)

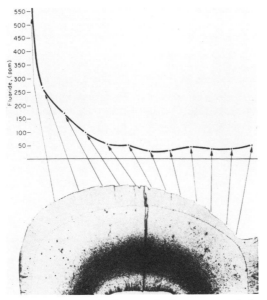

Fig. 35. Distribution of fluoride in enamel of a permanent incisor. (From Weatherell and Hargreaves, 1965.) (*Reproduced from 'Archives of Oral Biology', by kind permission of the Editor and Pergamon Press.*)

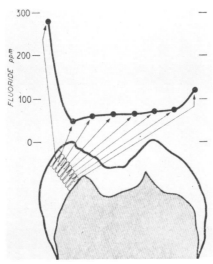

Fig. 36. Distribution of fluoride across the cuspal enamel of an unerupted mandibular third molar from a female aged 51 years. (From Hallsworth and Weatherell, 1969.) (*Reproduced by courtesy of the Editor, 'Caries Research'.*)

199

the marked gradient in fluoride content from surface inward of sound enamel, so often reported, was found to be primarily limited to discoloured enamel, characterized by a shallow micro radiolucent band just under the surface. The suggestion that fluoride tended to occur in enamel defects, including early carious cavities, was made by Dowse and Jenkins (1957), who applied ^{18}F to the surface of teeth. In a later report Jenkins (1963) stated that enamel ground from 'white spots' (which he equated with early carious lesions) contained over twice the fluoride content of similar boring from intact enamel in the same teeth (*Table* 54). Jenkins concluded that 'this suggests that under normal physiologic conditions fluoride might accumulate in early cavities and exert its effects just where it could be most beneficial'. Similarly Little et al. (1967) suggested that as most of the natural accumulation of fluoride is into the areas of lower mineral content, the beneficial effect of fluoride in reducing caries may be in preserving surfaces subject to demineralization.

Table 54. Fluoride Content of Normal and Carious Enamel from Towns with 0 ppm F and 2 ppm F in the Water Supply (*After Jenkins, 1963*)

	Non-carious enamel		Carious enamel	
	0 ppm	2 ppm	0 ppm	2 ppm
F ppm	250	440	640	850
No. of teeth	108	112	108	112

FLUORIDE IN BLOOD

Estimations of fluoride content of blood are normally made on blood plasma. Approximately three-quarters of the total blood fluoride is in the plasma and one-quarter in the red blood cells (Carlson et al., 1960b). Regulatory mechanisms operate within the body to maintain the plasma fluoride content within narrow limits (Singer and Armstrong, 1960, 1964; Smith et al., 1950). The mechanisms are effective under substantial variation of dietary fluoride intake (Carlson et al., 1960a). The regulation of plasma fluoride concentration is due, firstly, to the large volume of extracellular body fluid which dilutes the absorbed fluoride; secondly, to the deposition of fluoride in the skeleton; and thirdly, to the excretion of fluoride in the urine and, particularly in hot climates, to perspiration.

The fluoride content of blood plasma of residents in five areas where the fluoride content of drinking water varied from 0·15 to 5·4 ppm has been examined (Singer and Armstrong, 1960). In four centres where the drinking water contained 0·15–2·5 ppm F the mean plasma fluoride concentration lay within the range 0·14–0·19 ppm. In the community with

5·4 ppm F in the drinking water, the plasma fluoride concentration was 0·26 ppm. These quantities refer to total fluoride content of plasma. Work by Taves (1966) and Singer and Armstrong (1969) suggests that plasma contains two forms of fluoride: one form is free and ionic, the other is bound to albumin and is non-ionic. It is the free and ionic fluoride, which accounts for 15–20 per cent of the total plasma fluoride, which can be expected to participate in physiological reactions.

FLUORIDE IN PLACENTA AND FETUS

Evidence with regard to the extent of placental transfer in humans has been conflicting. Higher fluoride values were found in the maternal blood and placental tissue of pregnant women living an an area where the drinking water contained 1 ppm F than those living in a fluoride-free area (Gardner et al., 1952). Feltman and Kosel (1955) and Ziegler (1956) showed that in groups of women receiving fluoride tablets or fluoridated drinking water the full-term placental tissue contained much more fluoride than the fetal blood. These studies indicated that fluoride accumulates in the placenta, which therefore is acting as a partial barrier. However, Held (1954) reported about the same concentration of fluoride in maternal and fetal blood, and reported a similar increase in maternal and fetal blood levels after supplemental fluoride had been given. Gedalia et al. (1961, 1964) showed that when fluoride intake was low (0·1 ppm F in drinking water) the fluoride content of the placenta was lower than that of maternal or fetal blood, but when fluoride intake was raised the fluoride content of the placental tissue and of the maternal blood was higher than that of the fetal blood. This suggested that the placenta has a limited permeability to the increased concentration of fluoride ions and that the placenta plays a role in the transfer of fluoride from mother to fetus.

Ericsson and Malmnas (1962) studied the transfer of ^{18}F across the placenta of patients undergoing therapeutic abortions. The ^{18}F content of fetal blood was found to be very low 5–30 minutes after intravenous injection, always less than one-third of the simultaneous ^{18}F concentration in the maternal blood. The ^{18}F concentration of the placenta was between that of the maternal and that of the fetal blood. Certainly some fluoride does cross the placenta and is incorporated into fetal bones and teeth undergoing calcification (Gedalia et al., 1964), but it seems that the placenta may act as a partial barrier to fluoride, thus protecting the fetus from toxic amounts.

FLUORIDE IN SALIVA

The fluoride content of saliva has been found to be comparable with plasma levels. Carlson et al. (1960a, b) in their experiments with ^{18}F found that saliva from the parotid duct contained slightly lower concentration than plasma, but showed a similar but slower rise after ingestion of ^{18}F.

FLUORINE: AN ESSENTIAL MINERAL NUTRIENT?

Fluorine occurs naturally in a great number of foods and drinking water supplies and is universally present in the bodies of all higher animal species. The question has been raised as to whether fluorine plays a physiological role, or whether it is present in the tissues as an accidental constituent because it is ingested from food (Sharpless and McCollum, 1933). No human diet is free from fluoride ions and it is extremely difficult to prepare a diet for experimental animals which is very low in fluoride (a completely fluoride-free diet is virtually impossible to prepare—Jenkins, 1975).

Studies carried out between 1933 and 1957 on the effect of minimal fluoride intake in rats failed to show that fluorine was an essential nutrient (Sharpless and McCollum, 1933; Muhler, 1954; Maurer and Day, 1957), although in some cases the minimal diets employed contained fluorine, as judged by carcass fluoride analyses, and in others the purified diets employed were inadequate for support of normal reproductive performance. Doberenz et al. (1964) fed a minimal fluoride (< 0.005 ppm F) diet for a 10-week period to weanling rats and demonstrated significantly lower levels of bone fluoride in the study animals compared with a control group receiving the minimal diet plus 2 ppm F. More recently, Messer and co-workers have shown marked effects on haematocrit values and litter production in mice fed on a diet based on milk and cereals which had a very low fluoride content. Messer et al. (1972b) reported that the low fluoride intake did not influence the haematocrit values of non-pregnant adult female mice or of newborn pups. However, the stresses of pregnancy and rapid growth in the newborn period produced a severe anaemia in mice on the low fluoride intake. They suggested that fluoride may play a hitherto unidentified role in haemopoiesis which is manifested only during stress on the haemopoietic system. In another study, Messer, Armstrong and Singer (1972a) demonstrated that fluorine satisfies the major criteria for an essential trace element in the mouse. They reported that female mice maintained on a low fluoride diet over two generations showed a progressive decline in litter production, whereas mice receiving the same diet supplemented with fluoride reproduced normally and at constant intervals. Furthermore, this impaired reproductive capacity was prevented and cured by the addition of fluoride alone to the diet.

In man, the following statements have been made on the importance of fluoride as a mineral nutrient. The Food and Nutrition Board, National Research Council (1974), which includes fluoride in its recommended dietary allowances, concluded that extensive medical and public health studies have clearly demonstrated the safety and nutritional advantages that result from fluoridation of the water supply (American Academy of Pediatrics, 1972). The Food and Nutrition Board recommends fluoridation of public water supplies in areas where there are low natural fluoride levels.

The *Federal Register* of the United States Food and Drug Administration (1973) concerning the nutritional labelling of food and dietary supplements, lists fluorine as an essential nutrient, and the report by a WHO Expert Committee on Trace Elements in Human Nutrition (WHO, 1973) includes fluorine in its list of 14 trace elements which are believed to be essential for animal life.

REFERENCES

American Academy of Pediatrics, Committee on Nutrition (1972) Fluoride as a nutrient. *Pediatrics* **49**, 456–460.

Armstrong W. D. and Singer L. (1963) Fluoride contents of enamel of sound and carious teeth: a reinvestigation. *J. Dent. Res.* **42**, 133–136.

Barth T. F. W. (1947) The geochemical cycle of fluoride. *J. Geol.* **55**, 420–426.

Blayney J. R., Bowers R. C. and Zimmerman M. (1962) Evanston dental caries study, II. A study of fluoride deposition in bone. *J. Dent. Res.* **41**, 1037–1044.

Carlson C. H., Armstrong W. D. and Singer L. (1960a) Distribution and excretion of radio fluoride in the human. *Proc. Soc. Exp. Biol. Med.* **104**, 235–239.

Carlson C. H., Armstrong W. D. and Singer L. (1960b) Distribution, migration and binding of whole blood fluoride evaluated with radio fluoride. *Am. J. Physiol.* **199**, 187–189.

Chen P. S. jun., Smith F. A., Gardner D. E., O'Brien J. A. and Hodge H. C. (1956) Renal clearance of fluoride. *Proc. Soc. Exp. Biol. Med.* **92**, 879–883.

Cholak J. (1959) Fluorides: a critical review, I. The occurrence of fluoride in air, food and water. *J. Occup. Med.* **1**, 501–511.

Doberenz A. R., Kurnick A. A., Kurtz E. B., Kemmerer A. R. and Reid B. L. (1964) Effect of a minimal fluoride diet on rats. *Proc. Soc. Exp. Biol. Med.* **117**, 689–693.

Dowse C. M. and Jenkins G. N. (1957) Fluoride uptake in vivo in enamel defects and its significance. *J. Dent. Res.* **36**, 816.

Ericsson Y. (1958) The state of fluorine in milk and its absorption and retention when administered in milk: investigations with radioactive fluorine. *Acta Odontol. Scand.* **16**, 51–77.

Ericsson Y. and Malmnas C. L. (1962) Placental transfer of fluorine, investigated with F18 in man and rabbit. *Acta Obstet. Gynecol. Scand.* **41**, 144–158.

Feltman R. and Kosel G. (1955) Prenatal ingestion of fluorides and their transfer to the fetus. *Science* **122**, 560–561.

Fleischer M. (1953) Recent estimates of the abundance of the elements in the earth's crust. U.S. Geological Survey Circular No. 285. Washington, DC.

Food and Nutrition Board, National Research Council (1974) *Recommended Dietary Allowances*. Washington DC, National Academy of Sciences, pp. 98–99, 126.

Gardner D. W., Smith F. A., Hodge H. C. and Overton D. E. (1952) The fluoride content of placental tissue as related to the fluoride content of drinking water. *Science* **115**, 208–209.

Gedalia I., Brzezinski A., Bercovici B. and Lazarov E. (1961) *Proc. Soc. Exp. Biol. Med.* **106**, 147–149.

Gedalia I., Brzezinski A., Portuguese N. and Bercovici B. (1964) The fluoride content of teeth and bones of human fetuses. *Arch. Oral Biol.* **9**, 331–340.

Goodman L. S. and Gilman A. (1965) *The Pharmacological Basis of Therapeutics,* 3rd ed. New York, Macmillan.

Hallsworth A. S. and Weatherell J. A. (1969) The microdistribution, uptake and loss of fluoride in human enamel. *Caries Res.* **3**, 109–118.

Ham M. P. and Smith M. D. (1950) Fluoride studies related to the human diet. *Can. J. Res. F.* **28**, 227–233.

Ham M. P. and Smith M. D. (1954) Fluorine balance studies on four infants. *J. Nutr.* **53**, 215–223.

Heasman M. A. and Martin A. E. (1962) Mortality in areas containing natural fluoride in their water supplies. *Monthly Bull. Minist. Health* **21**, 150–160.

Held H. R. (1954) Fluormedikation und Blutfluor. *Schweiz. Med. Wochenschr.* **84**, 251–254.

Hodge H. C. and Smith F. A. (1965) Fluoride absorption: metabolism of inorganic fluorides. In: Simons J. H. (ed.), *Fluorine Chemistry,* Vol. 4. New York, Academic, pp. 137–176.

Isaac S., Brudevold F., Smith F. A. and Gardner D. E. (1958) Solubility rate and natural fluoride content of surface and sub-surface enamel. *J. Dent. Res* **37**, 254–263.

Jackson D. and Weidmann S. M. (1958) Fluorine in human bone related to age and the water supply of different regions. *J. Pathol. Bacteriol.* **76**, 451–459.

Jackson D. and Weidmann S. M. (1959) The relationship between age and the fluoride content of human dentine and enamel: a regional survey. *Br. Dent. J.* **107**, 303–306.

Jenkins G. N. (1963) Theories on the mode of action of fluoride in reducing dental decay. *J. Dent. Res.* **42**, 444–452.

Jenkins G. N. (1975) Recent advances in work on fluorides and the teeth. *Br. Med. Bull.* **31**, 142–145.

Jenkins G. N. and Speirs R. L. (1954) Some observations on the fluoride concentration of dental tissues. *J. Dent. Res.* **33**, 734.

Kappana A. N., Gadre G. T., Bhavnagary H. M. and Joshi J. M. (1962) Minor constituents of Indian sea-water. *Curr. Sci.* **31**, 273–274.

Largent E. J. (1960) Excretion of fluorine. In: Muhler J. C. and Hine M. K. (ed.), *Fluorine and Dental Health: the Pharmacology and Toxicology of Fluorine,* Bloomington, Indiana University Press, p. 132

Little M. F., Casciani F. S. and Rowley J. (1967) Site of fluoride accumulation in intact erupted human enamel. *Arch. Oral Biol.* **12**, 839–847.

Longwell J. (1957) Symposium on the fluoridation of public water supplies. (d) chemical and technical aspects. *R. Soc. Health J.* **77**, 361–370.

MacIntire W. H., Harden L. J. and Hester W. (1952) Measurement of atmospheric fluorine: analyses of rainwater and Spanish moss exposures. *Engng Chem.* **44**, 1365–1370.

McClure F. J. (1949a) Fluorine in foods. *Public Health Rep.* **64**, 1061–1074.

McClure F. J. (1949b) Fluorides and human health. *Public Health Rep.* **64**, 1061. Cited in *Fluorides and Human Health* (1970) *WHO Monogr. Ser.* No. 59. Geneva, WHO, p. 32.

McClure F. J. and Kinser C. A. (1944) Fluoride domestic waters and systemic effects; fluoride content of wine in relation to fluorine in drinking water. *Public Health Rep.* **59**, 1575–1591.

McClure F. J., Mitchell H. H., Hamilton T. S. and Kinser C. A. (1945) Balance of fluorine ingested from various sources in food and water by five young men. Excretion of fluorine through the skin. *J. Indust. Hyg.* **27**, 159–170.

Machle W. and Largent E. J. (1943) Absorption and excretion of fluoride. *J. Indust. Hyg. Toxicol.* **25**, 112–123.

Maurer R. L. and Day H. G. (1957) The non-essentiality of fluorine in nutrition. *J. Nutr.* **62**, 561–573.

Messer H. H., Armstrong W. D. and Singer L. (1972a) Fertility impairment in mice on a low fluoride intake. *Science* **177**, 893–894.

Messer H. H., Wong K., Wegner M., Singer L. and Armstrong W. D. (1972b) Effect of reduced fluoride intake by mice on haematocrit values. *Nature (New Biol.)* **240**, 218–219.

Ministry of Health (1962) The conduct of the fluoridation studies in the United Kingdom and the results achieved after five years. Reports on Public Health and Medical Subjects No. 105, London, HMSO.

Muhler J. C. (1954) Retention of fluorine in the skeleton of the rat receiving different levels of fluorine in the diet. *J. Nutr.* **54**, 481–490.

Neuman W. F. and Neuman M. W. (1958) *The Chemical Dynamics of Bone Mineral.* Chicago, University of Chicago Press.

Noguchi K., Ueno S., Kanuiya H. and Nishiido T. (1963) Chemical composition of the volatile matters emitted by the eruptions of Miyake Island in 1962. *Proc. Jpn Acad.* **39**, 364–369.

Sharpless G. R. and McCollum E. V. (1933) Is fluorine an indispensable element in the diet? *J. Nutr.* **6**, 163–178.

Singer L. and Armstrong W. D. (1960) Regulation of human plasma fluoride concentration. *J. Appl. Physiol.* **15**, 508–510.

Singer L. and Armstrong W. D. (1964) Regulation of plasma fluoride in rats. *Proc. Soc. Exp. Biol. Med.* **117**, 686–689.

Singer L. and Armstrong W. D. (1969) Total fluoride content of human serum. *Arch. Oral Biol.* **14**, 1343–1348.

Singer L., Ophang R. H. and Harland B. F. (1980) Fluoride intake of young male adults in the United States. *Am. J. Human Nutr.* **33**, 328–332.

Smith F. A., Gardner D. E. and Hodge H. C. (1950) Investigations on the metabolism of fluorine, II. Fluoride content of blood and urine as a function of the fluorine in drinking water. *J. Dent. Res.* **29**, 596–600.

Smith F. A., Gardner D. E. and Hodge H. C. (1953) Age increase in fluoride content in human bone. *Fed. Proc.* **12**, 368.

Smith F. A., Gardner D. E., Leone N. C. and Hodge H. C. (1960) The effects of the absorption of fluoride, V. The chemical determination of fluoride in human soft tissues following prolonged ingestion of fluoride at various levels. *Arch. Indust. Health* **21**, 330–332.

Stookey G. K., Crane D. B. and Muhler J. C. (1964) Further studies on fluoride absorption. *Proc. Soc. Exp. Biol. Med.* **115**, 295–298.

Tanganyika Goverment Chemist (1955) *Annual Report of the Government Chemist, 1954*. Dar es Salaam, Government Printer.

Taves D. R. (1966) Normal human serum fluoride concentrations. *Nature, Lond.* **211**, 192–193.

Thompson T. G. and Taylor H. J. (1933) Determination and occurrence of flourides in sea water. *Indust. Engng Chem. Analyt. Edn.* **5**, 87–89.

United States Food and Drug Administration (1973) *U.S. Federal Register* **38**, 20713, No. 148.

Vinogradov A. P. (1954) *Geochemie seltener und nur in Spuren vorhandener chemischer Elemente in Boden*. Berlin, Akademie Verlag. Cited in *Fluorides and Human Health* (1970), *WHO Monogr. Ser.* No. 59. Geneva, WHO, p. 21.

Wattenberg H. (1943) Zur chemie des Meerwassers: uber die in Spuren vorkommenden Alimente. *Z. Anorg. Allg. Chem.* **251**, 86–91.

Weatherell J. A. (1966) Fluoride and the skeletal and dental tissues. *Handb. Exp. Pharmak.* **20**(1), 141–172.

Weatherell J. A. (1969) Fluoride in bones and teeth and the development of fluorosis. In: Barltrop D. and Burland W. L. (ed.), *Mineral Metabolism in Paediatrics*. Oxford, Blackwell Scientific Publications, pp. 53–69.

Weatherell J. A. and Hargreaves J. A. (1965) The micro-sampling of enamel. *Arch. Oral Biol.* **10**, 139–142.

Weidmann S. M. and Weatherell J. A. (1959) The uptake and distribution of fluorine in bones. *J. Pathol. Bacteriol.* **78**, 243–255.

Weidmann S. M. and Weatherell J. A. (1970) Distribution in hard tissues. In: *Fluorides and Human Health* (1970), *WHO Monogr. Ser.* No. 59. Geneva, WHO, pp. 104–128.

Williamson M. M. (1953) Endemic dental fluorosis in Kenya: a preliminary report. *E. Afr. Med. J.* **30**, 217–233.

World Health Organisation (1970) *Fluorides and Human Health. WHO Monogr. Ser.* No. 59. Geneva, WHO.

World Health Organisation (1973) Trace elements in human nutrition. *WHO Tech. Rep. Ser.* No. 532. Geneva, WHO.

Yoon S. H., Brudevold F., Gardner D. E. and Smith F. A. (1960) Distribution of fluoride in teeth from areas with different levels of fluoride in the water supply. *J. Dent. Res.* **39**, 846–856.

Ziegler E. (1956) Untersuchungen lüber die Fluorierung der Milch zur Kariesprophylaxe. *Mitt. Naturw. Ges. Winterthur.* **28**, 1–63.

Zipkin I. and Leone N. C. (1957) Rate of urinary fluoride output in normal adults. *Am. J. Public Health* **47**, 848–851.

Zipkin I. and Likins R. C. (1957) Absorption of various fluorine compounds from the gastro-intestinal tract of the rat. *Am. J. Physiol.* **191**, 549–550.

CHAPTER 13

THE TOXICITY OF FLUORIDE

FLUORIDE INTOXICATION—EFFECT ON BONE

The manifestations of chronic fluoride intoxication depend upon the rate of ingestion, the duration of exposure and the age of the subject. The bone fluoride is roughly proportional to the water fluoride, due both to (1) exchange at the mineral surface, and (2) incorporation of fluoride in newly formed bone.

At water fluoride levels over 8 ppm, for example in South Africa (Ockerse, 1946) and India (Srikantia and Siddiqui, 1965), skeletal fluorosis may develop. This is characterized by an increase in the X-ray density of trabecular bone in the lumbar spine, pelvis and elsewhere, and an increase in the thickness of long bone cortices due to endosteal and periosteal apposition. In more advanced cases calcification of ligaments occurs, especially in the spine, and a clinical picture is observed which bears some resemblance to ankylosing spondylitis (Steinberg et al., 1955).

Histologically, fluorotic bone presents a very mixed picture. There may be a great increase in new bone formation, as well as increase in the width and number of osteoid borders (Weatherell and Weidmann, 1959). This apparent resemblance to osteomalacia has never been adequately explained, but it is reinforced by the finding that the plasma alkaline phosphatase level is raised. However, the plasma calcium is invariably normal and the plasma phosphate is believed to be the same. In addition, there are numerous resorption spaces with fibrous tissue replacement, which Faccini (1969) attributes to secondary hyperparathyroidism. He postulates that bone which has taken up fluoride becomes resistant to resorption which results in parathyroid overactivity and excessive turnover in less affected parts of the skeleton. If this secondary hyperparathyroidism led to hypophosphataemia the osteomalacic features of fluorotic bone would be explained, but such plasma phosphate values that are available do not suggest that this is the case. Although fluorotic bone is sclerotic, in the sense that there is more of it than normal, it is not as strong, weight for weight, as normal bone, and spontaneous fractures are common (Nordin, 1973).

Cases of severe chronic toxicity have occurred among cryolite workers studied by Roholm (1937). These men and women were absorbing 14–68 mg per day for a period of 20–30 years. A number of toxic effects were observed, principally gastric complaints, osteosclerosis, exostoses of long bones, vertebrae, jaw bones and other flat bones. Singh et al. (1962) studied the skeleton of a person living in an area where the fluoride content of the drinking water was 9·5 ppm. All the bones were heavy and irregular and were of a dull colour due to irregular deposition of fluoride. Irregular bone was laid down along the attachment of muscles and tendons and multiple exostoses developed. Continuous exposure to 20–80 mg of fluoride for 20–30 years results in deformities (Singh et al., 1962). The crippling deformities are partly due to mechanical factors and partly to the immobilization necessitated by pain and paraplegia.

The radiological changes of skeletal fluorosis were described by Roholm (1937). In stage 1 the spinal column and the pelvis show roughening and blurring of the trabeculae. In stage 2 the trabeculae merge together and the bone has a diffuse structureless appearance. In stage 3 the bone appears as marble white shadows; the configuration is woolly. The cortex of long bones is thick and dense and the medullary cavity is diminished.

The effects of exposure to fluoride at the level of 8 ppm has been studied in detail by Leone et al. (1954) in a survey of 116 persons in Bartlett (8 ppm) and 121 persons in Cameron (0·5 ppm). The study began in 1943, when each participant received a medical and dental examination and X-rays, blood and urine studies were performed. These were repeated 10 years later in 1953. No significant differences between the two towns were observed in the following characteristics measured: arthritic changes, blood pressure, bone changes, cataract and/or lens opacity, thyroid, hearing, tumours and/or cysts, fractures, urinary tract calculi and gall-stones. There was a slightly higher rate of cardiovascular abnormalities in Cameron and a marked predominance of dental fluorosis in Bartlett.

The effect of consuming drinking water containing up to 4·0 ppm F on bone has been investigated histologically, roentgenographically and chemically. Weidmann et al. (1963) examined histologically the ribs of individuals living in areas containing 0·5, 0·8 and 1·9 ppm F in the drinking water, for width of cortex and number and thickening of the cortical trabeculae. No differences were seen in resorption areas of the trabeculae or of the compacta among the three groups.

Schlesinger et al. (1956) examined children drinking water containing 1·2 ppm F in Newburgh, over a period of 10 years. Roentgenograms of the right hand, both knees and the lumbar spine were taken and bone density and bone age were estimated. No difference of any significance could be found in any of the roentgenographic studies.

Increased bone density or osteosclerosis was not apparent roentgeno-graphically when the concentration of fluoride in the drinking water was less than 4 ppm (Stevenson and Watson, 1957; Geever et al., 1958a, b; Morris, 1965), when the urinary fluoride concentration was less than 10 ppm (Largent et al., 1951) or when the bone contained less than about 5000 ppm F on a dry, fat-free basis (Weidmann et al., 1963).

The possible effect of fluoride on the chemical constituents of bone has been studied by Zipkin et al. (1960), using post-mortem specimens of the iliac crest, rib and vertebra of individuals exposed to drinking water containing up to 4·0 ppm F. Calcium, phosphorus and potassium in the bone ash were unaffected by mean concentrations of bone fluoride as high as 0·8 per cent. The carbonate content decreased by about 10 per cent, the citrate content decreased by about 30 per cent whereas the magnesium content increased by about 15 per cent when the fluoride showed an eightfold increase. An increase in bone fluoride is associated with an increase in the crystallinity of bone apatite (Posner et al., 1963).

THE USE OF SODIUM FLUORIDE IN BONE DISORDERS

Sodium fluoride has been used in doses of 50–75 mg daily (Schenk et al., 1970) in order to stimulate new bone formation in patients with osteoporosis. A combination of sodium fluoride therapy and supplementation of the diet with calcium and vitamin D has also been reported to be successful in treating cases of osteoporosis (Jowsey et al., 1972).

In cases of myelomatosis, once the myelomatosis is controlled by melphalan and corticosteroids (which correct the hypercalcaemia), sodium fluoride (30–60 mg/day) has been used to produce recalcification of the myeloma bone lesions without, as far as can be judged, affecting the underlying cellular abnormality (Carbone et al., 1968).

Sodium fluoride (30–60 mg/day) was reported by Rich and Ensinck (1961) to reduce bone resorption and improve calcium balance in one case of Paget's disease. This was confirmed by Bernstein et al. (1963) but later denied by Higgins et al. (1965) on the basis of balance studies in three cases.

Sodium fluoride (4–6 mg/day) was said to reduce the fracture rate in one 20-month-old girl (Kuzemko, 1970) suffering from osteogenesis imperfecta, but so little is known of the real nature of this disease that no rational therapy can be recommended.

FLUORIDE INTOXICATION: EFFECT ON TEETH

Dental fluorosis is a specific disturbance of tooth formation caused by excessive fluoride intake. The clinical features of dental fluorosis are extremely variable. It is characterized clinically by lustreless, opaque white patches in the enamel which may become mottled, striated and/or pitted. The mottled areas may become stained yellow or brown. The affected teeth may show a pronounced accentuation of the perikymata, or have multiple pits. Hypoplastic areas may also be present to such an extent in severe cases that the normal tooth form is lost (Pindborg, 1970).

EPIDEMIOLOGY OF DENTAL FLUOROSIS

The association between fluoride content of the drinking water and mottled enamel was established before the caries-inhibitory effect of the fluoride had been realized. In fact it was the observation of 'Colorado Brown Stain' by McKay and his realization that mottled enamel usually occurred in well-defined geographic areas (*Fig.* 37) that eventually led to the discovery of fluoride in drinking water (*see* Chapter 1).

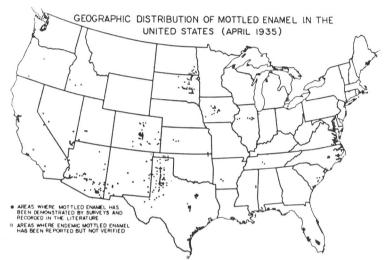

Fig. 37. Geographic distribution of mottled enamel in the United States (April 1935). (From Dean and Elvove, 1936.) (*Reproduced from 'Fluoride Drinking Waters', edited by McClure F. J., by kind permission of the US Department of Health, Education and Welfare, 1962.*)

H. Trendley Dean carried on McKay's pioneering work in America. He developed an index (Dean, 1934) to compare the severity of dental fluorosis in various communities. Each individual is allotted a value according to the following scale:

0	—	normal
0·5	—	questionable
1·0	—	very mild
2·0	—	mild
3·0	—	moderate
4·0	—	severe

The community fluorosis index is calculated in the following way:

$$\text{Fci} = \frac{\text{number of individuals} \times \text{statistical weight}}{\text{total number of individuals examined}}.$$

Møller (1965) suggested that three intermediate values should be introduced (1·5, 2·5, 3·5) to make Dean's index more sensitive. It is important to realize that very many factors other than fluoride can cause mottling or opacities to occur in enamel. This is recognized in Dean's index by the presence of the 'questionable' value. In some cases the term 'idiopathic enamel opacities' is used to describe mottling occurring in areas with a low-fluoride content of the water supply.

Dean (1936) showed that in America, in areas with 0·9 ppm F in the drinking water, less than 10 per cent of children displayed any opacities of teeth. However, as the concentration of fluoride in the drinking water increased, both the prevalence and severity of mottling increased rapidly, so that at a concentration of 2·5 ppm F in drinking water the incidence of mottling was approximately 70 per cent (*Fig. 38*).

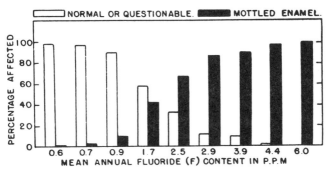

Fig. 38. The prevalence of mottled enamel in areas with differing concentrations of fluoride in the water supply. (From Dean, 1936.) (*Reproduced from 'Fluoride Drinking Waters', edited by McClure F. J., by kind permission of the US Department of Health, Education and Welfare, 1962.*)

Møller (1965) showed that a similar trend was evident in Danish schoolchildren although, for any given fluoride concentration, the severity of dental fluorosis was lower in Denmark than in the USA (*Fig. 39*).

In the United Kingdom Forrest (1956) carried out a study in four areas in which fluoride occurred naturally in the water supplies at concentrations of 5·8, 3·5, 2·0 and 0·9 ppm, and in two areas where there was no more than a trace of fluoride in the water. Her results are given diagrammatically in *Fig.* 40 and show that the index of mottling was lowest in the area (Slough) with 0·9 ppm F. As the fluoride concentration in the water supply increased beyond this figure, the incidence and severity of fluoride mottling were directly related to the amount of fluoride in the water. In the two areas with fluoride-free water supplies the index of mottling was higher than in Slough, thus supporting the view expressed by Cox (1954) that a certain amount of fluoride is necessary to prevent

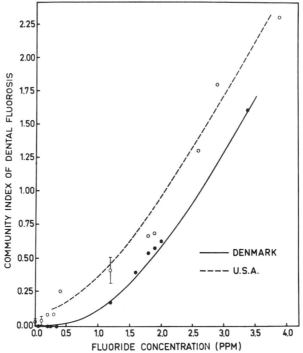

Fig. 39. Community index of dental fluorosis in USA and Denmark in relation to the fluoride content of the drinking water. (From Møller, 1965.) (*Reproduced from 'Dental Fluorose og Karies', by Møller I. J., Copenhagen, Rhodos, 1965.*)

enamel defects. In a further investigation Forrest and James (1965) carried out a blind study of enamel opacities in areas which had used artificially fluoridated drinking water for 8 years. In the fluoridated area, enamel opacities occurred in 36 per cent of the children; in 24 per cent they were of the idiopathic type and in only 12 per cent could they be classified as 'questionable' or 'very mild' fluorosis. In the control area idiopathic opacities occurred in 47 per cent of the children. This study highlights the problem of trying to determine whether opacities of enamel are due to excessive fluoride intake or are due to other disturbances, infectious, traumatic, metabolic or genetic, which can affect the developing tooth germ.

Studies in low-fluoride areas have shown that a high proportion of children have enamel opacities in permanent teeth. Zimmermann (1954) reported that 39·9 per cent of children had enamel opacities in Maryland, USA (0·2 ppm F in drinking water), and Jackson (1961) found a prevalence of 34·0 per cent in a study of 12-year-old children from Leeds,

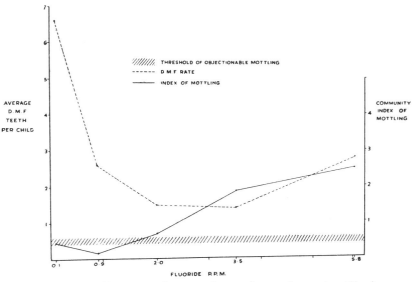

Fig. 40. Fluoride content of water, caries experience and enamel mottling in children aged 12–14 years. (From Forrest, 1956.) (*Reproduced by courtesy of the Editor, 'British Dental Journal'.*)

England (0·06 ppm F in drinking water). Jackson (1974) maintains that the clinical differentiation between the milder degrees of fluoride mottling and enamel opacities occurring in low-fluoride areas which cannot be attributed to fluoride ingestion is extremely difficult, if not impossible, and has the drawback that an assumption has to be made with regard to aetiology. He suggested a new approach based on the sound epidemiological principle that the recording of any condition once defined must be made on the basis of that definition and not on the basis of a presumed aetiology.

His index was also based on the principle that a simple descriptive index is preferable to a weighted one and he concluded that the following types of mottled enamel could be identified:

Type A: White areas less than 2 mm in diameter.

Type B: White areas of, or greater than, 2 mm in diameter.

Type C: Coloured (brown) areas less than 2 mm in diameter, irrespective of there being white areas.

Type D: Coloured (brown) areas of, or greater than, 2 mm in diameter, irrespective of there being any white areas.

Type E: Horizontal white lines, irrespective of there being any white non-linear areas.

Type F: Coloured (brown) or white areas or lines associated with pits or hypoplastic areas.

This classification is similar to that used by Young (1973).

This index has been employed in two recent surveys in fluoride and non-fluoride communities in Britain: 171 13–16-year-old Anglesey children who had received fluoridated drinking water (F = 0·9 ppm) all their lives were compared with 178 12–15-year-old children from Leeds, a low-fluoride area (F = 0·1 ppm) (Al-Alousi et al., 1975). The mouth prevalence of mottling was 39 per cent in Anglesey and 52 per cent in Leeds. The tooth prevalence of mottling was 9 per cent in Anglesey and 12 per cent in Leeds, thus confirming the finding by Forrest and James (1965) that the prevalence of enamel opacities in a community fluoridated near the optimal level of 1 ppm is smaller than that observed in a non-fluoride community. In a further study Jackson et al. (1975) assessed the level of fluoride mottling on incisor teeth of 15-year-old children from Anglesey and Bangor/Caernarvon (F < 0·01 ppm). Mouth prevalence of mottling was 35 per cent in Anglesey and 37 per cent in the control community. The proportion of standing teeth with mottling was 7·9 per cent in Anglesey and 7·7 per cent in Bangor/Caernarvon. It was concluded that 'the aetiology of the kind of mottling observed in Leeds, Anglesey, Bangor and Caernarvon, and in many other non-fluoride communities is independent of fluoride ingestion. It is quite erroneous to refer to this kind of mottling as dental fluorosis' (Jackson et al., 1975).

However, epidemiological studies have shown conclusively that high levels of fluoride in drinking water do interfere with the normal development of teeth and produce the clinical condition of 'dental fluorosis'.

HISTOPATHOLOGY OF DENTAL FLUOROSIS

The way in which fluoride might exert its effect has been studied principally using chemical and histopathological techniques. Information regarding the chemical aspects of the organic material in mottled enamel is limited (WHO, 1970). Bowes and Murray (1936) demonstrated a higher protein content in fluorosed enamel than in non-mottled enamel. This finding was confirmed by Bhussry (1959) who reported a higher nitrogen content in mottled enamel than in sound enamel. Chemical analysis of the inorganic content by Armstrong and Brekhus (1937), Bowes and Murray (1936), Smith and Lantz (1932) and Ockerse (1943) did not show any significant difference (ash basis) in the calcium, phosphorus, magnesium and carbonate content of mottled and non-mottled teeth.

An observation of great theoretical interest is that although the outermost layer of shark's teeth contains more than a hundred times the fluoride content of human mottled enamel, there are no signs of disturbance in its mineralization. Using biophysical and chemical methods, Glas (1962) demonstrated that the size and orientation of the apatite crystallites in the shark 'enamel' and its degree of mineralization were the same as in human enamel. In contrast to the hydroxyapatite occurring in human enamel, the inorganic phase of shark 'enamel' consists of an almost pure fluorapatite, which is formed during normal mineralization (Buttner, 1966). Unlike human enamel, which is of epithelial origin, the shark 'enamel' develops from mesodermal tissues (Kvam, 1950) and has been referred to as 'durodentin' and 'petrodentin' (Lison, 1941; Schmidt and Keil, 1958). This suggests that the epithelial enamel organ of human teeth demonstrates specific sensitivity to fluorides (WHO, 1970).

EXPERIMENTAL DENTAL FLUOROSIS

Developing human teeth are more sensitive to fluoride than are rat incisors; the threshold value for human dental fluorosis is 1–2 ppm F, whereas 8–9 ppm F is necessary to cause a loss of pigment from the rat incisors (Pindborg, 1970). Experimental dental fluorosis has been studied by peritoneal injections of fluoride (causing acute fluorosis) or by adding fluorides to drinking water or diet (causing chronic fluorosis). Acute fluorosis produces horizontal bands of pigment-free areas of the rat incisor enamel corresponding to the timing of injections. It is possible to detect histologic changes in the ameloblasts of the rat incisor as early as 1 hour after the injection of fluoride. The fluoride injections cause an accentuation of the incremental lines in enamel and dentine, a change which may be utilized in determining the amount of dentine formed during a given period (Schour and Smith, 1934).

Kruger (1970) used an electron microscope to determine the effect of different levels of fluoride on the ultrastructure of ameloblasts in the rat. Four-day-old Osborne-Mendel rats were given a single intraperitoneal injection of one of three fluoride solutions providing either 7 mg F/kg body weight or 3 mg F/kg body weight or 0·1 mg F/kg body weight. Animals from each of these treatment groups were decapitated at 30, 60 and 90 minutes after injection. At 30 minutes after the injection of the heaviest dose of fluoride there was no marked alteration to the ultra-structural morphology. By 60 minutes, however, a few large ribosome-free distensions were seen as isolated structures in the distal cytoplasm of an occasional cell and, by 90 minutes, these vacuolizations were much more prevalent and their continuity with the profiles of the rough endoplasmic reticulum could be seen. This confirmed a previous observation by Kruger (1968) that repeated doses of fluoride (7 mg F/kg body weight) produced large confluent distensions of the rough endoplasmic reticulum.

With the middle level of fluoride (3 mg F/kg body weight) some swelling of the rough-surfaced endoplasmic reticulum was observed after 30 minutes. By 60 minutes these swellings were still present, but had not progressed to the larger ribosome-free distensions which followed the administration of the heavy dose of fluoride. At 90 minutes after the injection of the 3 mg F dose the cytoplasm of the ameloblast was still morphologically different from that of a normal functional ameloblast in that the profiles of the intact rough-surfaced endoplasmic reticulum were few in number and there were numerous apparently free ribosomes in the cytoplasm. At the lowest level of fluoride used in Kruger's study (0·1 mg F/kg body weight) there was no discernible alteration to the ultrastructure of the ameloblast. Kruger concluded that over the range of mottling doses of fluoride used in his study there was a graded series of ultrastructural changes in the ameloblasts and stated that it would be interesting to know whether there is an associated change in protein synthesis by affected ameloblasts and if proteins are affected by a change in the dosage level of fluoride.

The effect of chronic fluorosis is dependent upon dosage and length of experimental period (Pindborg, 1950). The changes in the rat incisor enamel (on diets containing 0·125–0·5 per cent sodium fluoride) vary from loss of pigment to severe enamel hypoplasia. The ameloblasts are very sensitive to fluoride, reacting early by reducing height. Then follows proliferation of the enamel again, leading to formation of cysts in which amorphous calcified bodies are found. The enamel matrix does not mineralize normally and exhibits surface defects comprising accentuated incremental lines. Micro and radiographic studies of fluorosed rat incisor enamel have shown a hypermineralized surface layer similar to that found in human fluorosed teeth (Yaeger, 1966).

As a result of high dosages of fluoride four abnormalities may be seen in dentine: striations, hypoplastic defects, hypomineralized interglobular spaces, and gross deformations of the external outline of the dentine (Yaeger, 1966). Such changes have not been described in human fluorosed teeth (Pindborg, 1970).

Overall, the results of the experimental studies indicate that excessive fluoride levels do exert an effect at the cellular level. Whether this effect produces a change in the extracellular protein secreted by ameloblasts and odontoblasts is not yet known.

EFFECTS OF NATURAL FLUORIDE DRINKING WATER ON GENERAL HEALTH

Studies of the physiological manifestations in man of long exposure to high fluoride levels have been summarized in *Fluorides and Human Health* (WHO, 1970). The main conclusions were:

1. No impairment of or effect on the general health status could be detected among persons residing for an average of 37 years in areas where the water supply contains fluoride at the levels of 8 ppm, and no systemic abnormalities or abnormal laboratory findings were observed that might be associated with ingestion of fluorides (Leone et al., 1954, 1964).

2. Prolonged high fluoride intake up to 8 ppm does not affect morbidity or mortality (Leone et al., 1954; Geever et al., 1958a, b; Hagan, 1960). Studies of mortality from specific causes of death in 32 communities with 1 ppm F in drinking water have been compared with 32 communities with negligible fluoride in the water (Hagan et al., 1954). Death rates from heart disease, cancer, intracranial lesions, nephritis and cirrhosis of the liver were reported. No statistically significant differences were found between the mortality rates of the fluoride and non-fluoride cities, either for these five specific causes or from all causes combined.

3. Young males in high fluoride areas fail to reveal a relationship between bone fractures and fluoride exposure and their height/weight figures compare favourably with those of young men in other areas of the USA, indicating that fluoride exposure does not influence man's growth pattern (McClure, 1944; McCauley and McClure, 1954).

4. The prolonged ingestion of fluoride does not affect thyroid gland size or function in either man or animals (Shupe et al., 1963; Leone et al., 1964).

Martin (1970), in a review of the effect of fluorides on general health, concluded: 'By their wide distribution in nature, their inevitable presence in man's food and drink and their consequent presence in the tissues of the human body, fluorides form a natural part of man's environment, yet when present in excess they are known to be harmful. However, results have shown that a level of approximately 1 ppm F in temperate climates has no harmful effects on the community. The margin of safety is such that will cover any individual variation of intake to be found in such areas.'

ACUTE FLUORIDE POISONING

The acute lethal dose of fluoride for man is probably about 5 g of sodium fluoride (which yields 2·2 g F) (Goodman and Gilman, 1965). It would obviously be impossible for fluoridated water ever to cause acute fluoride poisoning: when water is fluoridated at a level of 1 ppm F, 1 litre of water contains 1 mg F. Thus in order to receive even 1 g F one would have to consume, over a very short period of time, 1000 litres of water.

However, topical fluoride agents commonly contain 1·23 per cent F. Thus a 250-ml bottle of APF gel contains approximately 3 g F, potentially a lethal dose if the whole bottle was consumed quickly by one person. One fatal case of acute fluoride poisoning due to consumption of topical fluoride agents has been reported; it is important for dentists to keep these agents safe and out of reach of young children (*see* p. 245).

Acute fluoride intoxication is very rare. Approximately 435 cases have been recorded (Roholm, 1937; Greenwood, 1940; WHO, 1970), but 236 cases of poisoning occurred in a single episode at the Oregon State Hospital (Lidbeck et al., 1943). Seventeen pounds of sodium fluoride were inadvertently added to a 10-gallon batch of scrambled eggs being prepared in the hospital kitchen and as a result 47 patients died. The main signs and symptoms of acute fluoride poisoning are diffuse abdominal pain, diarrhoea, vomiting and painful spasms in the limbs. If acute fluoride poisoning is suspected the contents of the stomach must be emptied as quickly as possible, by giving an emetic, in order to reduce the amount of fluoride absorbed.

REFERENCES

Al-Alousi W., Jackson D., Crompton G. and Jenkins O. C. (1975) Enamel mottling in a fluoride and in a non-fluoride community. *Br. Dent. J.* **138**, 9–15.

Armstrong W. D. and Brekhus P. J. (1937) Chemical constitution of enamel and dentine; principal components. *J. Biol. Chem.* **120**, 677–687.

Bernstein D. S. et al. (1963) The use of sodium fluoride in metabolic bone disease. *J. Clin. Invest.* **42**, 916.

Bhussry B. R. (1959) Chemical and physical studies of enamel from human teeth, IV. Density and nitrogen content of mottled enamel. *J. Dent. Res.* **38**, 369–373.

Bowes J. H. and Murray M. M. (1936) A chemical study of 'mottled teeth' from Malden, Essex. *Br. Dent. J.* **60**, 556–562.

Buttner W. (1966) In: James P. M. C. et al. (ed.), *Advances in Fluorine Research and Dental Caries Prevention. Proceedings 12th O.R.C.A. Congress, Utrecht,* 1965, vol. 4, pp. 193–200.

Carbone P. P., Zipkin I., Sokoloff L. et al. (1968) Fluoride effect on bone in plasma cell myeloma. *Arch. Intern. Med.* **121**, 130–140.

Cox G. J. (1954) In: Shaw J. H., *Fluoridation as a Public Health Measure.* Washington, American Association for the Advancement of Science, p. 36.

Dean H. T. (1934) Classification of mottled enamel diagnosis. *J. Am. Dent. Assoc.* **21**, 1421–1426.

Dean H. T. (1936) Chronic endemic dental fluorosis (mottled enamel). *J.A.M.A.* **107**, 1269–1272.

Dean H. T. (1942) The investigation of physiological effects by the epidemiological method. In: Moulton F. R. (ed.), *Fluorine and Dental Health.* Washington, American Association for the Advancement of Science, pp. 23–31.

Dean H.T. and Elvove E. (1936) Some epidemiological aspects of chronic endemic dental fluorosis. *Am. J. Public Health,* **26**, 567–575.

Faccini J. M. (1969) Fluoride and bone. *Calcif. Tissue Res.* **3**, 1–16.

Forrest J. R. (1956) Caries incidence and enamel defects in areas with different levels of fluoride in the drinking water. *Br. Dent. J.* **100**, 195–200.

Forrest J. R. and James P. M. C. (1965) A blind study of enamel opacities and dental caries prevalence after eight years of fluoridation of water. *Br. Dent. J.* **119**, 319–322.

Geever E. F., Leone N. C., Geiser P. and Lieberman J. E. (1958a) Pathological studies in man after prolonged ingestion of fluoride in drinking water. *Public Health Rep.* **73**, 721–731.

Geever E. F., Leone N. C., Geiser P. and Lieberman J. E. (1958b) Pathological studies in man after prolonged ingestion of fluoride in drinking water, I. Necropsy findings in a community with a water level of 2·5 ppm. *J. Am. Dent. Assoc.* **56**, 499–507.

Glas J. E. (1962) Studies on the ultrastructure of dental enamel, VI. Crystal chemistry of shark's teeth. *Odontol. Revy* **13**, 315–326.

Goodman L. S. and Gilman A. (1965) *The Pharmacological Basis of Therapeutics*, 3rd ed. New York, Macmillan.

Greenwood D. A. (1940) Fluoride intoxication. *Physiol. Rev.* **20**, 582.

Hagan T. L. (1960) Effects of fluoridation on general health as reflected in mortality data. In: Muhler J. C. and Hine M. K., *Fluorine and Dental Health: The Pharmacology and Toxicology of Fluorine*. Indiana University Press, pp. 157–165.

Hagan T. L., Pasternack M. and Scholz G. C. (1954) Waterborne fluorides and mortality. *Public Health Rep.* **69**, 451–454.

Higgins B. A., Nassim J. R., Alexander R. and Hilb A. (1965) Effect of sodium fluoride on calcium, phosphorus and nitrogen balance in patients with Paget's disease. *Br. Med. J.* **1**, 1159–1161.

Jackson D. (1961) A clinical study of non-endemic mottling of enamel. *Arch. Oral Biol.* **3**, 212–223.

Jackson D. (1974) Personal communication.

Jackson D., James P. M. C. and Wolfe W. B. (1975) Fluoridation in Anglesey: A clinical study. *Br. Dent. J.* **138**, 165–171.

Jowsey J., Riggs B. L., Kelly P. J. and Hoffman D. L. (1972) Effects of combined therapy with sodium fluoride, vitamin D and calcium in osteoporosis. *Am. J. Med.* **53**, 43–49.

Kruger B. J. (1968) Ultrastructural changes in ameloblasts from fluoride treated rats. *Arch. Oral Biol.* **13**, 969–977.

Kruger B. J. (1970) The effect of different levels on the ultrastructure of ameloblasts in a rat. *Arch. Oral Biol.* **15**, 109–114.

Kuzemko J. A. (1970) Osteogenesis imperfecta tarda treated with sodium fluoride. *Arch. Dis. Child.* **45**, 581–582.

Kvam T. (1950) *K. Norske Vidensk. Selskab. (Trondhjem)*.

Largent E. J., Bovard P. G. and Heyroth F. F. (1951) Roentgenographic changes and urinary fluoride excretion among workmen engaged in the manufacture of inorganic fluorides. *Am. J. Roentgenol. Radium Ther. Nucl. Med.* **65**, 42–48.

Leone N. C., Leatherwood E. C., Petrie I. M. and Lieberman L. (1964) Effect of fluoride on the thyroid gland: clinical study. *J. Am. Dent. Assoc.* **69**, 179–180.

Leone N. C., Shimkin M. B., Arnold F. A., Stevenson C. A., Zimmerman E. R., Geiser P. B. and Lieberman J. E. (1954) Medical aspects of excessive fluoride in a water supply. *Public Health Rep.* **69**, 925–936.

Lidbeck W. L., Hill I. B. and Beeman J. (1943) Acute sodium fluoride poisoning. *J.A.M.A.* **121**, 826–827.

Lison L. (1941) Sur la structure des dents poissons dipneustes. La petrodentine. *C. R. Séanc. Soc. Biol. (Paris)* **135**, 431–443.

McCauley H. B. and McClure F. J. (1954) Effect of fluoride in drinking water on the osseous development of the hand and wrist in children. *Public Health Rep.* **69**, 671–683.

McClure F. J. (1944) Fluoride domestic waters and systemic effects: relation to bone fracture experience, height and weight of high school boys and young selectees of the armed forces of the United States. *Public Health Rep.* **59**, 1543–1558.

McKay F. S. (1916) An investigation of mottled teeth: an endemic developmental imperfection of the enamel of the teeth, heretofore unknown in the literature of dentistry. *Dent. Cosmos* **58**, 477–484.

Martin A. E. (1970) Fluorides and general health: summary. In: *Fluorides and Human Health, WHO Monogr. Ser.* No. 59. Geneva, WHO, pp. 316–318.

Møller I. J. (1965) *Dental Fluorose og Karies.* Copenhagen, Rhodos.

Morris J. W. (1955) Skeletal fluorosis among Indians of the American South West. *Am. J. Roentgenol. Radium Ther. Nucl. Med.* 94, 608–615.

Nordin B. E. C. (1973) *Metabolic Bone and Stone Disease.* Edinburgh, Churchill Livingstone.

Ockerse T. (1943) The chemical composition of enamel and dentine in high and low caries area in South Africa. *J. Dent. Res.* 22, 441–446.

Ockerse T. (1946) *Endemic Fluorosis in South Africa.* Thesis, University of Witwatersrand. Pretoria, Government Printers.

Pindborg J. J. (1950) Den kroniske fluorog camidiumforgiftnings indfly-delse paa den huide rottes incisiver med saerligt henblik paa emaljeorganet. *Tandlaegebladet.* Suppl. 1.

Pindborg J. J. (1970) *Pathology of the Dental Hard Tissues.* Copenhagen, Munskgaard.

Posner A. S., Eanes E. D., Harper R. A. and Zipkin I. (1963) X-ray diffraction analysis of the effect of fluoride on human bone apatite. *Arch. Oral Biol.* 8, 549–570.

Rich C. and Ensinck J. (1961) Effect of sodium fluoride on calcium metabolism of human beings. *Nature (Lond.)* 191, 184–185.

Roholm K. (1937) *Fluorine Intoxication: A Clinical-hygienic Study with a Review of the Literature and some Experimental Investigations.* London, Lewis.

Russell A. L. (1964) In: Young W. O. and Striffer D. F. (ed.), *The Dentist, his Practice and his Community.* Philadelphia, Saunders.

Schenk R. K., Merz W. A. and Reutter F. W. (1970) Fluoride in osteoporosis: quantitative histological studies on bone structure and bone remodelling in serial biopsies of the iliac crest. In: Vischer T. L. (ed.), *Fluoride in Medicine.* Bern, Huber. pp. 153–168.

Schlesinger E. R., Overton D. E., Chase H. C. and Cantwell K. T. (1956) Newburgh–Kingston caries-fluorine study, XIII. Pediatric findings after ten years. *J. Am. Dent. Assoc.* 52, 296–306.

Schmidt W. J. and Keil A. (1958) *Die gesunden und die erkrankten Zahngewebe des Menschen und der Wirbeltiere im Polarisationsmikroskop.* Munich, Hanser.

Schour I. and Smith M. C. (1934) The histological changes in enamel and dentine of rat incisor in acute chronic experimental fluorosis. *Univ. Arizona Agric. Exp. Stat. Tech. Bull.* 52, 69–91.

Shupe J. L., Miner M. L., Greenwood D. A. et al. (1963) The effect of fluorine on dairy cattle, II. Clinical and pathological effects. *Am. J. Vet. Res.* 24, 964–979.

Singh A., Dass R., Hayreh S. S. and Jolly S. S. (1962) Skeletal changes in endemic fluorosis. *J. Bone Joint Surg.* 44B, 806–815.

Smith M. C. and Lantz E. M. (1932) Studies of the metabolism of fluorine, I. Effect of sodium fluoride in the diet upon the chemical composition of the incisors of albino rats. *J. Dent. Res.* 12, 552–554.

Srikantia S. G. and Siddiqui A. H. (1965) Metabolic studies in skeletal fluorosis. *Clin. Sci.* 28, 477–485.

Steinberg C. L., Gardner D. E., Smith F. A. and Hodge H. C. (1955) Comparison of rheumatoid (ankylosing) spondylitis and crippling fluorosis. *Ann. Rheum. Dis.* 14, 378–384.

Stevenson C. A. and Watson A. R. (1957) Fluoride osteosclerosis. *Am. J. Roentgenol. Radium Ther. Nucl. Med.* **78**, 13–18.

Weatherell J. A. and Weidmann S. M. (1959) The skeletal changes of chronic experimental fluorosis. *J. Pathol. Bacteriol.* **78**, 233–241.

Weidmann S. M., Weatherell J. A. and Jackson D. (1963) The effect of fluoride on bone. *Proc. Nutr. Soc.* **22**, 105–110.

World Health Organisation (1970) *Fluorides and Human Health, WHO Monogr. Ser.* No. 59. Geneva, WHO, pp. 278–279.

Yaeger J. A. (1966) The effects of high fluoride diets on developing enamel and dentine in the incisors of rats. *Am. J. Anat.* **118**, 665–683.

Young M. A. (1973) Ph.D. Thesis, University of London.

Zimmerman E. R. (1954) Fluoride and non-fluoride enamel opacities. *Public Health Rep.* **69**, 1115–1120.

Zipkin I., McClure F. J. and Lee W. A. (1960) Relation of the fluoride content of human bone to its chemical composition. *Arch. Oral Biol.* **2**, 190–195.

CHAPTER 14

MODES OF ACTION OF FLUORIDE IN REDUCING CARIES

In the preceding chapters we have seen that fluoride can reduce the occurrence of dental caries but that methods of delivering fluoride differ widely: the concentrations of fluoride have varied between 1 ppm F to over 1 per cent F, the frequency from several times a day to only once a year, and the fluoride compounds used, the pH of the solution and the length of exposure have all varied. How can it be that such widely different methods of application of fluoride are able to result in rather similar caries-preventive effects? In this chapter we shall consider the modes of action of fluoride in an attempt to answer this question. Although there is broad agreement that fluoride acts in several different ways to reduce caries and that this multiplicity of effects is the key to its caries-preventive action, the exact mechanisms and the relative importance of each are still unclear.

ENAMEL CRYSTAL STRUCTURE

The principal mineral substance in enamel (also in dentine and bone) is apatite which has the general formula $Ca_{10}(PO_4)_6X_2$. Hydroxyapatite (HA) is the most common apatite where X is OH. However, the fluoride ion has a strong affinity for mineralized tissues and HA can be readily converted to fluorapatite (FA) where F has replaced OH. The relative proportion of FA to HA in enamel varies, with a higher proportion of FA in outer enamel, in enamel exposed to fluoride solutions or covered with plaque for long periods (Weatherell et al., 1972). But even in enamel frequently exposed to fluoride, it is rare to find fluoride concentrations greater than 3000 ppm F, which represents less than a 10 per cent substitution of OH ions by F ions. Nevertheless, even modest changes in enamel fluoride concentration influence the susceptibility of enamel to dissolution.

The earliest studies investigating the action of fluoride showed that if enamel powder or whole teeth were exposed to fluoride solutions (even as dilute as 1 ppm), the dissolution of the enamel in acid buffer was reduced. In order to explain this effect, the position of the fluoride atom and its properties in the apatite crystal were investigated. It was found that the HA crystal tended to possess voids and that such voids were likely to increase the crystal's reactivity and it would therefore tend to dissolve more easily. These voids are due to the absence of an OH group which occurs because of the disordered arrangement of the other OH groups in relation to the columnar calcium triangles of the lattice (*Fig.* 41). The fluoride ion can fit perfectly in the centre of the triangular arrangement of calcium ions, replacing the missing OH group, thus eliminating the void and stabilizing the crystal structure.

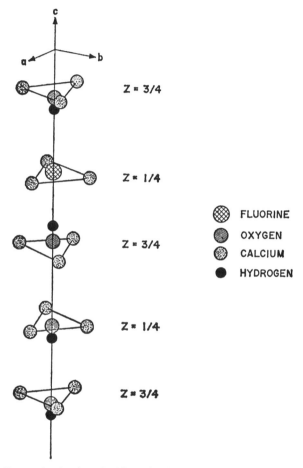

Fig. 41. Perspective drawing of calcium triangle arrangement indicates the two possible hydroxyl ion positions. A void (second triangle from the top) has been replaced by a fluoride ion. (From Young and Elliott, 1966.) (*Reproduced from 'Archives of Oral Biology', by kind permission of the Editor.*)

Ions in crystals frequently undergo exchange with ions in the environment. This can be either isoionic exchange (e.g. one Ca for another Ca ion) or heteroionic exchange so that an F ion might exchange with an OH group in the crystal. This exchange of F for OH appears to be a fairly simple diffusion-controlled process (Joyston-Bechal et al., 1973).

Apatite crystals tend to be surrounded by a hydration layer which may include other ions such as magnesium, carbonate and fluoride. But magnesium and carbonate, unlike fluoride, are associated with poor crystallinity and a further favourable action of fluoride would appear to be its ability to replace magnesium and carbonate in the apatite crystal, thus making the crystal more stable.

The mode of action of sodium monofluorophosphate in plaque and enamel remains obscure. There is good evidence that it is rapidly hydrolysed in plaque resulting in free fluoride, but it may also enter the apatite crystal as MFP (Ingram, 1972; Forward, 1980; de Rooij et al., 1981).

It is possible, therefore, to increase the fluoride concentration in enamel either while the apatite crystals of the tooth are forming (primarily systemic fluoride administration) or after the enamel is formed and the tooth erupted into the mouth (topical administration). Although differences in solubility of enamel with fairly modest changes in fluoride content have been observed, it has been calculated that the maximum cariostatic effect would be reached when about 50 per cent of the OH positions are reoccupied by F (Moreno et al., 1977).

Despite the evidence that incorporation of fluoride into enamel is associated with decreased solubility in vitro (Isaac et al., 1958) and that teeth from people in fluoride areas are less soluble than from fluoride-low areas (Healy and Ludwig, 1966), the importance attached to the above explanation for the caries-preventive effect of fluoride has lessened in recent years. It is now realized that the physiochemical changes at the plaque–enamel interface are much more complicated than changes which occurred in the original test-tube experiments. The main reasons for this change of view are: (1) in the mouth, the rate of change of conditions may be such that equilibria are seldom reached, (2) the type of acid and the pH reached are known to effect the ratio of HA to FA dissolved, and (3) the phase diagrams of the multitude of intermediate compounds resulting from apatite dissolution are very complex.

As well as assisting in the formation of more perfectly formed apatite crystals, incorporation of fluoride also tends to increase the size of the crystal (Grøn et al., 1963). Although this would result in a decrease in crystal surface area per unit volume and therefore reduce the rate of enamel dissolution, its relative importance in preventing caries progression remains uncertain.

If dietary intake of fluoride is too high during tooth formation, fluorosed enamel is formed (*see* pp. 209–14). The white flecks, lines or patches (which may brown with age) in these teeth are caused by changes in the optical properties of enamel due to hypomineralization. This is usually restricted to the outer one-third of enamel, although in more severe cases may involve the outer two-thirds. Mildly fluorosed enamel may have 1–5 per cent spaces, while this may rise to 10–25 per cent in more severely affected enamel. The surface layer of enamel, however, remains highly mineralized although pitting, which occurs in severe cases, is probably the result of a post-eruptive loss of surface contour. As discussed on pp. 214–16, it is not clear at what time during tooth development enamel formation is at greatest risk of fluorosis.

REMINERALIZATION OF ENAMEL

During the carious process of demineralization of enamel, apatite is reduced to simpler compounds or ions, but during a subsequent re-mineralization phase it is by no means certain that apatite will again be formed. Apatite is the most stable and least soluble of biological calcium phosphate compounds and its formation during mineralization is there-fore desirable. One of the more important actions of fluoride is likely to be its ability to increase the formation of apatite during remineralization at the expense of less stable, more soluble, calcium phosphate compounds such as brushite and amorphous calcium phosphate. Brown et al. (1977) have recently suggested that during remineralization the outer layer of the apatite crystal may take up F so that it acquires the property of FA.

Possibly due to fluoride's ability to enhance remineralization of carious enamel, fluoride becomes incorporated into the new crystal structure in increased amounts over many years—the extra fluoride coming presum-ably from the oral environment. This remineralized (or healed) enamel will thus be more resistant to future demineralization than the sur-rounding unaffected enamel (Koulourides et al., 1980). This cycle could occur many times, each time resulting in increased concentration of fluoride in the new enamel and a reduced susceptibility to future caries attack.

ALTERATION IN THE MORPHOLOGY OF TEETH

Forrest (1956) and Ockerse (1949) commented on the well-rounded cusps and shallow fissures of human teeth from fluoride areas in Great Britain and South Africa, but presented no statistical data. Wallenius (1957) reported that teeth found in a fluoride area were on average 1·7 per cent wider than those from a control area, whereas Cooper and Ludwig (1965), in New Zealand, measured the buccolingual and mesiodistal diameters and cusp depth of lower first permanent molars of children in fluoridated and control areas and found the diameters about 2 per cent smaller and the cusp depths 5 per cent smaller in the fluoridated area. Lovius and Goose (1969) reported no statistical difference in the size of teeth of children living in fluoridated and non-fluoridated areas of Anglesey.

Using experimental animals, Paynter and Grainger (1956) found that in rats fed 6 ppm F in their diet, the size of molar teeth was reduced, and the proportion of molars with rounded fissures was higher than in the controls. These results were confirmed by Kruger (1968, 1970) who observed a reduction in the thickness of enamel and dentine and this resulted in smaller teeth with wider fissures.

It is doubtful, though, if small differences in size and shape which may occur with fluoride ingestion could account for more than a minor part of the cariostatic effect of fluoride, especially in view of the fact that fluoride has its greatest effect on smooth surfaces and least effect on pit and fissure caries.

DELAYED ERUPTION OF TEETH

It has been postulated that the lower caries experience observed in children living in fluoridated areas compared with fluoride-low areas could, in part, be explained by the later eruption of their teeth. However, clinical data from areas with optimum fluoride levels do not support this hypothesis. In a large study involving 56 000 children aged 4–15 years in East Germany, Künzel (1976) found that the only clear difference in eruption times between the children in the fluoride-low and the fluoridated areas related to the premolar teeth. He concluded that the difference probably represents a normalization of the dental development in the fluoride areas due to the retention of caries-free deciduous molars, rather than a genuine retardation of tooth eruption. A positive correlation between early loss of deciduous molars and early eruption of first permanent molars was observed by Rugg-Gunn et al. (1977), who also found that for children with all deciduous molars present, there was no difference in eruption times of first permanent molars in 5-year-olds living in fluoridated and non-fluoridated areas of North-East England. It would seem impossible, therefore, for the caries-preventive action of fluoride to be accounted for by delayed eruption of teeth, especially in view of the fact that the caries-preventive effect is observed even in adult life (Murray, 1971).

INHIBITION OF PLAQUE BACTERIA

It has been known for about 50 years that certain enzymes are sensitive to fluoride (Lohmann and Mayerhof, 1934, quoted by Hamilton, 1977): early experiments suggested that enolase in bacteria was particularly sensitive and its inhibition responsible for reduced carbohydrate metabolism in the presence of fluoride (Stone and Werkman, 1937). Since anaerobic glycolysis by plaque bacteria is almost universally accepted as an essential step in caries aetiology, the possibility that fluoride might reduce glycolysis has received widespread attention. Research has tended to follow two main pathways: first, determination of the fluoride concentration which will significantly reduce the fall in plaque pH after sugar ingestion and, second, to determine whether such a fluoride concentration occurs in dental plaque.

Most studies investigating the fluoride concentration necessary for reduction of acid production have been undertaken using either cultures of one particular organism or mixtures of saliva sediment and sugar solution, and extrapolation of these findings to what occurs in vivo is not easy. Nevertheless, it would seem that even low concentrations of fluoride (1–2 ppm F) are able to produce detectable reductions in acid production; 10 ppm F produces a moderately large reduction and 100 ppm F completely inhibits bacterial growth (Jenkins, 1978). The pH of the medium is of very great importance and at pH 5, fluoride levels of only 6–8 ppm will completely inhibit acid production in vitro.

The actual metabolic processes in plaque inhibited by fluoride are still uncertain, although it is likely that extracellular enzymes (e.g. those concerned with extracellular polysaccharide production are unaffected, and that intracellular inhibition is much more important. It may be that the important site is the cell wall, and glucose transport into the cell has been shown to be inhibited by fluoride. Intracellular glycogen production and breakdown is also reduced by fluoride and the final stages of glycolysis involving breakdown of 2-P-glycerate to P-enolypyruvate (hence to pyruvate and lactic acid) are also inhibited. The reason that the metabolisms of many bacteria are much more sensitive to fluoride at low pH might be due to the increased permeability of their cell walls to fluoride at low pH.

The first estimations of fluoride concentration in plaque were very high (up to 179 ppm) (Hardwick and Leach, 1963). With more accurate methods, concentration (wet plaque) of about 8 ppm F have been recorded in adolescent children (Birkeland et al., 1971) and about 4 ppm F in 5-year-old children (Edgar and Rugg-Gunn, 1975). Since saliva contains only about 0·02 ppm F (Shannon, 1977) and plaque several hundred times more than this, it is clear that much of the fluoride in plaque must be bound. The ionic fluoride in plaque fluid has been estimated to be between 0·08 and 0·8 ppm, while the rest is either loosely or tightly bound in plaque (Jenkins and Edgar, 1977). The loosely bound fluoride is probably of greatest metabolic importance since its activity increases as the plaque pH falls. Although there is evidence that fluoride is bound to inorganic constituents in plaque, this is thought to be an intermediate step to its more important site on or in the plaque bacteria.

Whatever the exact mechanism of action, fluoride does appear to successfully reduce acid production and pH fall in plaque in vivo. Jenkins et al. (1969) found that the final pH reached by plaque samples incubated with sucrose was less in children living in Hartlepool (1·8 ppm F in drinking water) (0·15 pH unit less) or Newcastle (1 ppm F) (0·05 pH unit less) than in children living in a fluoride-low area. Likewise, Edgar et al. (1970) showed that the final pH of a plaque/glucose incubate was higher in young adults after fluoridation was introduced into Newcastle than before it, while no change was observed in control subjects living in a neighbouring non-fluoridated community. Inhibition of acid production has also been observed in vivo after topical application of more concentrated fluoride solution (Wooley and Rickles, 1971). Although the effect of F inhibiting the fall in plaque pH may be small in terms of pH units, it should be appreciated that even small differences near the critical pH at which enamel may begin to dissolve may have a large effect on the amount of demineralization which occurs.

It has been suggested that (1) amine fluorides have a number of additional benefits in that plaque quantity is reduced and fluoride retention in enamel is enhanced (Muhlemann et al., 1957), and (2) the stannous ion inhibits the bacterial cell wall transport mechanisms (Svatun and Attramadal, 1978). But since amine fluoride and stannous fluoride do not appear to have a greater caries-inhibiting effect compared with sodium fluoride, these actions are likely to be unimportant.

It is clear that plaque can accumulate fluoride, but where does this fluoride come from? It is very unlikely that the fluoride comes from enamel (except during periods of demineralization) since Weatherell et al. (1972) have shown the reverse—that plaque-covered enamel has a higher fluoride level than enamel not covered by plaque. The concentration of F in foods and drinks is generally low and their brief contact with the plaque makes this source unlikely. However, raised plaque F levels observed in the fluoridated areas (Dawes et al., 1965; Edgar and Rugg-Gunn, own data) are probably due to the fairly frequent contact between the fluoridated water and the plaque (Jenkins and Edgar, 1977). In low fluoride areas, at least, it would appear that the majority of plaque F originates from saliva, and perhaps also from gingival fluid, during constant contact throughout the day and night. Elevation of plaque F concentration after fluoride mouthrinsing is fairly short-lived—most being lost within 24 hours (Birkeland et al., 1971)—indicating the importance of frequency of application of fluoride to the plaque.

INHIBITION OF PLAQUE FORMATION

After a tooth is thoroughly cleaned, the exposed tooth mineral is covered by a cell-free protein layer (dental pellicle) within a matter of minutes. These proteins are derived from saliva and adhere to the enamel surface by electrostatic forces (Jenkins, 1978). Fluoride (and other ions with a high affinity for calcium) inhibit adsorption of salivary proteins (presumably by competitive inhibition of the acidic side groups of the proteins) to the calcium of the crystal surface. Since calcium bridges are important in binding plaque bacteria, it is conceivable that fluoride might also reduce the agglutination of bacteria and so reduce plaque formation. Despite impressive theoretical and in vitro data, there is no clear evidence for reduction of dental plaque in vivo by fluoride, and the importance of this potential cariostatic action of fluoride remains speculative.

IMPORTANCE OF VARIOUS FACTORS IN THE CARIES-INHIBITORY ACTION OF FLUORIDE

The principal variables in fluoride therapy are: the concentration of fluoride in the environment of the tooth, the fluoride compound used and adjunctive ion, the pH of the solution, duration of each application, frequency of application, the continuity of the therapy throughout life and whether or not plaque is removed before application.

In many methods of fluoride therapy, and certainly from the historical viewpoint, the principal objective has been to increase the fluoride concentration in enamel to as great a depth as possible. For this, concentrated solutions of fluoride for topical application have been favoured and much work has been done to discover ways of increasing uptake. For example, greater F uptake was observed when the pH of the solution was low—hence the development of the APF system by Brudevold et al. (1963)—and, secondly, priming the enamel surface with substances such as aluminium, which would bind F tightly, has been investigated. Since the main product deposited after application of concentrated fluoride solutions—CaF_2—is undersaturated in saliva, methods for reducing its formation or prolonging its contact with the enamel surface have been developed. But in spite of the large amount of research effort expended in trying to improve topical fluoride agents, the most important variable in respect of the caries-preventive effectiveness of fluoride is frequency of application. Even at the very low concentration of 1 ppm F, fluoridated water would appear to have a substantial topical effect: this is almost certainly due to the fact that the water has contact with the teeth and plaque many times a day. It would seem, therefore, that the important factor is to maintain an adequate fluoride level at the plaque/enamel interface, and that this 'adequate level' may in fact be fairly low and achieved by 1 ppm F in drinking water. If frequent applications are impossible, increasing fluoride levels in enamel might create a reservoir of fluoride and allow adequate levels at the plaque–enamel interface to be maintained for some time. Although systemic administration of fluoride improves enamel crystallinity and raises the enamel fluoride level, two of the more important actions of fluoride are currently thought to be fluoride's ability to (1) assist in remineralization to form apatite, and (2) depress the glycolytic activity of plaque bacteria.

Because the role of plaque in the caries-preventive action of fluoride has become more important, it has been questioned whether it is desirable that plaque should be removed. McNee et al. (1980) have shown that NaF diffuses rapidly through plaque, which is in agreement with the observations of Joyston-Bechal et al. (1976) that plaque is no barrier to fluoride deposition in enamel from topical solutions. Also, it is in plaque-covered areas that enamel acquires the most fluoride. But while plaque removal prior to topical fluoride application may not alter the clinical effectiveness of the application, it is prudent at this stage to conclude that the harmful effect of plaque as a major cause of caries and gingivitis far outweighs its beneficial effect as a vehicle in which fluoride may act, and that it should be removed.

Although the post-eruptive action of fluoride is currently thought to be of very great importance, the advantages of adequate fluoride ingestion during enamel formation before eruption should not be ignored. Evidence from public water fluoridation and school fluoridation schemes have clearly shown that systemic fluoride administration leads to substantial caries reductions in addition to any topical effect. It is known that the caries-preventive effect of topical fluoride diminishes rapidly after the fluoride therapy ceases. It may be, although there is lack of data either way, that teeth which have received fluoride sytemically during formation, as well as topically, lose their protection much less rapidly than if they had only been exposed to topical fluorides.

REFERENCES

Birkeland J. M., Jorkjend L. and von der Fehr F. R. (1971) The influence of fluoride rinses on the fluoride content of dental plaque in children. *Caries Res.* 5, 169–179.

Brown W. E., Gregory T. M. and Chow L. C. (1977) Effects of fluoride on enamel solubility and cariostasis. *Caries Res.* 11, suppl. 1, 118–141.

Brudevold F., Savory A., Gardner D. E., Spinelli M. and Spiers R. (1963) A study of acidulated fluoride solutions. *Arch. Oral Biol.* 8, 167–177.

Cooper V. K. and Ludwig T. G. (1965) Effect of fluoride and of soil trace elements on the morphology of permanent molars in man. *N. Z. Dent. J.* 61, 33–40.

Dawes G., Jenkins G. N., Hardwick J. L. and Leach S. A. (1965) The relation between the fluoride concentrations in the dental plaque and in drinking water. *Br. Dent. J.* 119, 164–167.

de Rooij J. F., Arends J. and Kolar Z. (1981) Diffusion of monofluorophosphate in whole bovine enamel at pH 7. *Caries Res.* 15, 363–368.

Edgar W. M. and Rugg-Gunn A. J. (1975) Own data.

Edgar J. M., Jenkins G. N. and Tatevossian A. (1970) The inhibitory action of fluoride on plaque bacteria: further evidence. *Br. Dent. J.* 128, 129–132.

Forrest J. R. (1956) Caries incidence and enamel defects in areas with different levels of fluoride in the drinking water. *Br. Dent. J.* 100, 195–200.

Forward G. C. (1980) Action on and interaction of fluoride in dentifrices. *Community Dent. Oral Epidemiol.* **8**, 257–266.

Grøn P., Spinelli M., Trautz O. and Brudevold F. (1963) The effect of carbonate on the solubility of hydroxapatite. *Arch. Oral Biol.* **8**, 251–263.

Hamilton I. R. (1977) Effects of fluoride on enzymatic regulation of bacterial carbohydrate metabolism. *Caries Res.* **11**, suppl. 1, 262–291.

Hardwick J. L. and Leach S. A. (1963) The fluoride content of the dental plaque. *Adv. Flu. Res. Dent. Caries Prev.* **1**, 151–158.

Healy W. B. and Ludwig T. G. (1966) Enamel solubility studies on New Zealand teeth. *N. Z. Dent. J.* **62**, 276–278.

Ingram G. S. (1972) The reaction of monofluorophosphate with apatite. *Caries Res.* **6**, 1–15.

Isaac S., Brudevold F., Smith F. A. and Gardner D. E. (1958) Solubility rate and natural fluorine content of surface and subsurface enamel. *J. Dent. Res.* **37**, 254–263.

Jenkins G. N. (1978) *The Physiology and Biochemistry of the Mouth.* 4th ed. Oxford, Blackwell.

Jenkins G. N. and Edgar W. M. (1977) Distribution and forms of F in saliva and plaque. *Caries Res.* **11**, suppl. 1, 226–242.

Jenkins G. N., Edgar W. M. and Ferguson D. B. (1969) The distribution and metabolic effects of human plaque fluorine. *Arch. Oral. Biol.* **14**, 105–119.

Joyston-Bechal S., Duckworth R. and Braden M. (1973) The mechanism of uptake of ^{18}F by enamel from sodium fluoride and acidulated phosphate fluoride solutions labelled with [18]F. *Arch. Oral. Biol.* **18**, 1077–1089.

Joyston-Bechal S., Duckworth R. and Braden M. (1976) The effect of artificially produced pellicle and plaque on the uptake of ^{18}F by human enamel 'in vitro'. *Arch. Oral Biol.* **21**, 73–78.

Koulourides T., Keller S. E., Manson-Hing L. and Lilley V. (1980) Enhancement of fluoride effectiveness by experimental cariogenic priming of human enamel. *Caries Res.* **14**, 32–39.

Kruger B. J. (1968) Ultrastructural changes in ameloblasts from fluoride treated rats. *Arch. Oral Biol.* **13**, 969–977.

Kruger B. J. (1970) The effect of different levels of fluoride on the ultrastructure of ameloblasts in the rat. *Arch. Oral Biol.* **15**, 109–114.

Künzel W. (1976) Influence of water fluoridation on the eruption of permanent teeth. *Caries Res.* **10**, 96–103.

Lovius B. B. J. and Goose D. H. (1969) The effect of fluoridation of water on tooth morphology. *Br. Dent. J.* **127**, 322–324.

McNee S. G., Geddes D. A. M., Main C. and Gillespie F. C. (1980) Measurement of the diffusion coefficient of NaF in human dental plaque 'in vitro'. *Arch. Oral Biol.* **25**, 819–823.

Moreno E. C., Kresak M. and Zahradnik R. T. (1977) Physicochemical aspects of fluoride-apatite systems relevant to the study of dental caries. *Caries Res.* **11**, suppl. 1, 142–171.

Muhlemann H. R., Schmid H. and Konig K. G. (1957) Enamel solubility reduction with inorganic and organic fluorides. *Helv. Odontol. Acta* **1**, 23–33.

Murray J. J. (1971) Adult dental health in fluoride and non-fluoride areas. *Br. Dent. J.* **131**, 391–395.

231

Ockerse T. (1949) *Dental Caries: Clinical and Experimental Investigations.* Pretoria, South Africa, Department of Health.

Paynter K. J. and Grainger R. M. (1956) The relation of nutrition to the morphology and size of rat molar teeth. *J. Can. Dent. Assoc.* **22**, 519–531.

Rugg-Gunn A. J., Carmichael C. L., French A. D. and Furness J. A. (1977) Fluoridation in Newcastle and Northumberland. *Br. Dent. J.* **142**, 395–402.

Shannon I. L. (1977) Biochemistry of fluoride in saliva. *Caries Res.* **11**, suppl. 1, 206–225.

Stone R. W. and Werkman C. H. (1937) The occurrence of phosphoglyceric acid in the bacterial dissimulation of glucose. *Biochem. J.* **31**, 1516–1523.

Svatun B. and Attramadal A. (1978) The effect of stannous fluoride on human plaque acidogenicity in situ (Stephan curve). *Acta Odontol. Scand.* **36**, 211–218.

Wallenius B. (1957) Die Zahnbreite in relation zum Fluorgehalt im Trinkwasser. *Odontol. Revy* **8**, 429–434.

Weatherell J. A., Robinson C. and Hallsworth A. S. (1972) Changes in the fluoride concentration of the labial enamel surface with age. *Caries Res.* **6**, 312–324.

Wooley L. H. and Rickles N. H. (1971) Inhibition of acidogenesis in human dental plaque 'in situ' following the use of topical sodium fluoride. *Arch. Oral Biol.* **16**, 1187–1194.

Young R. A. and Elliott J. C. (1966) Atomic-scale bases for several properties of apatites. *Arch. Oral Biol.* **11**, 699–707.

CHAPTER 15

HEALTH AND WATER FLUORIDATION

It has been suggested over the years that many different disorders can be caused or aggravated by fluoridation. A summary of these disorders, compiled by the Royal College of Physicians (1976), is given in *Table 55*.

Table 55. Disorders claimed to be caused or aggravated by Fluoridation (*Royal College of Physicians, 1976*)

Gastro-intestinal disorders:	Flatulence Nausea Abdominal pain Vomiting Haematemesis Peptic ulcer	Diarrhoea Constipation Gingivitis Stomatitis Oral ulcers
Neurological and mental disorders:	Headache Migraine Depression Paraesthesiae Painful numbness in the limbs	Mental deterioration Convulsions Personality change Deafness
Urinary tract disorders:	Urethritis Cystitis Pyelitis	Nephritis
Skin disorders:	Urticaria Rashes Dermatoses	Furunculosis Brittle nails Alopecia
Musculo-skeletal disorders:	Skeletal Fluorosis Backache Pain or muscular assertion of the ribs (sic)	Arthritis Renal osteodystrophy Scheuermann's disease
Dental disorders:	Mottling of the teeth	
Ocular disorders:	Optic neuritis	
Endocrine disorders:	Thyroid enlargement Diabetes mellitus	Parathyroid disorders Adrenal disorders
Cardiovascular disorders:	Heart disease Arteriosclerosis	
Congenital malformations:	Mongolism Anencephalus Spina bifida	
Non-specific disorders:	Lethargy Exhaustion after sleep Muscular weakness	

Recently, further information on urban mortality, cancer mortality and congenital malformation in relation to fluoridation has been published and these data will be reviewed.

URBAN MORTALITY

Rogot et al. (1978) sampled 473 urban areas of the United States that had populations of over 25 000 in 1950. These cities had a combined population of 61 million in 1950 and 71 million in 1970, constituting 40·6 per cent and 35 per cent respectively of the total US population in those years. Numbers of deaths from all causes and from cardiovascular, renal and heart disease and cancer separately in each urban area were obtained from official vital statistics for the years 1949–1950, 1959–1961 and 1969–1971. To allow comparison of mortality in cities whose age, race and sex compositions varied, the method of indirect adjustment was employed using the US 1960 mortality rates as standard.

For the three census years 1950, 1960 and 1970, each city's population in each of 76 age–race–sex subgroups was multiplied by the US 1960 standard rates and by the number of years in the peri-censal period to give the expected number of deaths in that city for the particular census period. The ratio of the number of deaths which occurred to the number of deaths expected was called the 'mortality ratio'. The Average Mortality Ratio (AMR) was obtained for groups of cities by summing individual mortality ratios for each city and dividing by the number of cities in the group. (This gives cities equal weight to one another. In preliminary analyses, average mortality ratios weighted by city size were also used. The results of the two sets of analyses were similar.)

Of the 473 study cities, 260 had fluoridated sometime before 1970 and 213 had not. Of the fluoridated cities, 26 had discontinued fluoridation at some time before 1970, 4 had incomplete coverage and 3 had been on water with a high natural F content before switching sources and fluoridating. These 33 cities were considered of uncertain fluoridation status, leaving for analysis 227 cities which originally received water with a low F content, then fluoridated, and maintained complete and continuous coverage until 1970. Of the cities which never fluoridated, 187 were using water with an average F content of less than 0·7 ppm and 26 had water ranging from 0·7 to 2·7 ppm F.

The findings for total deaths is given in *Table* 56. The average mortality ratio (AMR) for the 227 cities which had fluoridated declined from 1·13 to 0·97 over the 20-year period; the corresponding figures for the 187 non-fluoridated cities were 1·16 to 0·99. For the F cities 11 cities showed increases in their MR; for the NF group 10 cities showed increases in their MR. Overall the basic trend showed a decline in mortality over the

Table 56. Populations and Average Mortality Ratios (AMR) for 1950, 1960 and 1970 Periods and Average Per cent Change from 1950 to 1970, 1950 to 1960, and 1960 to 1970 for cities by Fluoridation Status: US, selected study cities (*Rogot et al., 1978*)

Fluoridation group	Combined population (millions)			AMR			Average % change from		
	1950	1960	1970	1950	1960	1970	1950–1970	1950–1960	1960–1970
F	37·7	39·6	40·5	1·13	1·03	0·97	−14	−8	−6
NF	17·9	20·7	22·4	1·16	1·07	0·99	−14	−7	−7
H	2·1	3·1	4·0	1·19	1·02	0·96	−19	−14	−6
U	3·6	4·2	4·4	1·15	1·02	0·97	−15	−10	−5
T	61·2	67·5	71·1	1·15	1·05	0·98	−14	−8	−6

F, 227 cities that fluoridated in the period 1945–1969; NF, 187 cities with low natural fluoride (less than 0·7 ppm), that had not fluoridated by 1970; H, 26 cities with high natural fluoride (0·7 ppm or greater); U, 33 cities of uncertain fluoridation status; T, Total of 473 cities.

20 years of the study—a mean per cent drop of 13·5 in fluoridated cities compared with 13·6 in the non-fluoridated cities. The overall findings clearly showed no consistent relation between fluoridation and observed changes in mortality over the 20-year period studied.

CANCER MORTALITY

Data purporting to show the age dependence of cancer mortality related to artificial fluoridation have been put forward by Yiamouyiannis and Burk (1977). The ten largest fluoridated cities in the United States were taken as the experimental group. The ten largest cities in the United States which had not fluoridated as of 1969 but had a cancer death rate greater than 155 per 100 000 per year were taken as the control group. The results show that the crude cancer death rates of both groups of cities had a strikingly similar trend between 1940 and 1950. Subsequent to fluoridation, however, a divergence could be observed that was maintained up to 1969, the last year of the study. The authors deduced from their data that 25 000 excess cancer deaths per year would be caused by fluoridation of all US water supplies (*Fig.* 42).

The US National Cancer Institute asserted that the rise in cancer deaths could be explained by the different age–sex–race structures of the population in the two groups of cities, and this aspect was considered further by Oldham and Newell (1977), on behalf of the Royal Statistical Society (England) at the request of the Royal College of Physicians, London. They reported: 'Our analysis shows that the two groups of 10 cities differed in their age–sex–race structure in 1950. The cities which were to be fluoridated started with many fewer elderly white females, somewhat fewer elderly white males and more non-whites at all ages below 50. By

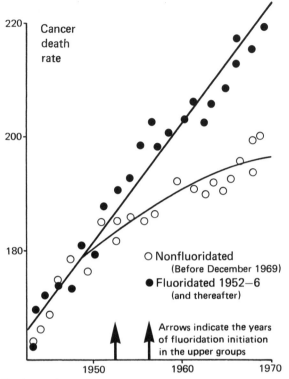

Fig. 42. Comparison of cancer death rates in the 10 largest American cities fluoridated since 1952–1956 with 10 American cities which had not fluoridated before 1969. (From Yiamouyiannis and Burk, 1977.) *See text for discussion of these data.*

1970, the two sets of cities differed much more in their demographic structure than they had in 1950. The fluoridated cities now had many more non-whites of all ages in their populations, and many fewer whites under the age of 55. When the demographic changes are taken into account we find, in proportional terms, that the excess cancer rate increased by 1 per cent over the 20 years in the fluoridated cities, but it also increased by 4 per cent in the unfluoridated control cities, giving a difference of 3 per cent to the advantage of the fluoridated cities.' This point is also made by Newbrun (1977), who showed that although Yiamouyiannis and Burk (1977) claimed that the death rate from cancer increased in San Francisco after fluoridation, their supporting data were not adjusted for age. The US Census shows a steady increase in the older population residing in San Francisco. The per cent of the population of people over 65 was 9·7 in 1950 but had risen to 14·1 per cent by 1970; as cancer mortality rate increases dramatically with advancing age it is not surprising that San Francisco cancer mortality rates rose during the 20-year period. However, if the change in the age distribution is taken into account there is no trend in the cancer mortality rate in San Francisco (*Table* 57).

Table 57. San Francisco—Population and Cancer Mortality Rates 1950–1970
(*Newbrun, 1970*)

		Age 65 and over		Cancer mortality rates (per 100 000)	
Year	Total population	No.	% of total	Unadjusted	Age adjusted*
1950	762 082	74 050	9·7	239	239
1960	727 898	91 603	12·6	249	216
1970	706 601	99 738	14·1	266	230

* San Francisco's water supply has been fluoridated since 25 August 1952. Adjusted for age 5 and over, based on 1950 San Francisco population.

In Great Britain, the incidence of cancer has recently been investigated in relation to water fluoride level. By means of the national cancer registration scheme it was possible to compare cancer incidence in areas with contrasting levels of fluoride in the water.

For each local authority district with a water fluoride level of 1 mg/litre or over ('high'), one or more nearby district of similar size with a fluoride level of 0·2 mg/litre or less ('low'), was selected for comparison. For areas with a fluoride level in the range 0·5–0·99 mg/litre ('high'–'medium'), control areas were chosen with fluoride levels of 0·1 mg/litre or less ('very low'). The numbers of cancers of each anatomical site were arranged by age group, sex and water fluoride level. For each anatomical site, the numbers of cancers observed were then compared, within each age group, sex and area, with the numbers expected if the incidence of the disease had been uniform throughout the four areas (Royal College of Physicians, 1976). *Table* 58 shows, for cancers of the thyroid, kidney, stomach, oesophagus, colon, rectum, bladder, bone and breast, the numbers observed in each of the four sets of districts grouped by water fluoride level, together with the ratios of observed to expected numbers. It will be seen that there is no tendency for the ratio for any cancer to be greater in the high-fluoride areas than in the low-fluoride areas.

CONGENITAL ANOMALIES

The suggestion that fluoride is a cause of mongolism derives from two studies by Rapaport (1959, 1963) in the USA. His results are summarized in *Table* 59, and at first sight the correlation between the incidence of

Table 58. Ratios of Observed to Expected Numbers of Cancers in Certain Organs in Areas with Different Levels of Fluoride in Water in Great Britain (*Royal College of Physicians, 1976*)

Site of cancer	High F (1 ppm)	High–medium F (0·5–0·99 ppm)	Low F (0·2 ppm)	Very low F (0·1 ppm)
Thyroid	1·05 (45)*	0·79 (54)	1·27 (57)	1·02 (84)
Kidney	1·01 (129)	1·00 (198)	1·02 (131)	0·98 (233)
Stomach	0·88 (375)	1·15 (733)	0·90 (327)	1·05 (815)
Oesophagus	0·87 (73)	1·02 (131)	0·87 (73)	1·13 (177)
Colon	0·96 (386)	1·03 (618)	0·99 (385)	1·00 (719)
Rectum	0·93 (273)	1·11 (486)	0·94 (264)	0·99 (519)
Bladder	1·00 (430)	0·96 (632)	1·06 (444)	1·00 (786)
Bone	1·00 (18)	1·06 (30)	1·02 (19)	0·94 (31)
Breast	0·92 (567)	1·06 (999)	1·08 (650)	0·97 (1105)
Total population	482 398	779 054	510 045	896 625

* The total numbers of cancers observed are given in parentheses.

Table 59. Incidence of Mongolism in Illinois (*After Rapaport, 1959, 1963*) (*Royal College of Physicians, 1976*)

Size of towns	No. of towns	Fluoride in water (mg/litre)	Mongols	
			No. of cases	Frequency per 1000 births
10 000	15	0·0	15	0·24
to	24	0·1–0·2	52	0·39
100 000	17	0·3–0·7	33	0·47
inhabitants	12	1·0–2·6	48	0·72
5000				
to	—	0·0–0·2	10	0·40
10 000	—	0·3–2.6	19	0·78
inhabitants				

mongolism and the fluoride content of the water is impressive. But, as the report by the Royal College of Physicians (1976) shows, the highest rates found by Rapaport are only about half those that are normally reported after intensive case finding, while the lowest rates are only about one-sixth as high. Intensive investigation has shown that the incidence of mongolism is remarkably constant, the rate ranging from 1·15 to 1·92 per 1000 births (median value of 1·5 per 1000) in Denmark, Great Britain, Switzerland and the USA. Rates at this level are universally accepted by paediatricians as compatible with complete ascertainment. To obtain such a level of ascertainment, however, it is usually necessary to utilize, in addition to the sources used by Rapaport (1959, 1963), a range of further information, including the records of community physicians, school doctors, midwives, health visitors, social workers and others concerned with the welfare of mongols. It is difficult to attach any meaning to Rapaport's limited enquiry, missing, as it would, most surviving children with mongolism who were cared for at home.

Berry (1958) undertook a similar study in nine English towns, making the sort of intensive enquiries that are needed for complete ascertainment. His results are summarized in *Table* 60, along with those obtained by other British investigators (*see* R.C.P. Report, 1976). These data provide no evidence that the incidence of mongolism bears any relationship to the fluoride content of the drinking water. The absence of any relationship is, moreover, confirmed by the experience in Birmingham where fluoridation has been practised since 1964.

Table 60. Incidence of Mongolism in England (*After Berry, 1958, 1962*) (*Royal College of Physicians, 1976*)

Place	Fluoride in water (ppm)	Mongols	
		No. of cases	Frequency per 1000 live births
High Wycombe		9	1·31
Reading	Less	30	1·53
Tynemouth	than	24	1·90
Carlisle	0·2	19	1·64
Gateshead		37	1·65
Stockton		16	1·08
Slough	0·9	13	1·37
South Shields	0·7–1·1	33	1·59
W. Hartlepool	1·9–2·0	16	1·23
6 towns	Less than 0·2	135	1·53
3 towns	More than 0·7	64	1·42
Liverpool	—	18	1.29*
UK	—	7	1·69
London	—	107	1·50*
Rural Northants	—	86	1·63*

* Live and still births.

Further evidence that mongolism (Down's syndrome) and other selected congenital malformations are not associated with water fluoridation is given by Erickson et al. (1976) in a very large study of 1 387 027 births using two sources: the Metropolitan Atlanta Congenital Malformation Surveillance Program and the National Cleft Lip and Palate Intelligence Service. Their results are given in *Table* 61 and show no association between water fluoridation and the incidence of congenital malformations.

Table 61. Incidence of Selected Common Congenital Malformations in Areas with and without Fluoridated Water (*Erickson et al., 1976*)

Malformation	Metropolitan Atlanta, 1967–1973					NIS surveillance areas, 1961–1966					
	Fluoride (95 254 total births)		Non-fluoride (25 373 total births)			Fluoride (234 300 total births)		Non-fluoride (1 032 100 total births)			
	No. cases	Rate/10000 white births	No. cases	Rate/10000 white births	χ^2	No. cases	Rate/10000 white births	No. cases	Rate/10000 white births	χ^2	
Anencephaly	101	10·6	33	13·0	0·83	70	3·0	275	2·7	0·62	
Cardiac and other circulatory system defects	379	39·8	78	30·7	4·11	120	5·1	456	4·4	1·93	
Cleft lip with/without cleft palate	107	11·2	35	13·8	0·91	185	7·9	784	7·6	0·19	
Cleft palate	50	5·2	20	7·9	1·96	94	4·0	331	3·2	3·45	
Clubfoot	414	43·5	96	37·8	1·38	303	12·9	1642	15·9	10·84	
Down's syndrome	166	9·9	86	8·5	1·41	115	4·9	524	5·1	0·08	
Hydrocephalus	77	8·1	34	13·4	5·59	70	3·0	299	2·9	0·03	
Hypospadias	237	24·9	47	18·5	3·18	198	8·5	736	7·1	4·33	
Reduction deformities	82	8·6	14	5·5	2·03	79	3·4	358	3·5	0·03	
Spina bifida	149	15·6	37	14·6	0·09	146	6·2	535	5·2	3·71	
All malformation cases	2787	292·6	685	270·0	3·58	2264	96·6	10526	102·0	5·43	

Degree of freedom corrected for continuity; P 0·05 = 3·84.
Data given here refer to a 1% sample of NIS records.

240

CONCLUSIONS

Schemes for the fluoridation of public water supplies have now been operated for over 30 years, although in the last few years the progress of water fluoridation has been slow, especially in Western Europe. The main obstacles to further implementation seem to be sociopsychological and political factors which are determining attitudes, rather than technical or economic problems. The results of our review of 95 community water fluoridation schemes show, beyond reasonable doubt, that artificial fluoridation is effective in reducing caries experience by approximately 50 per cent, regardless of climate, race or social conditions (p. 68). The effect of water fluoridation on general health has been thoroughly investigated in a series of population studies. There is no evidence that the consumption of water containing approximately 1 ppm F (in a temperate climate) is associated with any harmful effect.

REFERENCES

Berry W. T. C. (1958) Study of incidence of mongolism in relation to fluoride content of water. *Am. J. Ment. Defic.* **62**, 623–636.

Erickson J. D., Oakley G. P., Flynt J. W. and Hay S. (1976) Water fluoridation and congenital malformations: no associations. *J. Am. Dent. Assoc.* **93**, 981–984.

Newbrun E. (1977) The safety of water fluoridation. *J. Am. Dent. Assoc.* **94**, 301–304.

Oldham P. D. and Newell D. J. (1977) Fluoridation of water supplies and cancer— a possible association. *J. R. Statist. Soc. Ser. C (Appl. Statist.)* **26**, 125–135.

Rapaport I. (1959) Nouvelles recherches sur le mongolisme à propos du rôle pathogénique du fluor. *Bull. Acad. Nat. Med. (Paris)* **143**, 367–370.

Rapaport I. (1963) Oligophrénie mongolienne et caries dentaires. *Rev. Stomatol. (Paris)* **46**, 207–218.

Rogot E., Sharrett A. R., Feinleib M. and Fabsitz R. R. (1978) Trends in urban mortality in relation to fluoridation status. *Am. J. Epidemiol.* **107**, 104–112.

Royal College of Physicians (1976) *Fluoride Teeth and Health.* London, Royal College of Physicians.

Yiamouyiannis J. and Burk D. (1977) *Fluoridation and Cancer: Age dependence of cancer mortality related to artificial fluoridation.* Presented at the 8th International Society for Fluoride Research Conference, Oxford, England, May 29–31.

CHAPTER 16

FLUORIDE THERAPY PLANNING FOR THE INDIVIDUAL AND THE COMMUNITY

Although the previous chapters provide the dental practitioner with information on the efficacy of various methods of delivering fluoride for caries prevention, the choice between the various methods and their place in the total treatment plan of an individual patient has not been fully discussed. Planners of dental services will also wish to compare the merits of the various methods of fluoride therapy in relation to the levels of caries experience and resources available in their community. In recent years much information has been published to assist the dental practitioner in choosing fluoride therapy for the individual patient and the planner in the use of fluoride in the community: this will now be brought together in this chapter.

FLUORIDE THERAPY FOR THE INDIVIDUAL

The dental practitioner is faced with a large number of methods for administering fluoride, often capable of being used at different concentrations and amounts and frequencies. In the first place it is helpful to divide these into those methods primarily aimed at systemic administration and those formulated for topical oral use only (*Table* 62). In general, methods of systemic fluoride administration will provide fluoride at an optimal dosage level. If the dosage is optimal, then only one method of systemic fluoride therapy should be given to any one individual. For example, if a child lives in an area of England supplied with drinking water containing about 1 ppm F, this will provide the child with a sufficient amount of ingested fluoride and no other systemic fluoride (e.g. drops or tablets) should be prescribed. If a young child did ingest both fluoride tablets and adequately fluoridated water, there would be a risk of fluorosis in developing enamel. Very occasionally this rule of 'only one method of

Table 62. Methods of Fluoride Administration

Systemic	Topical
Public water fluoridation	Clinical topical application
School water fluoridation	Fluoride mouthrinse
Fluoridized salt	Fluoride toothpaste
Fluoridized milk	
Fluoride drops/tablets	

systemic administration' might be broken, if prevention of caries is more important than aesthetics: this might be so in the case of several medically handicapped children in whom a carious tooth might be a threat to life or the severely mentally handicapped in whom topical fluoride therapy and treatment may be very difficult. Systemic fluoride administration is usually considered desirable only when enamel is forming before the teeth erupt, and is considered no longer beneficial in adults. While the possibility that the slightly raised fluoride level in saliva and gingival fluid after fluoride ingestion may have a caries-preventive effect should be investigated, it is likely that this action is much less important than the local effect of fluoride (e.g. in water, toothpaste, rinse, etc.) in the mouth. So, although there would appear to be no harm in continuing with systemic administration of fluoride in adulthood, the caries-preventive effect is likely to be limited to the local action in the mouth.

In practical terms, the only method of systemic fluoride therapy under the control of the dental practitioner is the prescription of fluoride drops or tablets, since there are no UK school fluoridation schemes and fluoridized salt and milk are not on sale in the UK.

Although a patient should receive only one source of systemic fluoride, this restriction does not apply to those methods aimed solely at a topical effect. If no fluoride is ingested there is no toxological reason why all three of the topical methods (*Table* 62) should not be given in combination. However, some mouthrinse or toothpaste may be swallowed, especially in children, so that restriction in the use of fluoride mouthrinses and toothpastes is desirable in young children who are also at the greatest risk of developing enamel fluorosis. The amount of fluoride ingested during and immediately after a clinical topical application of fluoride should be low if the technique is good. Applications tend to be infrequent, lessening the risk of chronic fluoride ingestion.

Ekstrand et al. (1981) recently reported that the average quantity of fluoride ingested, in 8 children, was $31 \cdot 2$ mg F after a mean of $3 \cdot 33$ g of gel ($1 \cdot 23$ per cent F) was applied in a pair of custom-fitted trays. This indicates that 78 per cent of the gel was swallowed and only 22 per cent removed with the tray or spat out. The 1-hour plasma fluoride level ranged from 300 to 1443 ng/ml ($0 \cdot 3$–$1 \cdot 4$ ppm F in plasma) in these children. In adults, who received 5 g gel in commercially available disposable trays, plasma levels ranged from 300 to 980 ng/ml, but levels were reduced to a maximum of 230 ng/ml in these adults when custom-fitted trays were used. The authors point out that plasma F levels in excess of 950 ng/ml are likely to be nephrotoxic and warn against the frequent use at home of gels containing fluoride concentrations as high as $1 \cdot 23$ per cent F.

Saliva ejectors do not appear to have been used in Ekstrand et al.'s study, and the results highlight the need for some salivary removal system during application (especially since highly flavoured acid gels induce high salivary flow) and the use of accurately fitting trays. It is likely that fluoride-ingestion would be much less if application of solution were made (either on a quadrant or half-mouth basis) with a cotton bud, where the mouth is isolated with saliva ejector and cotton-wool rolls.

Apart from ingestion of fluoride, there are three factors which should be considered. First, the level of cooperation expected from the patient and parent. The daily use of fluoride drops, tablets or mouthrinse at home requires considerable effort and a high level of motivation. The daily use of a toothpaste is a better established practice but, as long as the patient attends the surgery, only minimum cooperation is required for clinical topical fluoride application. Therefore, if cooperation is in doubt, topical application in the surgery may be first choice.

The second consideration is the risk:benefit ratio. This involves predicting how much caries the patient is likely to develop over the next few years. If the patient is expected to develop many carious lesions, it would be justified to recommend the high level of fluoride therapy to try to prevent the carious lesions developing. But if little or no caries development is expected it would not be justified in recommending extensive fluoride therapy for so little gain. It is especially important in a country like the UK today, where children's teeth may be filled at no cost to the parent but the parent is expected to pay for any fluoride therapy, that adequate information is given about the likely benefit from the therapy. The best predictors of future caries increment, at the present time, are the past caries experience of the patient and the number of pre-cavitation ('white spot') carious lesions; microbiological tests have not yet been shown to be superior (Klock and Krasse, 1979). Patients about to wear fixed or removable orthodontic appliances or partial dentures can also be considered to be at increased risk. So, for a cooperative child, over about 8 years, living in an area with a fluoride-low water supply and considered to be at high caries risk, one could recommend the daily ingestion of fluoride tablets, the use of a fluoride mouthrinse and toothpaste at home and clinical topical applications in the surgery—the greater the caries risk the more frequent could be the clinical applications of fluoride as long as precautions are taken to reduce ingestion of the fluoride solution or gel.

The third consideration is the age of the patient. We have already said that there appears to be little point in recommending systemic fluorides after about 18 years of age; the younger end of the age range is more important. Fluoride tablet dosage at various ages has been discussed in Chapter 6. There would appear to be no lower age limit on clinical topical application of fluoride, although it is usually limited by lack of cooperation for such a lengthy procedure. It has already been noted that adequate removal of excess solution and gel is essential. On the other hand, because control of swallowing is poor in young children the use of mouthrinses should not be recommended below about 6 years, and parental supervision of the amount of fluoride toothpaste used (so that it does not exceed the size of a small pea) would also be prudent below this age.

It is usually recommended that a prophylaxis be carried out to clean the teeth before topical application in the surgery. Recent data suggest that the efficacy of the application is unaltered by the omission of plaque removal, although this may only be relevant to application of solution, and plaque may reduce the efficacy of gel application (Horowitz et al., 1974). However, plaque removal is so important as far as gingival health is concerned that it is necessary to include it, for this reason, in the treatment plan.

The point at which various fluoride therapies occur in a treatment plan should be considered. As mentioned earlier, the home use of tablets and mouthrinses requires considerable cooperation and it may be sensible to delay recommending these until the degree of cooperation expected is assessed. If it is planned to fissure-seal teeth, topical fluoride application should be delayed until after this has been completed, since, in theory, the raised enamel fluoride level resulting from the topical fluoride application might lessen the effectiveness of enamel etching prior to sealing. This precaution might not be completely necessary, as it is known that the retention of fissure sealants is as good in fluoridated as in fluoride-low areas.

Clinical trials have shown that the use of fluoride can greatly assist the dental practitioner in preventing the occurrence of dental caries in patients. The choice of régimes can be tailor-made to the needs of the patient. However, as with all materials, caution is needed to avoid untoward side-effects and, as a warning, it is relevant to recall that a 3-year-old child died a few years ago as the result of fluoride treatment in the dental surgery. Undoubtedly, the materials were misused. A prophylaxis was given with a mixture of pumice and 4 per cent SnF_2 applied to the teeth with a cotton swab. The excess pumice was removed with a swab dipped in 4 per cent SnF_2 solution, and the child then instructed to rinse his mouth with 4 per cent SnF_2. He died about 3 hours later. It was estimated that he swallowed about 45 ml of the solution and ingested about 435 mg F from the rinse alone (Horowitz, 1977). As Horowitz says, this is not an indictment against stannous fluoride, for the results might have occurred with any fluoride compound, but it is a warning that all agents should be handled with care and intelligence.

FLUORIDE THERAPY IN THE COMMUNITY

Treatment of an individual patient involves explanation by the dental practitioner of the alternatives available and agreement between the two parties on the proposed treatment plan. In some cases, a patient may be prepared to pay more for having caries-preventive therapy than he would have to pay to have restored the teeth which would have become carious without the preventive therapy. This is perfectly ethical as long as the patient is fully informed. But decisions in public health about different health-care strategies are usually made solely on a monetary basis. The community will demand that the health planner provides the best possible health services for their money. Since the planner will have to decide between various strategies he will have to be able to estimate (1) the cost of the proposed measure and (2) the benefit likely to accrue from that measure—both in monetary terms. This is called cost-benefit analysis and is a well-recognized procedure in public health planning. However, we will leave a discussion of the cost and benefit of various fluoride procedures until after a review of community preventive schemes which have been in operation in various countries for many years, since cost-benefit decisions are, in part, based on findings from these studies. The extent and effectiveness of public water fluoridation has already been discussed and this review will not cover this aspect of community fluoride therapy.

Sweden

Sweden is without artificial water fluoridation but virtually all Swedish schoolchildren participate in some school-based fluoride preventive programme. While in and around Stockholm children brush with fluoride solutions 4 times per year (Berggren and Welander, 1960, most children in the rest of Sweden rinse with 0·2 per cent NaF either weekly or fortnightly. Supervised fortnightly fluoride mouthrinsing began in Göteborg in 1960 and by 1963 all schoolchildren in the city were involved. Because dental services in Göteborg are so comprehensive, the record of the number of fillings inserted per child per year provides an excellent estimate of the

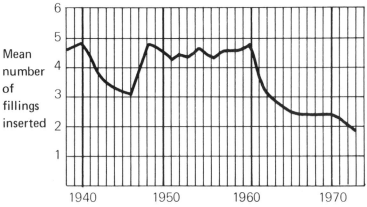

Fig. 43. The mean number of fillings inserted for each child, 6–15 years of age, by the Public Dental Service of Göteborg, Sweden between 1938 and 1973 (about 40 000 children). (From Torell and Ericsson, 1974.) (*Reproduced by courtesy of the authors.*)

effectiveness of the caries-preventive programme. The number of fillings inserted fell from nearly 5/child/year in 1960 to 2/child/year in 1973 (*Fig.* 43). During the same period, the number of extractions per 100 children/year fell from 13 to 4, and the number of endodontic treatments fell from 4 to 1 per 100 children/year (Torell and Ericsson, 1974). Torell and Ericsson (1974) also showed that the cost-benefit ratios for the fluoride rinse schemes were favourable in four Swedish communities (*Table* 63).

Table 63. Cost–benefit Analysis of Supervised School-based Fluoride Mouthrinsing in Sweden (*Torell and Ericsson, 1974*)

Community	No. of children involved in 1971	Cost–benefit ratio*
Fortnightly rinsing Goteborg	40 000	1 : 6
Weekly rinsing Halland County	59 000	1 : 8
Norrbotten	39 000	1 : 2·7
Kronberg County	20 000	1 : 3·5

* The ratio of the cost of the fluoride mouthrinsing scheme to the estimated cost of dental treatment prevented.

Norway

Like Sweden, Norway has no artificial water fluoridation but has

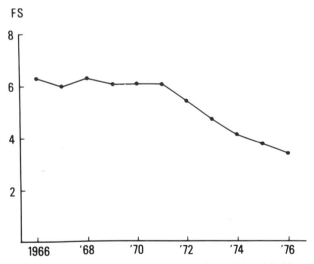

FS

Fig. 44. The mean number of fillings (filled surfaces) inserted in Norwegian 6–17-year-olds between 1966 and 1976. (From Lokken and Birkeland, 1978.) (*Reproduced by courtesy of the Editor, 'Community Dent. Oral Epidemiol'.*)

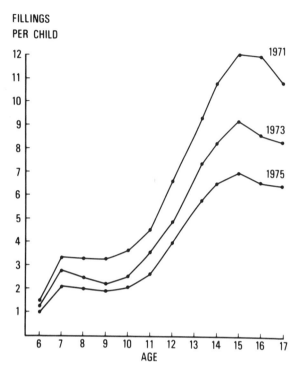

FILLINGS
PER CHILD

Fig. 45. The mean number of fillings (filled surfaces) inserted in Norwegian children in 1971, 1973 and 1975, by age (6–17 years). (From Lokken and Birkeland, 1978.) (*Reproduced by courtesy of the Editor, 'Community Dent. Oral Epidemiol.'.*)

developed alternative fluoride schemes (Lokken and Birkeland, 1978). While less than 1 per cent of Norwegian children received fluoride tablets in 1971, by 1976 about 50 per cent of children aged 0–5 years and 20 per cent of children aged 6–11 years were receiving them. Likewise, fluoride toothpastes were almost non-existent before 1970 but constituted 60 per cent of the toothpaste market by 1976, equivalent to 216 g of fluoride toothpaste/person/year. The number of schoolchildren taking part in fluoride brushing or rinsing programmes in school has continuously risen since 1965 to reach 60 per cent of children aged 7–15 years by 1970 and 90 per cent in 1977 (Rise and Haugejorden, 1980).

The effect of this increase in fluoride prophylaxis and increasing emphasis on prevention can be seen in *Fig.* 44. These data are based upon records of 200 000–300 000 children per year, and record a reduction in the

FILLED SURFACES (n)

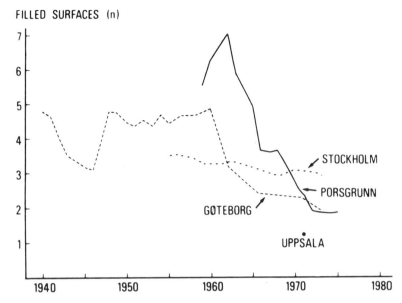

Fig. 46. The mean number of fillings inserted in 6–15-year-old Swedish children in Göteborg, Stockholm and Uppsala. (Torell and Ericsson, 1974) and in 6–14-year-old Norwegian children in Porsgrunn (filled surfaces). (From Birkeland et al., 1977.) (*Reproduced by courtesy of the Editor, 'Scand. J. Dent. Res.'.*)

need for fillings of about 45 per cent between 1966 and 1976 (Norway also has a comprehensive school dental service). These figures indicate a saving of about 880 000 fillings in 1976 compared with 1966, corresponding to the working capacity of about 220 dentists (Lokken and Birkeland, 1978). Over that same period the number of teeth extracted fell from 8/100 children to less than 1/100 children/yr. The observation that the need for fillings decreased consistently for all ages (*Fig. 45*). indicates real benefits rather than just a delay in the need for treatment.

Two régimes of fluoride prophylaxis operate in Norwegian schools—fluoride rinsing with 0·2 per cent NaF and brushing with 0·5 per cent NaF 4–5 times per year. While the latter has been very effective in some communities (Hope, 1979), greater benefits have been claimed for the rinsing programme (Birkeland and Jorkjend, 1975).

In a comprehensive analysis of the effect of the caries-preventive programme in the community of Porsgrunn for the 10 years after its inception in 1964–1965, a fall in the need for fillings of 70 per cent was observed (*Fig. 46*) (Birkeland et al., 1977). Over 95 per cent of children take part in the school rinsing programme which cost, in 1976, about 15 Nor Kr/child/year. An important observation in this study was that considerably more fillings were inserted per child per year than were reflected in the DMFS index, indicating that the standard DMF index under-records the amount of work done on children during their school years.

Switzerland

Basel is the only fluoridated city in Switzerland, but in 1963 a caries-preventive programme was started in the canton of Zurich. It is mainly fluoride-based and, although the methods of fluoride therapy have changed, progressively larger reductions in caries experience have been recorded (Marthaler, 1972a, 1974; Marthaler and Loosli, 1980). The caries-preventive programme has included the following factors:

1. The general introduction of fluoridated domestic salt (at 90 mg F/kg). It is now known that this dosage was far too low, giving a fluoride intake equal to only 35 per cent of the optimal intake. To increase the level of ingested fluoride, since 1970 fluoride tablets (0·7 mg F) have been distributed to children daily at school.

2. Supervised toothbrushing in school 4–6 times per year with 0·5 per cent NaF (5–9-year-olds) or 1 per cent NaF (over 9 years old) solutions. In 1970 1–3 rinsing tablets (7 mg F each) were substituted for the solutions, to simplify administration.

3. Ten-minute instruction on toothbrushing and eating habits given at each of the 4–6 brushing sessions per year.

4. The use of fluoride-containing toothpastes rapidly increased in the period 1960–1963 and has remained at a high level. In some small communities fluoride toothpastes are sold at a reduced price in school.

The caries experience of children aged 8, 10, 12 and 14 years has been reported every 4 years: *Table 64* gives the DMFT and DMFS data for 14-year-old children. A continuous fall in caries experience can be observed so that in 1975–1976, after 12 years of the programme, caries experience was only slightly higher than that recorded in fluoridated Basel. Unfortunately there appear to be no data on the cost of the caries-preventive programme in Zurich canton to compare with the published cost of

Table 64. Caries Experience of 14-year old Children in the Canton of Zurich Following Commencement in 1963 of the Caries-preventive Programme, and in Fluoridated Basel in 1977 (*Marthaler and Loosli, 1980*)

	DMFT		DMFS	
	Mean	% Fall	Mean	% Fall
1963–1964	12·8		28·7	
1967–1968	10·2	20	21·0	27
1971–1972	8·1	37	15·0	48
1975–1976	6·3	51	9·6	67
Basel (1977)	5·7		9·1	

fluoridation in Basel (Künzel, 1974). An improvement in the gingival health was also observed in Zurich children after 8 years of the caries-preventive programme (*Fig. 47*). Evidence from other countries (Birkeland and Jorkjend, 1975) suggests that the improvement is unlikely to be primarily due to the supervised brushing in school, but is a result of the improved caries state and the greater awareness of preventive measures.

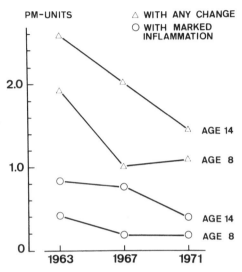

Fig. 47. The mean number of gingival (PM) units inflamed (out of a maximum of 6 units) in 8- and 14-year-old children in Zurich Canton in 1963, 1967 and 1971, after commencement of the Caries Preventive Program in 1963. (From Marthaler, 1972b.) (*Reproduced by courtesy of the Editor, 'Helv. Odont. Acta'.*)

The USA

The USA is the birthplace of water fluoridation. Progress in fluoridating public water supplies has been steady since its conception in 1945 so that in 1979, 50 per cent of Americans were consuming optimally fluoridated water. Largely because of the emphasis on water fluoridation, alternative (or complementary) community measures were not widely investigated until the advent of the National Caries Program in 1972. Since then, under the direction of Dr H. S. Horowitz, the US public health service has tested a wide variety of alternative community preventive schemes—virtually all of them fluoride based. Many schemes have been implemented, so that by 1980 some 10 million American children took part in school-based fluoride preventive programmes, although it is recognized that this accounts for only 20 per cent of the total school population (Horowitz,

1980). Unique to the USA is the implementation of fluoridation of school water supplies, which in 1979 operated in more than 400 schools in 14 US states. The 40 per cent caries reduction observed is encouraging, especially since a greater effectiveness on late erupting teeth appears to indicate an important systemic effect on developing teeth in addition to the topical effect on teeth already erupted. Most of the remaining school-based fluoride programmes involve mouthrinsing and by 1979 8 million American children were involved in fluoride rinsing schemes (Horowitz, 1980; Horowitz and Horowitz, 1980). Averaged over 17 community clinical trials, organized by the National Institute of Health, involving 75 000 children, the cost of supplies for weekly mouthrinsing with 0·2 per cent NaF was calculated at 50c/child/year, although including the cost of salaries of paid personnel increased the cost to $3.49/child/year (Brunelle and Miller, 1979).

Because (1) rinsing produces only a topical effect (which may be quickly lost if the rinsing is stopped), (2) the caries-preventive effect of a school-based fluoride tablet programme did not diminish quickly after cessation (Driscoll et al., 1979), and (3) the systemic effect of school water fluoridation has been observed, it is probably advantageous to combine fluoride tablets with fluoride rinsing in a school programme. Such a scheme is currently being tested in Nelson County, Virginia, with encouraging results after 6 years (Horowitz et al., 1980). The children slowly chew a 1 mg F tablet in school each day and rinse with 0·2 per cent NaF each week in school, as well as using a fluoride toothpaste at home. Twelve-year-old children, who had taken part in the programme since the age of 6 years, showed a 45 per cent reduction in DMFS compared with baseline scores, and an 80 per cent reduction in approximal carious surfaces. A strong post-treatment effect was observed for up to 5 years after the children left the scheme at the age of 12 years. The cost per child per year was $1.77 for tablets and rinse and their distribution, although distribution of toothpaste and brushes for home use cost a further $5.10.

COST–BENEFIT ANALYSIS

Horowitz and Heifetz (1979) have pointed out that cost–benefit analysis is of value in deciding between alternative public health programmes where the primary objective differs (e.g. comparing a day-stay unit for dental procedures with an orthodontic screening service in schools). Here, both the cost of the benefits and the cost of implementation have to be calculated. In caries prevention it is frequently necessary to decide between alternative ways of achieving the same primary objective of caries prevention. It then becomes unnecessary to calculate the benefit in monetary terms and this can then be expressed in terms of the number of carious teeth or surfaces prevented. This is cost-effectiveness analysis which enables the planner to determine the least expensive of several alternatives of achieving a stated objective.

It must be recognized that all such calculations are imperfect and serve only as the best available information for the planner. Of particular relevance is our lack of long-term knowledge of the caries-preventive effect of various fluoride procedures. Many procedures are school based and the benefits may be lost soon after the participants leave school. Public water fluoridation is the only fluoride therapy for which there is information on its lifelong effectiveness. Almost all the studies reported in the previous chapters have been short-term clinical trials, or what O'Mullane (1976) has classed as 'experimental clinical trials', where the agent or procedure is given the greatest chance of showing its effectiveness. The effectiveness of a preventive régime may differ when implemented on a community basis from that observed in an experimental clinical trial, although the limited amount of data available (mainly from Scandinavia) seems to indicate that percentage reductions in community preventive schemes and experimental clinical trials are substantially similar.

The most thorough review of cost-effectiveness of methods of caries prevention was achieved at a conference in Ann Arbor, Michigan, in 1978 (Burt, 1978). *Table* 65 is taken from this publication and provides a guide to the order of efficiency of fluoride programmes. The table is compiled with the assumption of a caries increment of 2 DMFS per child per year in a fluoride-low area, and the costing is given in US dollars as calculations were made on US wages and material costs. For further details of how the costs were calculated, the reader is referred to the workshop report (Burt, 1978). To emphasize how difficult it is to calculate the cost-benefit and cost-effectiveness of community programmes, *Table* 66 lists factors which may be excluded from analyses. For example, the estimation of the cost of weekly fluoride mouthrinsing (*Table* 65) excluded the cost of the teachers' time, which may have to be included in some communities. It is probable that in many estimates both the cost and the benefit are underestimated, although benefits are more likely to be underestimated than costs (Burt, 1978). Because disease levels and resources will vary from community to community, a public health planner must estimate cost-effectiveness ratios based as much as possible on local information.

The size of the caries increment will considerably alter the cost-effectiveness of a caries-preventive measure. For example, in a community with optimum water fluoride level, the cost-effectiveness of any topical fluoride régimes will be halved. Alternatively, if only children at high risk of developing caries are included, the ratio becomes more favourable to the preventive measure, although the organization becomes much more difficult.

As mentioned earlier, lack of information on the effectiveness of school-based fluoride schemes after the child leaves school (post-treatment effect)

Table 65. Ranking of Alternative Fluoride Therapies According to Estimated Cost-effectiveness (*From Newbrun, 1978 and Heifetz, 1978*)

Procedure	Estimated per cent caries reduction	Annual cost ($) per capita	Cost ($) per 1 DMFS saved	Rank
Systemic				
Public water fluoridation	50	0·20	0·20	1
Fluoride tablet distribution	35	0·40	0·57	3
School water fluoridation	40	1·50	1·88	3
Topical				
Weekly mouthrinse (0·2 per cent NaF)	25	0·50	1·00	1
Clinical application (multiple chair) (2 per cent NaF)	40	2·06	2·60	2
Clinical application (annual) (1·23 per cent F APF gel in tray)	40	3·50	4·40	3
Toothbrushing in school (5 × /yr) (0·6 per cent F solution)	20	2·23	5·60	4
Toothbrushing at home (0·1 per cent F toothpaste)	20	4·00	10·00	5
Daily self-application by tray (0·5 per cent F APF gel)	80	34·09	21·30	6

Table 66. Factors which are frequently excluded from Cost–benefit Analysis

Cost	Benefit
1. Teachers' time supervising preventive measure 2. Subjects' time doing preventive measure 3. Discounting of costs (benefits accrue later)	1. Repeat treatment (e.g. fillings) of teeth not included in DMF index 2. Subjects' (and parents') time and cost of attending surgery for treatment 3. Freedom from pain, infection, etc. 4. Post-treatment benefit 5. Benefit to deciduous teeth 6. Effect on gingival health of a complete dentition and unrestored teeth

is a serious gap. It would be especially useful to be able to compare the post-treatment effect of, say, the Swedish school programme (based largely on fluoride mouthrinsing) with the Zurich programme (involving both systemic and topical fluoride therapy). It is possible that the latter may produce the greater post-treatment effect.

In the UK, apart from water fluoridation, few community preventive schemes have been implemented, although Bennie et al. (1978) reported a substantial caries reduction after 5 years of a programme (largely fortnightly fluoride rinsing) in the county of Sutherland, Scotland. In spite of this absence of organized school preventive programmes, caries severity seems to be falling in the UK (Palmer, 1980). Although other factors (such as dietary changes) may also be involved, the increasing use of fluoride toothpastes in the UK in the 1970s seems to be a factor in this welcome occurrence.

CONCLUDING REMARKS

The inspired observations by McKay in Colorado Springs at the very beginning of this century, followed by his persistent search for the cause of enamel mottling and caries inhibition, led eventually to the discovery of fluoride in drinking water. McKay's work was continued by H. Trendley Dean and other researchers who showed that the adjustment of water fluoride levels could reduce dental caries, and the effectiveness of water fluoridation has now been documented in twenty countries throughout the world. The study of the systemic and topical effects of fluoride has produced a tremendous outpouring of research, particularly over the last fifty years and our knowledge of dental epidemiology, clinical trials, community dental health, dental plaque, physiology, biochemistry, toxicity and aspects of general health has increased enormously as a result. Our aim has been to review the development of these various strands and to try to draw them together in order to give the reader a perspective of the vital part that fluorides can play in caries prevention.

REFERENCES

Bennie A. M., Tullis J. I., Stephen K. W. and MacFadyen E. E. (1978) Five years of community preventive dentistry and health education in the County of Sutherland, Scotland. *Community Dent. Oral Epidemiol.* **6**, 1–5.

Berggren H. and Welander E. (1960) Supervised toothbrushing with a sodium fluoride solution in 5000 Swedish schoolchildren. *Acta Odontol. Scand.* **18**, 209–234.

Birkeland J. M. and Jorkjend L. (1975) Effect of mouthrinsing and toothbrushing with fluoride solutions on caries among Norwegian schoolchildren. *Community Dent. Oral Epidemiol.* **3**, 201–207.

Birkeland J. M., Broch L. and Jorkjend L. (1977) Benefits and prognoses following 10 years of a fluoride mouthrinsing program. *Scand. J. Dent. Res.* **85**, 31–37.

Brunelle J. A. and Miller A. J. (1979) Cost analysis of school-based mouthrinse programs in 17 communities in the U.S. and Guam. *J. Dent. Res.* **58A**, 388 (abstr.).

Burt B. A. (1978) *The Relative Efficiency of Methods of Caries Prevention in Dental Public Health.* Proceedings of a workshop at the University of Michigan, June 5–8, 1978. Ann Arbor, University of Michigan, 1978.

Dowell T. B. (1976) The economics of fluoridation. *Br. Dent. J.* **140**, 103–106.

Driscoll W. S., Heifetz S. B. and Brunelle J. A. (1979) The use of fluoride tablets by schoolchildren: treatment and post-treatment effects on dental caries. *J. Dent. Res.* **58A**, 294 (abstr.).

Ekstrand J., Koch G., Lindgren L. E. and Petersson L. G. (1981) Pharmacokinetics of fluoride gels in children and adults. *Caries Res.* **15**, 213–220.

Heifetz S. B. (1978) Cost-effectiveness of topically applied fluorides. In: Burt B. A. (ed.), *The Relative Efficiency of Methods of Caries Prevention in Dental Public Health.* Ann Arbor, University of Michigan, pp. 69–104.

Hope T. (1979) Results of 10 years of supervised fluoride toothbrushing in Rygge, Norway. *Community Dent. Oral Epidemiol.* **7**, 330–334.

Horowitz A. M. and Horowitz H. S. (1980) School-based fluoride programs: a critique. *J. Prev. Dent.* **6**, 89–94.

Horowitz H. S. (1977) Abusive use of fluoride. Editorial. *J. Public Health Dent.* **37**, 106–107.

Horowitz H. S. (1980) Established methods of prevention. *Br. Dent. J.* **149**, 311–318.

Horowitz H. S. and Heifetz S. B. (1979) Methods for assessing the cost-effectiveness of caries preventive agents and procedures. *Int. Dent. J.* **29**, 106–117.

Horowitz H. S., Heifetz S. B., Meyers R. J., Driscoll W. S. and Li S.- H. (1980) A program of self-administered fluorides in a rural school system. *Community Dent. Oral Epidemiol.* **8**, 177–183.

Horowitz H. S., Heifetz S. B., McClendon J., Viegas A. R., Guimaraes L. O. C. and Lopes E. S. (1974) Evaluation of self-administered prophylaxis and supervised toothbrushing with acidulated phosphate fluoride. *Caries Res.* **8**, 39–51.

Klock B. and Krasse B. (1979) A comparison between different methods for prediction of caries activity. *Scand. J. Dent. Res.* **87**, 129–139.

Künzel W. (1974) The cost and economic consequences of water fluoridation. *Caries Res.* **8**, suppl. 1, 28–35.

Lokken P. and Birkeland J. M. (1978) Acceptance, caries reduction and reported adverse effects of fluoride prophylaxis in Norway. *Community Dent. Oral Epidemiol.* **6**, 110–116.

Marthaler T. M. (1972a) Decrease of DMF levels 4 years after the introduction of a caries preventive program; observations in 5819 schoolchildren of 20 communities. *Helv. Odontol. Acta* **16**, 45–68.

Marthaler T. M. (1972b) Reduction of caries, gingivitis and calculus after eight years of preventive measures—observations in seven communities. *Helv. Odontol. Acta* **16**, 69–83.

Marthaler T. M. (1974) Improved oral health of schoolchildren of 16 communities after 8 years of prevention. I. Combining DMF data from the communities. *Helv. Odontol. Acta* **18**, 119–142.

Marthaler T. M. and Loosli U. (1980) Caries at age 14 in schoolchildren with either small or large amounts of dental plaque in a community with well organised prevention. *Caries Res.* **14**, 168–169 (abstr.).

Newburn E. (1978) Cost-effectiveness and practicality features in the systemic use of fluorides. In: Burt B. A. (ed.), *The Relative Efficiency of Methods of Caries Prevention in Dental Public Health.* Ann Arbor, University of Michigan, pp. 27–48.

O'Mullane D. M. (1976) Efficiency in clinical trials of caries preventive agents and methods. *Community Dent. Oral Epidemiol.* **4**, 190–194.

Palmer J. D. (1980) Dental health in children—an improving picture? *Br. Dent. J.* **149**, 48–50.

Rise J. and Haugejorden O. (1980) Monitoring and evaluation of results of community fluoride programs in Norway during the 1960's and 1970's. *Community Dent. Oral Epidemiol.* **8**, 79–83.

Torell P. and Ericsson Y. (1974) The potential benefits to be derived from fluoride mouthrinses. In: Forrester D. J. and Schulz E. M. (eds), *International Workshop on Fluorides and Dental Caries Reductions.* Baltimore, University of Maryland, pp. 113–176.

INDEX